Anterior Cruciate Ligament (ACL) Injuries: Clinical Treatment and Rehabilitation

Anterior Cruciate Ligament (ACL) Injuries: Clinical Treatment and Rehabilitation

Guest Editor

Young-Jin Seo

MDPI

Basel • Beijing • Wuhan • Barcelona • Belgrade • Novi Sad • Cluj • Manchester

Guest Editor
Young-Jin Seo
Department of Orthopaedic Surgery
Dongtan Sacred Heart Hospital
Hallym University College of Medicine
Hwaseong
Republic of Korea

Editorial Office
MDPI AG
Grosspeteranlage 5
4052 Basel, Switzerland

This is a reprint of the Special Issue, published open access by the journal *Journal of Clinical Medicine* (ISSN 2077-0383), freely accessible at: https://www.mdpi.com/journal/jcm/special_issues/68Y6AV5X59.

For citation purposes, cite each article independently as indicated on the article page online and as indicated below:

Lastname, A.A.; Lastname, B.B. Article Title. *Journal Name* **Year**, *Volume Number*, Page Range.

ISBN 978-3-7258-7585-6 (Hbk)
ISBN 978-3-7258-7586-3 (PDF)
https://doi.org/10.3390/books978-3-7258-7586-3

Contents

About the Editor vii

Preface ix

Joo Hyung Han, Sung-Hwan Kim, Min Jung, Hyun-Soo Moon and Kwangho Chung
Combined Anterior Cruciate Ligament and Anterolateral Ligament Reconstruction Shows Reduced Graft Failure Rates and Superior Residual Rotational Stability Regardless of Anterolateral Ligament Reconstruction Graft: A Systematic Review
Reprinted from: *J. Clin. Med.* **2025**, *14*, 2237, https://doi.org/10.3390/jcm14072237 1

Han-Kook Yoon, Chang-Min Lee, Hyun-Cheol Oh, Taemi Youk and Sang-Hoon Park
The Risk of Secondary Knee Procedures After Anterior Cruciate Ligament Reconstruction—A Nationwide Retrospective Cohort Study
Reprinted from: *J. Clin. Med.* **2025**, *14*, 3823, https://doi.org/10.3390/jcm14113823 18

Young Jin Seo, Si Young Song and Dongju Kim
Propensity Score-Matched Comparison of Six-Strand All-Inside and Conventional Four-Strand Hamstring Autografts for ACL Reconstruction
Reprinted from: *J. Clin. Med.* **2025**, *14*, 6010, https://doi.org/10.3390/jcm14176010 26

Roberto Ricupito, Rosalba Castellucci, Filippo Maselli, Marco Bravi, Fabio Santacaterina, Riccardo Guarise and Florian Forelli
Early Open Kinetic Chain Hamstring Exercise After ACL Reconstruction: A Retrospective Safety and Efficacy Study
Reprinted from: *J. Clin. Med.* **2025**, *14*, 6871, https://doi.org/10.3390/jcm14196871 41

Grant M. Pham
Biologic Augmentation in Anterior Cruciate Ligament Reconstruction and Beyond: A Review of PRP and BMAC
Reprinted from: *J. Clin. Med.* **2025**, *14*, 6959, https://doi.org/10.3390/jcm14196959 56

Sultan A. Alanazi, Samia A. Alamrani, Sarah S. Bajuaifer, Layan Alhammad, Nouf Alotaibi, Naif Z. Alrashdi, et al.
"Returning to Sport Is Not Just About the Knee": Physiotherapists' Experiences of the Management of Anterior Cruciate Ligament Injury: A Qualitative Study
Reprinted from: *J. Clin. Med.* **2025**, *14*, 7301, https://doi.org/10.3390/jcm14207301 69

Roxana Mihaela Munteanu, Andrei Marian Feier, Bogdan Voicu, Arpad Solyom, Pia Simona Făgăraș and Tudor Sorin Pop
Can PRP Enhance Hamstring Recovery Post-ACL Reconstruction? Retrospective Insights from Non-Professional Athletes
Reprinted from: *J. Clin. Med.* **2025**, *14*, 8266, https://doi.org/10.3390/jcm14238266 86

Chieh-An Chuang, You-Hung Cheng, Cheng-Pang Yang, Chen-Heng Hsu, Chung-Yu Chen, Yi-Hsuan Lin and Huan Sheu
Short-Term Outcome of Combined Anterior Cruciate Ligament Reconstruction and Anterolateral Ligament Reconstruction with Suture Tape Augmentation
Reprinted from: *J. Clin. Med.* **2025**, *14*, 8283, https://doi.org/10.3390/jcm14238283 99

Simone Giusti, Angelo Matteucci, Simone Pavone, Ciro Mignano and Ezio Adriani
Does Adding LEAP to ACL Reconstruction Reduce Graft Failure? A Systematic Review and Meta-Analysis of Comparative Studies with Minimum Two-Year Follow-Up
Reprinted from: *J. Clin. Med.* **2025**, *14*, 8499, https://doi.org/10.3390/jcm14238499 110

Hyun-Soo Moon, Sungjun Kim, Min Jung, Kwangho Chung, Se-Han Jung, Junhee Cho, et al.
Combined ACL and ALL Reconstruction Using Allografts as the ACL Graft Source Reduces Surgical Failure and Improves Graft Maturity Compared with Isolated ACL Reconstruction
Reprinted from: *J. Clin. Med.* **2026**, *15*, 735, https://doi.org/10.3390/jcm15020735 . . . . **127**

About the Editor

Young-Jin Seo

Young-Jin Seo, MD, PhD, is an orthopedic surgeon specializing in knee surgery and sports medicine. He is affiliated with a medical college and has extensive experience in anterior cruciate ligament reconstruction, with particular interest in surgical techniques, graft configuration, and biomechanical optimization. His research focuses on improving clinical outcomes through advanced imaging analysis and comparative studies of reconstruction methods. He is actively involved in editorial activities in international peer-reviewed journals and continues to contribute to both clinical practice and academic research.

Preface

As Guest Editor, I am pleased to present this Reprint, which brings together selected contributions from the Special Issue entitled "Anterior Cruciate Ligament Injuries: Clinical Treatment and Rehabilitation" published in the *Journal of Clinical Medicine*. The field of ACL reconstruction and rehabilitation continues to evolve, driven by ongoing discussions regarding optimal surgical techniques, graft selection, and the role of adjunctive procedures. In this context, it is essential to critically interpret emerging evidence while maintaining relevance to real-world clinical decision-making.

This Reprint has been developed with the aim of providing a balanced and clinically meaningful perspective that reflects both established principles and evolving concepts. Particular attention has been given to factors that directly influence surgical strategy, patient outcomes, and long-term joint health, including the integration of biological and rehabilitative considerations.

It is my hope that this Reprint will serve as a valuable resource for orthopedic surgeons, sports medicine specialists, and researchers, supporting thoughtful interpretation of the literature and ultimately contributing to improved care for patients with ACL injuries.

Young-Jin Seo
Guest Editor

Journal of
Clinical Medicine

MDPI

Systematic Review

Combined Anterior Cruciate Ligament and Anterolateral Ligament Reconstruction Shows Reduced Graft Failure Rates and Superior Residual Rotational Stability Regardless of Anterolateral Ligament Reconstruction Graft: A Systematic Review

Joo Hyung Han [1,†], Sung-Hwan Kim [2,3,†], Min Jung [2,4], Hyun-Soo Moon [2,4] and Kwangho Chung [2,5,*]

1 Yonsei University College of Medicine, Seoul 03722, Republic of Korea; hanjh93@gmail.com
2 Arthroscopy and Joint Research Institute, Yonsei University College of Medicine, Seoul 03722, Republic of Korea; orthohwan@gmail.com (S.-H.K.); oshsdesu@gmail.com (H.-S.M.)
3 Department of Orthopedic Surgery, Gangnam Severance Hospital, Yonsei University College of Medicine, Seoul 03722, Republic of Korea
4 Department of Orthopedic Surgery, Severance Hospital, Yonsei University College of Medicine, Seoul 03722, Republic of Korea
5 Department of Orthopedic Surgery, Yongin Severance Hospital, Yonsei University College of Medicine, Yongin 16995, Republic of Korea
* Correspondence: khchung85@gmail.com; Tel.: +82-31-5189-8482
† These authors contributed equally to this work.

Abstract: Objectives: The aim of this study is to evaluate the literature for comparing clinical outcomes of anterior cruciate ligament reconstruction (ACLR) with concomitant anterolateral ligament reconstruction (ALLR) versus isolated ACLR, with a primary focus on analyzing differences in outcomes based on the type of graft used for ALLR. **Methods**: We identified comparative studies involving primary ACLR performed in conjunction with ALLR. Graft failure rates, residual pivot shift, residual anterior–posterior (AP) laxity at follow-up, and patient-reported outcome measures were determined. Variables associated with isolated ACLR and ACLR combined with ALLR were compared based on the type of graft used for ALLR. **Results**: This systematic review included nine studies involving 2740 patients. Combined ACLR with ALLR using hamstring tendon (HT) autografts or tibialis allografts showed lower graft failure rates than isolated ACLR (HT autograft: rate, 0–5.9%, odds ratio [OR], 2.16–12.91; tibialis allograft: rate, 0%, OR, 2.00–5.27). Similarly, the combined procedure showed reduced residual pivot shift rates (HT autograft: rate, 0–9.1%, OR, 2.00–12.16; tibialis allograft: rate, 0%, OR, 7.65–15.33) compared to isolated ACLR. Residual AP laxity and patient-reported outcomes were similar or more favorable for the combined procedure; however, the results were heterogeneous. Complications related to the type of graft used for ALLR or the presence of ALLR itself were not reported. **Conclusions**: Regardless of the graft type used for ALLR, the combination of ACLR with ALLR showed better clinical outcomes, including reduced graft failure rates and superior residual rotational stability compared to isolated ACLR. However, the high heterogeneity observed across studies suggests that these findings should be interpreted with caution, and further research is needed to draw more definitive conclusions.

Keywords: anterior cruciate ligament reconstruction; anterolateral ligament reconstruction; graft failure; residual rotational stability; systematic review

1. Introduction

Anterior cruciate ligament (ACL) rupture, one of the most frequently injured ligaments in the knee joint, is effectively treated using ACL reconstruction (ACLR) [1,2]. However, graft failure requiring revision surgery remains an unresolved issue. It is reported in 4–25% of patients who have undergone ACLR, with the majority of cases noted within two years after surgery [3–7]. Persistent rotational instability following ACLR is recognized not only as a frequent cause of graft failure but also as a factor that adversely affects patient outcomes [8].

Anterolateral ligament (ALL) reconstruction (ALLR), in conjunction with ACLR, has been proposed to address residual rotational instability that cannot be controlled by ACLR alone. The biomechanics and functions of the ALL have been investigated in several studies. The results indicate that the ALL acts as a secondary stabilizer to the ACL, especially in resisting anterior tibial translation and internal rotation, thus playing a vital role in preserving rotational stability and preventing knee instability [9,10]. Compared with isolated ACLR, combined ACLR and ALLR enhances rotational stability, assessed through the pivot shift test [9]. Furthermore, the combination reduces graft rates and enhances subjective function scores [11].

Graft selection for ACL is one of the most extensively discussed topics to date, with substantial evidence supporting various graft options, leading to different outcomes depending on the type of graft utilized [12–14]. When comparing autografts and allografts for ACLR, autografts, such as hamstring grafts and bone–patellar tendon–bone (BPTB) grafts, are generally considered superior to allografts in terms of graft failure rates, which can be up to six times higher with allografts, particularly in younger more active patients [15–18].

Several systematic reviews and meta-analyses have consistently shown that combining ACLR with anterolateral ligament reconstruction (ALLR) results in improved outcomes compared to isolated ACLR [11,19,20]. While the integration of ALLR into ACLR has become increasingly prevalent, with various graft types being utilized for ALLR [12], there remains a lack of evidence and literature to support specific graft choices and their impact on clinical outcomes.

This systematic review sought to assess the available literature for a comparison of the clinical outcomes of combined ACLR and ALLR versus isolated ACLR, with a primary focus on assessing differences in outcomes based on the type of graft used for ALLR. We hypothesize that ACLR combined with ALLR will consistently yield superior clinical outcomes compared to isolated ACLR, regardless of the graft type used for ALLR.

2. Materials and Methods

2.1. Search Strategy

The review was registered in advance in the PROSPERO prospective register of systematic reviews (ID: CRD42023482821) and was carried out according to a predefined protocol following the PRISMA (Preferred Reporting Items for Systematic Reviews and Meta-analyses) guidelines. A thorough search strategy was developed to identify relevant studies. We conducted a systematic search of PubMed, Embase, the Cochrane Library, and Google Scholar for articles published up to 11 September 2024. The search was conducted utilizing the following search parameters: [("antero lateral ligament" OR "anterolateral ligament" OR "ALL") AND ("anterior cruciate ligament" [mesh] OR "anterior cruciate ligament" OR "ACL") AND "reconstruction"]. The search was restricted to studies published in the English language.

2.2. Identification of Eligibility

The inclusion criteria were as follows: (1) skeletally mature patients aged 15 to 50 years diagnosed with ACL rupture; (2) studies involving the intervention of primary single-bundle ACLR with ALLR; (3) comparative studies with levels of evidence I to III, published in English; (4) studies with a minimum follow-up period of 24 months; and (5) studies specifying the graft type used for ALLR. The exclusion criteria were as follows: (1) articles not in English; (2) studies with incomplete data; (3) studies involving revision ACLR; and (4) studies including lateral extra-articular tenodesis; and (5) level IV to V studies, including cadaveric, animal studies, case reports, systematic reviews, or biomechanical studies. Eligibility was determined by two independent reviewers who screened the search results.

2.3. Data Extraction

Two independent reviewers extracted data including the following factors: primary author, publication year, country of origin, study design, level of evidence, type of graft used for ALLR, sample size, duration of follow-up, sex distribution, age, body mass index, reported ACLR graft failure rate, residual pivot shift at follow-up, residual anterior–posterior (AP) laxity, and patient-reported outcome measures, such as pre-and postoperative International Knee Documentation Committee (IKDC) scores, Lysholm scores, and Tegner scores, along with documented complications. In the case of disagreement between the reviewers, discrepancies were resolved via discussion until a consensus was reached. If no agreement could be reached, a third reviewer was consulted.

To assess the risk of bias, randomized controlled trials (RCTs) were evaluated using the Cochrane Collaboration's Risk of Bias 2 tool [21]. Each study was categorized with a low, unclear, or high risk of bias. The risk of bias for non-randomized studies was assessed using the Methodological Index for Non-Randomized Studies (MINORS), which includes 12 criteria for comparative studies [22]. Each category was rated as 0 (if not reported), 1 (if reported but inadequate), or 2 (if reported and considered adequate). The risk of bias was independently assessed by two reviewers, with disagreements resolved via consultation with a third reviewer.

2.4. Statistical Analysis

Descriptive statistics, including the mean and standard deviation for numerical variables, were recorded. For studies that did not provide the standard deviation, we calculated it using other available statistical values, following the method outlined by Furukawa et al. [23].

In cases where results were presented only as graphs without numerical values, we employed the approach described by Gheibi et al. to derive numerical data for analysis [24]. For each investigated variable, we calculated the differences in clinical efficacy between ACLR with concomitant ALLR and isolated ACLR. Residual AP laxity was represented by the side-to-side difference in millimeters as reported in each study, while residual pivot shift was defined as cases exhibiting a grade 2 or 3 pivot shift. For continuous outcome measures, mean differences (MDs) with 95% confidence intervals (CIs) were utilized. Odds ratios (ORs) were calculated for dichotomous outcomes, with 95% CIs. Studies from the same research group, where there was a potential overlap of patients in the intervention groups, were excluded from the analysis, with the exception of the study with the largest sample size. Heterogeneity between studies was assessed using the Q statistic and the I^2 statistic. While a meta-analysis was considered, its feasibility was limited by the relatively low level of evidence and high heterogeneity across studies. As a result, pooled synthesis was avoided. Instead, Forest plots were generated for outcomes including graft failure rate, residual AP laxity, residual pivot shift, and patient-reported outcome measures, with subgroup analysis based on the type of graft utilized in ALLR. All statistical analyses and data visualizations were performed using R software (version 4.2.1; R Foundation, Vienna, Austria).

3. Results

3.1. Characteristics of Included Studies

This systematic review identified 1623 relevant studies from multiple databases. After eliminating duplicates and assessing the full texts, 37 studies were considered for eligibility. Ultimately, nine studies, involving 2740 patients in total, fulfilled our inclusion criteria and were included in the analysis (Figure 1) [25–33]. The characteristics of these included studies are detailed in Tables 1 and 2. Based on the graft utilized in ALLR, seven studies [25,27–32] used a hamstring tendon (HT) autograft, and two studies [26,33] employed a tibialis allograft.

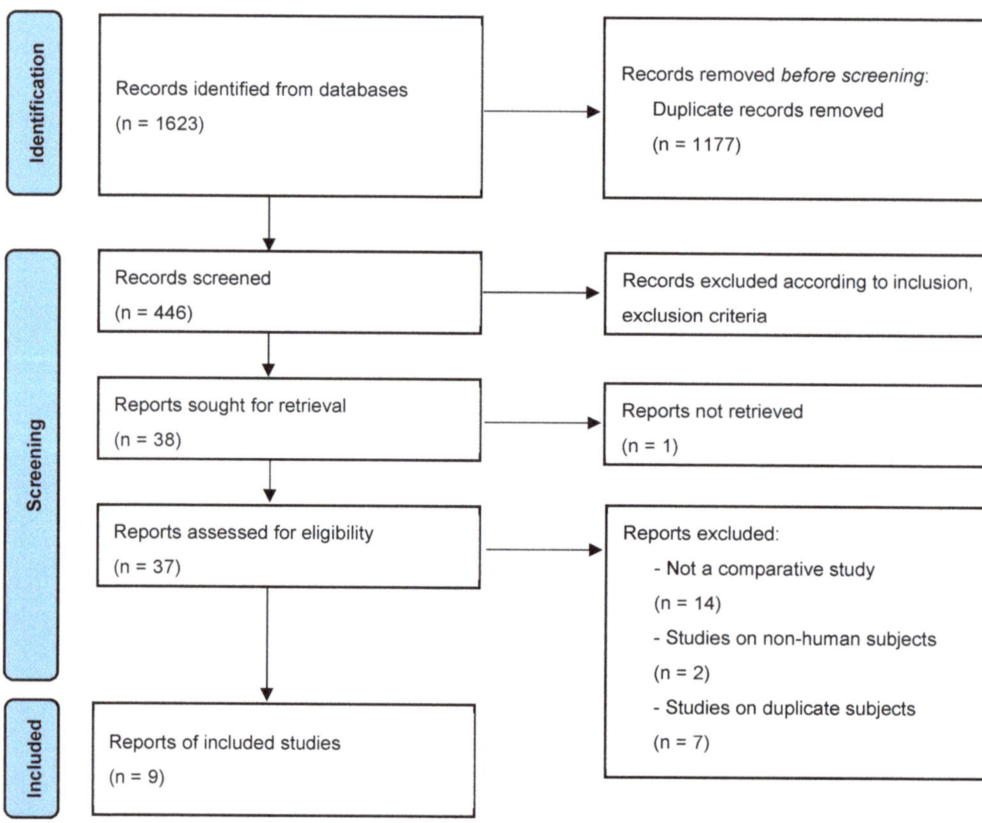

Figure 1. PRISMA flow diagram for the systematic review.

Table 1. Overview of included studies.

Study	Year	Journal	Country	Study Design	Level of Evidence	Number of Patients	Graft Used for ACLR	Graft Used for ALLR
Torkaman et al. [33]	2024	*BMC Musculoskeletal. Disord.*	Iran	Prospective comparative study	2	41	4 strand ST	1 strand GT
Gonnachon et al. [27]	2023	*Eur. J. Orthop. Surg. Traumatol.*	France	Cohort study	3	79	3 or 4 strand ST + GT	1 strand ST
Lee et al. [26]	2023	*Orthop. J. Sports Med.*	Republic of Korea	Cohort study	3	78	4 strand ST	TA allograft
Yang et al. [25]	2023	*Arthroscopy*	Republic of Korea	Cohort study	3	70	4 strand ST + GT	Tibialis allograft
Laboudie et al. [29]	2022	*Knee Surg. Sports Traumatol. Arthrosc.*	France	Retrospective comparative study	3	203	4 strand ST	1 strand GT
Pioger et al. [28]	2022	*Am. J. Sports Med.*	France	Cohort study	3	2018	4 strand ST + GT	1 strand GT
Hamido et al. [30]	2021	*Knee Surg. Sports Traumatol. Arthrosc.*	Kuwait	Randomized controlled trial	1	102	4 strand ST	2 strand GT
Goncharov et al. [31]	2019	*Int. Orthop.*	Russia	Prospective comparative study	2	48	BPTB Autograft	ST + GT
Helito et al. [32]	2018	*Knee Surg. Sports Traumatol. Arthrosc.*	Brazil	Cohort study	3	101	4 strand ST + GT	1 strand GT

ACLR, anterior cruciate ligament reconstruction; ALLR, anterolateral ligament reconstruction; ST, semitendinosus tendon; GT, gracilis tendon; BPTB, bone patellar tendon bone; TA, tibialis anterior.

Table 2. Demographics of patients in included studies.

Graft Used for ALLR	Study	Follow-Up Duration (Mean ± SD)	Sex (n, Male/Female)	Age (Years, Mean ± SD)	BMI (kg/m^2, Mean ± SD)
HT Autograft	Torkaman et al., 2024 [33]	39.8 ± 14.1 (isolated ACLR), 41.3 ± 15 (ACLR + ALLR) months	17/4 (isolated ACLR), 18/2 (ACLR + ALLR)	26.7 ± 8.9 (isolated ACLR), 25.9 ± 6.9 (ACLR + ALLR)	24.5 ± 2.2 (isolated ACLR), 24.2 ± 2.1 (ACLR + ALLR)
	Gonnachon et al., 2023 [27]	54 months	67/16	24 ± 7.2	NR
	Laboudie et al., 2022 [29]	4.8 ± 0.9 years	57/44 (isolated ACLR), 62/40 (ACLR + ALLR)	16.5 ± 2.2 (isolated ACLR), 16.8 ± 1.9 (ACLR + ALLR)	21.8 ± 3 (isolated ACLR), 22.1 ± 3 (ACLR + ALLR)
	Pioger et al., 2022 [28]	101.3 ± 59.9 months	840/169 (isolated ACLR), 845/163 (ACLR + ALLR)	25.8 ± 7.5 (isolated ACLR), 25.8 ± 7.9 (ACLR + ALLR)	24.4 ± 3.4 (isolated ACLR), 24.3 ± 3.4 (ACLR + ALLR)
	Hamido et al., 2021 [30]	median 60 months (range 55–65)	52/0 (isolated ACLR), 50/0 (ACLR + ALLR)	26 (isolated ACLR), 24 (ACLR + ALLR)	NR
	Goncharov et al., 2019 [31]	24 months	NR	NR	NR
	Helito et al., 2018 [32]	26 (isolated ACLR), 25 (ACLR + ALLR) months	59/9 (isolated ACLR), 30/3 (ACLR + ALLR)	33.9 ± 6.1 (isolated ACLR), 33.1 ± 8.8 (ACLR + ALLR)	NR
Tibialis Allograft	Lee et al., 2023 [26]	30.4 ± 3.9 (isolated ACLR), 29.3 ± 3.5 (ACLR + ALLR) months	0/39 (isolated ACLR), 0/39 (ACLR + ALLR)	31.1 ± 5.7 (isolated ACLR), 30.4 ± 6.1 (ACLR + ALLR)	19.4 ± 2.5 (isolated ACLR), 19.7 ± 2.7 (ACLR + ALLR)
	Yang et al., 2023 [25]	46.6 months, 42.5 months	31/4 (isolated ACLR), 29/6 (ACLR + ALLR)	26.8 ± 9.9 (isolated ACLR), 26.1 ± 10.8 (ACLR + ALLR)	26.2 ± 4.6 (isolated ACLR), 26.6 ± 4.5 (ACLR + ALLR)

ALLR, anterolateral ligament reconstruction; SD, standard deviation; BMI, body mass index; HT, hamstring tendon, ACLR, anterior cruciate ligament reconstruction; NR, not reported.

3.2. Methodological Quality Assessment of Included Studies

Among the included studies, one study [30] was classified as level I evidence, two studies [31,33] as level II evidence, and six studies [25–29,32] as level III evidence. One study [30], classified as an RCT, was evaluated using the Cochrane Collaboration's Risk of Bias 2 tool, and the results are presented in Figure A1. The remaining eight studies [25–29,31–33] were assessed using the MINORS tool, with a mean score of 21.4 ± 1.5 out of a maximum of 24 points, indicating generally high methodological quality. Further details on the MINORS scores are provided in Table A1. The inclusion criteria used in each study are summarized in Table A2.

3.3. Graft Failure

Graft failure rates have been reported in eight studies (Table 3) [25–30,32,33]. Combined ACLR with ALLR had a lower graft failure rate (0–5.9%) compared to isolated ACLR (2.9–14.3%), with an OR ranging from 2.16 to 12.91. The comparison of combined ACLR with ALLR to isolated ACLR based on the graft used for ALLR showed that HT autograft [27–30,32,33] had an OR of 2.16–12.91, whereas tibialis allograft [25,26] had an OR of 2.00–5.27 (Figure 2a). Both HT autograft (I^2 = 0%, τ^2 = 0.0, p = 0.74) and tibialis allograft (I^2 = 0%, τ^2 = 0.0, p = 0.81) exhibited low heterogeneity.

Table 3. Graft failure rate, residual pivot shift rate, and residual AP laxity reported in included studies.

Graft Used for ALLR	Study	Graft Failure		Residual Pivot Shift		Residual AP Laxity (mm, Mean ± SD)		
		Isolated ACLR	ACLR + ALLR	Isolated ACLR	ACLR + ALLR	Isolated ACLR	ACLR + ALLR	Method
HT Autograft	Torkaman et al., 2024 [33]	3/21 (14.3%)	0/20 (0%)	2/21 (9.5%)	1/20 (5.0%)	1.9 ± 1.9	1.7 ± 0.9	KT-1000
	Gonnachon et al., 2023 [27]	5/39 (12.8%)	0/40 (0%)	NR	NR	NR	NR	NR
	Laboudie et al., 2022 [29]	12/101 (11.9%)	6/102 (5.9%)	NR	NR	1.3 ± 1.3	1 ± 1.3	GNRB
	Pioger et al., 2022 [28]	100/1009 (9.9%)	35/1009 (3.5%)	NR	NR	0.6 ± 1.2	0.4 ± 1.1	Rolimeter
	Hamido et al., 2021 [30]	5/52 (9.6%)	0/50 (0%)	5/52 (9.6%)	0/50 (0%)	2.5 ± 0.7	1.2 ± 0.7	KT-1000
	Goncharov et al., 2019 [31]	NR	NR	NR	NR	NR	NR	NR
	Helito et al., 2018 [32]	5/68 (7.4%)	0/33 (0%)	24/68 (35.3%)	3/33 (9.1%)	2 (95% CI 1.5–2.1)	1 (95% CI 1.14–1.6)	KT-1000
Tibialis Allograft	Lee et al., 2023 [26]	2/39 (5.1%)	0/39 (0%)	6/39 (15.4%)	0/39 (0%)	2.3 ± 1.2	1.4 ± 1.2	KT-2000
	Yang et al., 2023 [25]	1/35 (2.9%)	0/35 (0%)	3/35 (8.6%)	0/35 (0%)	4.2 ± 2.2	3.5 ± 2.8	Telos stress

ALLR, anterolateral ligament reconstruction; ACLR, anterior cruciate ligament reconstruction; AP, anterior–posterior; SD, standard deviation; HT, hamstring tendon; NR, not reported; CI, confidence interval.

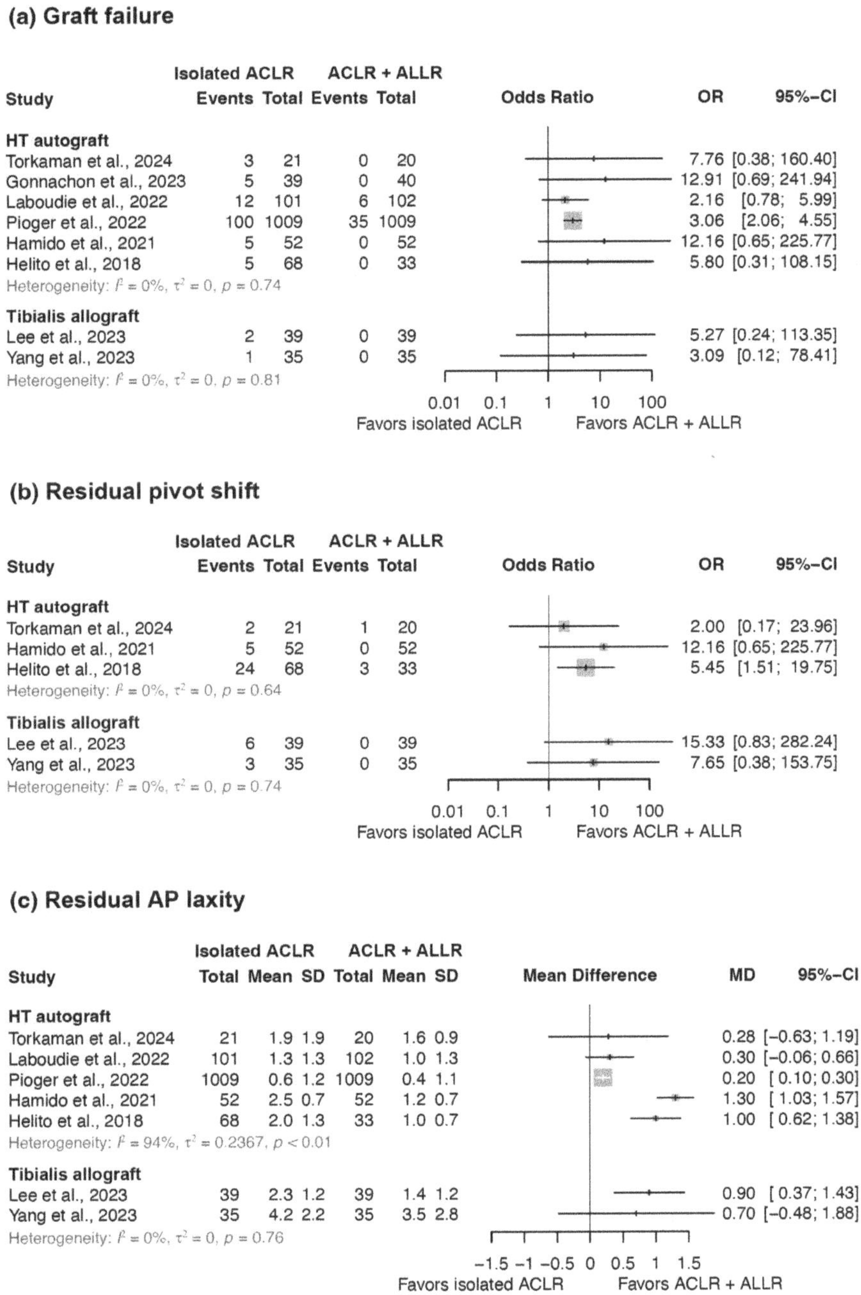

Figure 2. Forest plot illustrating the differences in treatment effects between isolated ACLR and cases in which ACLR and ALLR were performed concurrently, divided into subgroups according to the ALLR graft used. The results for (**a**) the failure rate of the ACLR graft, (**b**) residual pivot shift, and (**c**) residual anterior–posterior (AP) laxity are presented. Gray squares indicate the effect estimates for each study, with their size representing the study's weight in the analysis. ACLR, anterior cruciate ligament reconstruction; ALLR, anterolateral ligament reconstruction; SD, standard deviation; MD, mean difference; CI, confidence interval; HT, hamstring tendon [25–30,32,33].

3.4. Residual Pivot Shift

Residual pivot shift rates have been reported in five studies (Table 3) [25,26,30,32,33]. Combined ACLR with ALLR had a lower residual pivot shift rate (0–9.1%) compared to isolated ACLR (8.6–35.3%), with an OR ranging from 2.00 to 15.33. The comparison of combined ACLR with ALLR to isolated ACLR based on the graft used for ALLR showed that HT autograft [30,32,33] had an OR of 2.00–12.16, whereas tibialis allograft [25,26] had an OR of 7.65–15.33 (Figure 2b). Both HT autograft ($I^2 = 0\%$, $\tau^2 = 0.0$, $p = 0.64$) and tibialis allograft ($I^2 = 0\%$, $\tau^2 = 0.0$, $p = 0.74$) exhibited low heterogeneity.

3.5. Residual Anterior–Posterior Laxity

Residual AP laxity has been reported in seven studies (Table 3) [25,26,28–30,32,33]. The comparison of combined ACLR with ALLR with isolated ACLR based on the graft used for ALLR showed that for HT autografts [28–30,32,33], MDs ranged from 0.20 to 1.30, whereas for tibialis allografts [25,26], MDs ranged from 0.70 to 0.90 (Figure 2c). HT autografts ($I^2 = 94\%$, $\tau^2 = 0.2367$, $p < 0.01$) exhibited high heterogeneity, whereas tibialis allografts ($I^2 = 0\%$, $\tau^2 = 0.0$, $p = 0.76$) exhibited low heterogeneity.

3.6. Patient-Reported Outcome Measures

Patient-reported outcome measures included the Lysholm and IKDC scores and the Tegner activity scale (Table 4). The Lysholm score has been reported in eight studies [25–27,29–33]. The comparison of combined ACLR with ALLR with isolated ACLR based on the graft used for ALLR showed that for HT autografts [27,29–33], MDs ranged from −0.40 to 5.40, whereas for tibialis allografts [25,26], MDs ranged from 0.10 to 3.40 (Figure 3a). HT autografts ($I^2 = 49\%$, $\tau^2 = 2.9088$, $p = 0.08$) exhibited moderate heterogeneity, whereas tibialis allografts ($I^2 = 0\%$, $\tau^2 = 0.0$, $p = 0.43$) exhibited low heterogeneity.

Table 4. Patient-reported outcome measures of included studies.

Graft Used for ALLR	Study	Lysholm Score (Mean ± SD)		IKDC Score (Mean ± SD)		Tegner Activity Scale (Mean ± SD)	
		Isolated ACLR	ACLR + ALLR	Isolated ACLR	ACLR + ALLR	Isolated ACLR	ACLR + ALLR
HT Autograft	Torkaman et al., 2024 [33]	89.1 ± 8.7	90.2 ± 9.3	79 ± 9.2	81.5 ± 8.8	NR	NR
	Gonnachon et al., 2023 [27]	80.5 ± 11.7	82.05 ± 14.6	85.6 ± 12.3	85.8 ± 13.8	6.2 ± 1.3	6.6 ± 1.6
	Laboudie et al., 2022 [29]	83.3 ± 14.3	82 ± 14.4	86.4 ± 15.2	86 ± 16.8	7	7
	Hamido et al., 2021 [30]	NR	NR	94 ± 4.5	96 ± 5	7.8 ± 1.4	7.9 ± 0.8
	Goncharov et al., 2019 [31]	90.3 ± 10	96.3 ± 3.6	92.1 ± 10.5	97.4 ± 2.3	NR	NR
	Helito et al., 2018 [32]	87.1 ± 9	92.7 ± 5.9	90 ± 7.1	95.4 ± 5.3	NR	NR
Tibialis Allograft	Lee et al., 2023 [26]	82.9 ± 8.8	87.1 ± 9.8	87.3 ± 7.9	90.7 ± 8.1	5.6 ± 1.3	6.1 ± 1.4
	Yang et al., 2023 [25]	84.3 ± 15.9	84.7 ± 12.2	89.6 ± 17.6	89.7 ± 13.3	5.5 ± 2.1	6 ± 1.7

ALLR, anterolateral ligament reconstruction; ACLR, anterior cruciate ligament reconstruction; SD, standard deviation; HT, hamstring tendon; NR, not reported; IKDC, Internation Knee Documentation Committee.

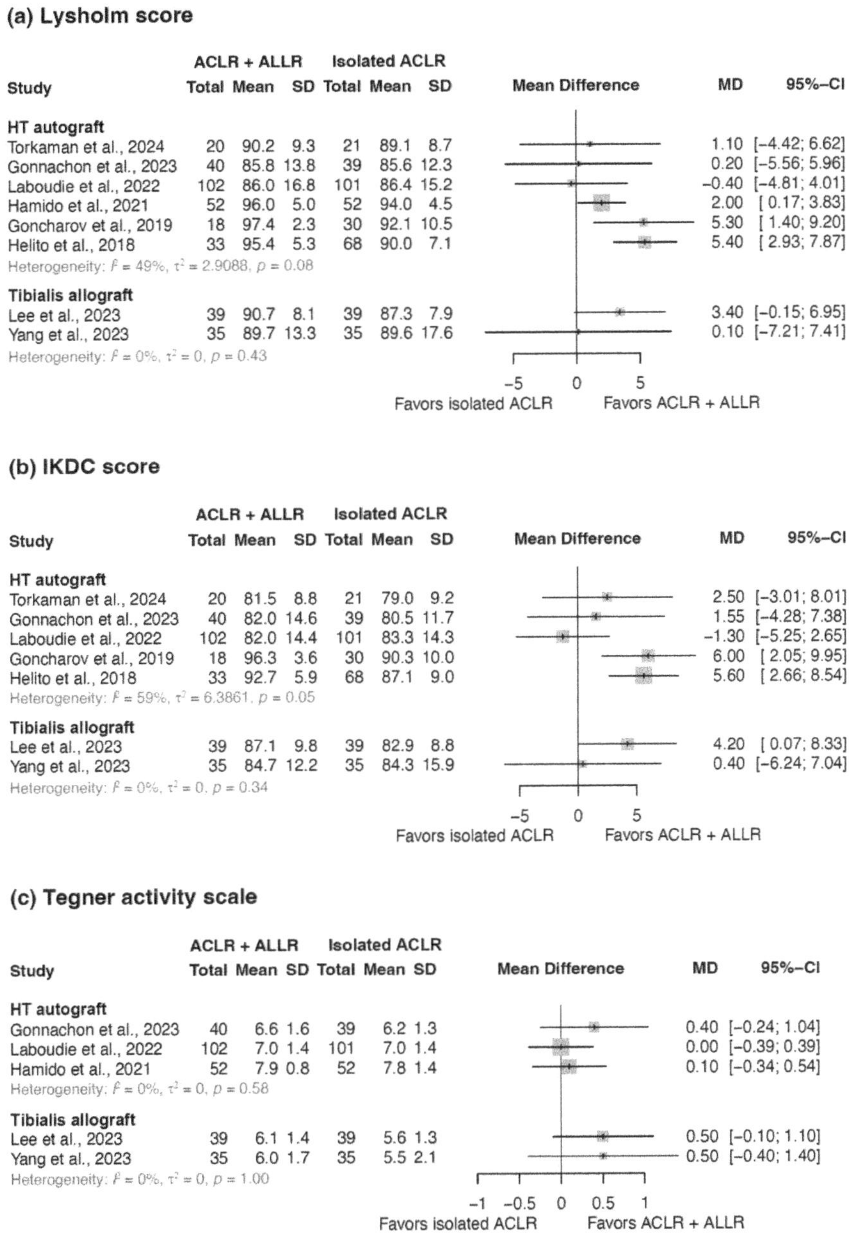

Figure 3. Forest plot illustrating the differences in treatment effects between isolated ACLR and cases in which ACLR and ALLR were performed concurrently, divided into subgroups according to the ALLR graft used. The results for (**a**) Lysholm score, (**b**) IKDC score, and (**c**) Tegner activity scale are presented. Gray squares indicate the effect estimates for each study, with their size representing the study's weight in the analysis. ACLR, anterior cruciate ligament reconstruction; ALLR, anterolateral ligament reconstruction; SD, standard deviation; MD, mean difference; CI, confidence interval; HT, hamstring tendon; IKDC, International Knee Documentation Committee [25–27,29–33].

The IKDC score has been reported in seven studies [25–27,29,31–33]. The comparison of combined ACLR with ALLR with isolated ACLR based on the graft used for ALLR showed that for HT autografts [27,29,31–33], MDs ranged from −1.30 to 6.00, whereas for tibialis allografts [25,26], MDs ranged from 0.40 to 4.20 (Figure 3b). HT autografts (I^2 = 59%, τ^2 = 6.3861, p = 0.05) exhibited high heterogeneity, whereas tibialis allografts (I^2 = 0%, τ^2 = 0.0, p = 0.34) exhibited low heterogeneity.

The Tegner activity scale has been reported in five studies [25,26,29–31]. The comparison of combined ACLR with ALLR with isolated ACLR based on the graft used for ALLR showed that for HT autografts [27,29,30], MDs ranged from 0.00 to 0.40, whereas for tibialis allografts [25,26], the MD of 0.50 was reported (Figure 3c). Both HT autografts (I^2 = 0%, τ^2 = 0.0, p = 0.58) and tibialis allografts (I^2 = 0%, τ^2 = 0.0, p = 1.00) exhibited low heterogeneity.

3.7. Complications

Complications have been reported in seven studies [25–30,32]. For HT autografts for ALLR, Gonnachon et al. [27] and Hamido et al. [30] reported no major complications in either the isolated ACLR group or the combined ACLR and ALLR group. Laboudine et al. [29] observed no difference in occasional knee pain, hardware problems, stiffness, swelling, or cyclops lesion between the two groups two years after surgery. Pioger et al. [28] reported that reoperations for symptomatic cyclops lesions and secondary meniscectomy were more frequent in the isolated ACLR group. Helito et al. [32] reported that one patient in the isolated ACLR group had a hypertrophic scar on the thigh due to the outside-in technique, and one patient had a pretibial cyst. In the ACLR with ALLR group, one patient experienced femoral anchor loosening with irritation of the lateral soft tissue of the knee, requiring removal. Torkaman et al. [33] reported that one patient in the isolated ACLR group and one patient in the combined ACLR and ALLR group developed postoperative arthrofibrosis, but both regained full range of motion within six months. Additionally, eight patients in the isolated ACLR group and seven in the combined group experienced anterior knee pain, with no statistically significant difference in complications between the groups.

For studies using tibialis allografts for ALLR, Lee et al. [26] reported no sustained pain, bioabsorbable screw protrusion, stiffness, or swelling at a minimum two-year follow-up. Yang et al. [25] noted that in the ACLR with ALLR group, one patient had a cyclops-type lesion and one patient had a superficial wound infection. However, all patients in both groups recovered by the final follow-up without specific complications.

4. Discussion

The primary findings of this systematic review revealed that regardless of the graft type used for ALLR, combining ACLR with ALLR resulted in reduced graft failure rates and superior residual rotational stability compared to isolated ACLR. Additionally, residual AP stability and patient-reported outcome measures were generally favorable or comparable for the combined procedure; however, the results were heterogeneous across studies. Notably, no complications related to the specific graft type used for ALLR or the presence of ALLR were reported. Future research, particularly studies directly comparing graft types for ALLR, is needed to better define the influence of graft selection on the outcomes of combined ACLR and ALLR procedures.

The primary objective of introducing ALLR was to address persistent rotatory instability, a common issue associated with isolated ACLR, which ultimately aims to prevent ACL graft failure [34]. Several systematic reviews and meta-analyses have consistently reported that the combined ACLR and ALLR procedure is superior to isolated ACLR in terms of graft failure, residual pivot shift, and clinical outcomes [11,19,20]. Consistent with other reviews, our study also demonstrates that combined reconstruction is superior to isolated ACLR in terms of graft failure and residual pivot shift.

Graft selection, whether autografts or allografts, is recognized as one of the critical modifiable factors that influence surgical outcomes, such as graft failure, following ACLR [5]. In their randomized controlled trial comparing tibialis posterior allografts and hamstring autografts for ACLR, Bottoni et al. [15] demonstrated that the allograft had a failure rate over three times higher than the autograft at a minimum ten-year follow-up. Similarly, data from the Kaiser Permanente ACLR Registry indicated that BPTB allografts had an overall 4.5-fold higher risk of revision compared to BPTB autografts for ACLR [35]. However, these higher failure rates of allografts compared to those of autografts have not been consistent in some recent studies, possibly due to the use of fresh frozen allografts instead of irradiated allografts [36]. The ACL grafts used in the studies included in this review are predominately autologous hamstring grafts, with only one study using a BPTB graft. The impact of the included BPTB autograft is considered negligible, as there is no statistically significant difference in graft failure rates, even though HT grafts tend to exhibit a higher failure rate [37–39].

Given the impact of graft selection on ACLR outcomes, it is essential to examine how graft choice may similarly affect ALLR and, consequently, influence the overall outcomes of ACLR. Despite this, limited research exists regarding the optimal graft choice for ALLR, with few studies investigating this issue. Previous meta-analyses related to our study topic have explored ALLR, lateral extra-articular procedures, and their various clinical outcomes [11,19,20]. However, none have conducted a detailed analysis of differences based on ALLR graft selection. Therefore, this study aims to provide insights into this aspect, which has not been addressed in prior systematic reviews or meta-analyses. While various autograft candidates for ALLR, including the iliotibial band and the gracilis, semitendinosus, plantaris longus, quadriceps, and patellar tendons, have been proposed [40], the HT, predominantly the one-strand gracilis tendon, was the most commonly used autograft for ALLR performed concurrently with ACLR in this review [27–33].

In their cadaveric study, Wytrykowski et al. [41] compared the mechanical properties of ALL with potential graft candidates for ALLR, including the gracilis tendon and iliotibial band. They observed that the two-strand gracilis tendon exhibited the highest maximum load to failure at 201 N compared to the native ALL at 141 N and the iliotibial band at 161 N. Considering that a four-strand gracilis tendon has a maximum load to failure of 416 N, which is double that of a two-strand gracilis, it can be inferred that a one-strand gracilis would have half or less than half of the maximum load that a two-strand gracilis construct can withstand [42]. Consequently, the one-strand gracilis tendon used in most of the included studies may not attain the strength of the native ALL, as it is estimated to have a maximum load of approximately 100 N. This insufficient graft strength may limit its ability to recapitulate the role of the ALL, potentially leading to no significant difference in graft failure or residual pivot shift between autografts and allografts in the current review; however, it may still yield superior outcomes than isolated ACLR. Additionally, while it is difficult to determine the exact properties of the grafts used in each study included in this review, reports suggest that tibialis allografts can serve as substitutes for hamstring tendons based on their mechanical properties [43]. This supports the finding that there was no clear difference between autografts and allografts in the review.

Allografts can be a viable graft option for ALLR, particularly when autograft options have been exhausted in multi-ligament or revision reconstructions or when performing both ACLR and ALLR with a hamstring autograft results in suboptimal ACL or ALL graft characteristics [40]. In cases of combined ACLR and ALLR using a hamstring autograft, as in the studies included in our review, most grafts, such as a three-strand semitendinosus tendon and one-strand gracilis tendon or a three- or four-strand semitendinosus tendon, are used for ACLR, leaving only a one- or two-strand gracilis tendon for ALLR [25–33]. These graft constructs present a potential risk of a small ACL graft diameter, even with a three- or four-strand ACL graft. In an attempt to compensate by creating a three- or four-strand construct, the ACL graft tunnel length may become shortened, often leaving only a one-strand gracilis tendon available for use as the ALL graft [44]. The ACL graft diameter has considerable implications for graft failure, as every 0.5 to 1.0 mm increase in diameter is associated with an approximately 20% decrease in the graft failure rate [45,46]. Furthermore, short graft tunnel length raises concerns regarding graft fixation, stability, and the risk of tunnel enlargement [47,48]. Given that our study revealed no significant differences in graft rupture rates, rotational stability, or patient-reported outcomes between autografts and allografts, using an allograft for ALLR may be particularly useful for surgeons who wish to utilize hamstring autograft for ACLR without compromising graft characteristics.

Common issues associated with the use of allografts include concerns regarding disease transmission and increased cost [49]. However, the studies included in this review did not report complications specific to allografts or ALLR. This absence of complications could be attributed to the rarity of disease transmission today due to more stringent donor screening and testing protocols [49]. Furthermore, unlike lateral extra-articular tenodesis, ALLR demonstrates a lower risk of overconstraint-related issues, such as knee stiffness, which may account for the lack of reported complications [11]. However, the increased cost associated with its use should be thoroughly discussed with the patient prior to decision-making. Our findings may serve to guide surgeons in selecting the most appropriate graft type based on the specific clinical scenario and the unique characteristics of each graft, thereby potentially optimizing patient outcomes.

The residual AP laxity reported in several studies included in this review generally demonstrated either more favorable or comparable results for combined ACLR and ALLR compared to those for isolated ACLR. This finding aligns with previous research suggesting that the ALL works synergistically with the ACL to maintain both rotatory and AP stability of the knee [50]. However, in this review, a subgroup analysis based on the type of ALLR graft utilized revealed that HT autografts ($I^2 = 94\%$, $\tau^2 = 0.2367$, $p < 0.01$) exhibited high heterogeneity. Consequently, there is insufficient evidence to draw definitive conclusions regarding AP laxity differences related to ALLR graft types.

Patient-reported outcome measures, including the Lysholm and IKDC scores, and the Tegner activity scale demonstrated similar or higher outcome scores when both ACLR and ALLR were performed compared to isolated ACLR. However, for HT autografts, the Lysholm score showed moderate heterogeneity ($I^2 = 49\%$, $\tau^2 = 2.9088$, $p = 0.08$) and the IKDC score exhibited high heterogeneity ($I^2 = 59\%$, $\tau^2 = 6.3861$, $p = 0.05$).

The observed heterogeneity across studies may stem from differences in surgical techniques, graft preparation and fixation methods, rehabilitation protocols, and indications for ALLR. Variations in patient demographics, follow-up durations, and outcome assessment methods also likely contributed to inconsistencies. Additionally, the risk of bias for each study was assessed, but it is important to note that there is only one study with a level-I-evidence RCT, and differences in the inclusion criteria used across studies may also contribute to potential sources of bias. Given these factors, the results should be interpreted with caution.

Limitations

Our study has some limitations. First, a few high-level evidence studies are available in this domain, particularly those focusing on the outcomes of using allografts in ALLR, which prevents the possibility of conducting a pooled synthesis. To address this, we presented the results by dividing the grafts into subgroups and providing a range of effect sizes through a forest plot. Second, only ALLR performed with primary ACLR was included, excluding studies involving other lateral extra-articular procedures or revision cases. Different lateral procedures may introduce heterogeneity due to anatomical differences from ALLR, and revision cases could represent a distinct clinical entity, potentially affecting outcomes such as graft failure. Therefore, our inclusion criteria were deemed appropriate for evaluating the specific function of the ALLR graft. Third, indications for ALLR differ across studies, which may have introduced heterogeneity in the analysis. Fourth, study design limitations made it impossible to directly compare the outcomes of autografts and allografts. Fifth, surgical outcomes can also be influenced by patient-specific factors such as age, activity level, and concomitant procedures, which necessitates caution when interpreting the results. Sixth, many studies in the analysis had relatively short- to medium-term follow-up periods, underscoring the need for future studies assessing long-term outcomes. Lastly, the number of studies using allografts as the ALLR graft was relatively small. Future studies should focus on directly comparing autografts and allografts or conducting a systematic review that includes more studies to enable more definitive conclusions.

5. Conclusions

Regardless of the graft type used for ALLR, the combination of ACLR with ALLR showed better clinical outcomes, including reduced graft failure rates and superior residual rotational stability compared to isolated ACLR. However, the high heterogeneity observed across studies suggests that these findings should be interpreted with caution, and further research is needed to draw more definitive conclusions.

Author Contributions: Conceptualization, K.C. and S.-H.K.; methodology, K.C. and S.-H.K.; data curation, J.H.H. and K.C.; software, J.H.H.; visualization, J.H.H.; writing—original draft preparation, J.H.H., S.-H.K. and K.C.; writing—review and editing, M.J. and H.-S.M.; supervision, S.-H.K., M.J. and K.C. All authors have read and agreed to the published version of the manuscript.

Funding: This research received no external funding.

Data Availability Statement: The data presented in this study are available upon request from the corresponding author.

Conflicts of Interest: The authors declare no conflicts of interest.

Abbreviations

The following abbreviations are used in this manuscript:

ACLR	Anterior cruciate ligament reconstruction
ALLR	Anterolateral ligament reconstruction
AP	Anterior–posterior
HT	Hamstring tendon
OR	Odds ratio
ACL	Anterior cruciate ligament
ALL	Anterolateral ligament
BPTB	Bone–patellar tendon–bone
PRISMA	Preferred Reporting Items for Systematic Reviews and Meta-analyses
IKDC	International Knee Documentation Committee
RCT	Randomized controlled trial
MINORS	Methodological Index for Non-Randomized Studies
MD	Mean difference
CI	Confidence interval

Appendix A

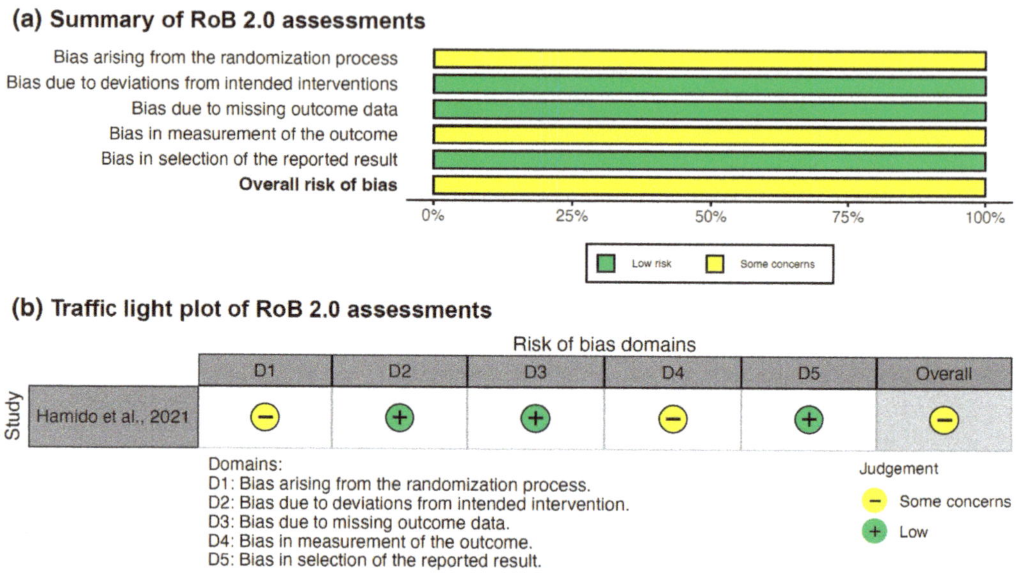

Figure A1. Summary of the risk of bias assessment for included studies. (**a**) Summary of the RoB 2.0 assessment. (**b**) Traffic light plot for the RoB 2.0 assessment. RoB, risk of bias [30].

Table A1. Risk of bias was assessed using the MINORS score.

Study	Torkaman et al. [33]	Gonnachon et al. [27]	Lee et al. [26]	Yang et al. [25]	Laboudie et al. [29]	Pioger et al. [28]	Goncharov et al. [31]	Helito et al. [32]
Year	2024	2023	2023	2023	2022	2022	2019	2018
Level of evidence	2	3	3	3	3	3	2	3
1. A stated aim of the study	2	2	2	2	2	2	2	2
2. Inclusion of consecutive patients	2	2	2	2	2	2	2	2
3. Prospective collection of data	2	2	2	2	2	2	2	2
4. Endpoint appropriate to the study aim	2	2	2	2	2	2	2	2
5. Unbiased evaluation of endpoints	2	2	2	2	2	2	2	2
6. Follow-up period appropriate to the major endpoint	2	2	2	2	2	2	2	2
7. Loss to follow up not exceeding 5%	2	2	0	0	1	2	2	0
8. Prospective calculation of the sample size	2	0	0	2	1	0	0	1
9. A control group having the gold standard intervention	2	2	2	2	2	2	2	2
10. Contemporary groups	2	1	1	2	2	2	2	1
11. Baseline equivalence of groups	2	2	2	2	2	2	1	2
12. Statistical analyses adapted to the study design	2	2	2	2	2	2	2	2
Total scores	24	21	19	22	22	22	21	20

Table A2. Inclusion criteria of studies.

Study	Year	Graft Used for ALLR
Torkaman et al. [33]	2024	Patients had unilateral ACL injury, underwent ACLR using a quadruple-bundle semitendinosus tendon autograft, had an intact meniscus, exhibited a pivot shift test grade of 2+ or 3+, and had a minimum follow-up of two years.
Gonnachon et al. [27]	2023	Patients had ACL rupture and participated in pivot contact sports such as team sports or martial arts, regardless of competition level.
Lee et al. [26]	2023	Female patients had ACL rupture and a high-grade pivot shift (grade 2) and underwent combined ACLR and ALLR.
Yang et al. [25]	2023	Patients undergoing primary ACLR + ALLR met one or more of the following criteria: participation in high-level sporting activities (training at least twice a week, competing to win, professional or elite players), involvement in pivoting sports, presence of ligamentous hyperlaxity/genu recurvatum based on the modified Beighton scale, or a grade 3 pivot shift.
Laboudie et al. [29]	2022	Patients had a pivot shift grade ≥2, hyperlaxity (knee recurvatum >10°), were high-level athletes, or had a Segond fracture.
Pioger et al. [28]	2022	Patients underwent combined ACLR + ALLR due to high-grade pivot shift, chronic injuries, hyperlaxity, or participation in pivoting sports at a young age.
Hamido et al. [30]	2021	Patients had a high-grade pivot shift (grade III), a Segond fracture, participated in high-level sports, or engaged in sports involving frequent pivoting.
Goncharov et al. [31]	2019	Patients trained at least three times a week, participated in competitions, were involved in professional sports, and were aged between 16 and 40 years.
Helito et al. [32]	2018	Patients had an ACL injury for more than 12 months, confirmed by clinical and imaging examinations, and had no associated peripheral ligament injuries apart from the anterolateral corner.

The inclusion criteria presented in each study were summarized, and cases where specific criteria for combined ACLR and ALLR were provided were separately indicated. ACL, anterior cruciate ligament; ACLR, anterior cruciate ligament reconstruction; ALLR, anterolateral ligament reconstruction.

References

1. Sanders, T.L.; Maradit Kremers, H.; Bryan, A.J.; Larson, D.R.; Dahm, D.L.; Levy, B.A.; Stuart, M.J.; Krych, A.J. Incidence of anterior cruciate ligament tears and reconstruction: A 21-year population-based study. *Am. J. Sports Med.* **2016**, *44*, 1502–1507. [PubMed]
2. Diermeier, T.; Rothrauff, B.B.; Engebretsen, L.; Lynch, A.D.; Ayeni, O.R.; Paterno, M.V.; Xerogeanes, J.W.; Fu, F.H.; Karlsson, J.; Musahl, V.; et al. Treatment after anterior cruciate ligament injury: Panther symposium acl treatment consensus group. *Knee Surg. Sports Traumatol. Arthrosc.* **2020**, *28*, 2390–2402. [PubMed]
3. Lind, M.; Menhert, F.; Pedersen, A.B. Incidence and outcome after revision anterior cruciate ligament reconstruction: Results from the danish registry for knee ligament reconstructions. *Am. J. Sports Med.* **2012**, *40*, 1551–1557.
4. Kamath, G.V.; Redfern, J.C.; Greis, P.E.; Burks, R.T. Revision anterior cruciate ligament reconstruction. *Am. J. Sports Med.* **2011**, *39*, 199–217.
5. Koga, H.; Engebretsen, L.; Fu, F.H.; Muneta, T. Revision anterior cruciate ligament surgery: State of the art. *J. ISAKOS* **2017**, *2*, 36–46.
6. Bae, B.S.; Yoo, S.; Lee, S.H. Ramp lesion in anterior cruciate ligament injury: A review of the anatomy, biomechanics, epidemiology, and diagnosis. *Knee Surg. Relat. Res.* **2023**, *35*, 23.
7. Yoon, K.H.; Lee, S.M.; Park, J.Y.; Lee, H.S.; Hwang, S.H. A comparison of results in older, middle-aged, and younger patients after primary anterior cruciate ligament reconstruction: Minimum 10-year follow-up. *Clin. Orthop. Surg.* **2024**, *16*, 57–65.
8. Ayeni, O.R.; Chahal, M.; Tran, M.N.; Sprague, S. Pivot shift as an outcome measure for acl reconstruction: A systematic review. *Knee Surg. Sports Traumatol. Arthrosc.* **2012**, *20*, 767–777.
9. Littlefield, C.P.; Belk, J.W.; Houck, D.A.; Kraeutler, M.J.; LaPrade, R.F.; Chahla, J.; McCarty, E.C. The anterolateral ligament of the knee: An updated systematic review of anatomy, biomechanics, and clinical outcomes. *Arthroscopy* **2021**, *37*, 1654–1666.
10. Morgan, A.M.; Bi, A.S.; Kaplan, D.J.; Alaia, M.J.; Strauss, E.J.; Jazrawi, L.M. An eponymous history of the anterolateral ligament complex of the knee. *Knee Surg. Relat. Res.* **2022**, *34*, 45.
11. Na, B.R.; Kwak, W.K.; Seo, H.Y.; Seon, J.K. Clinical outcomes of anterolateral ligament reconstruction or lateral extra-articular tenodesis combined with primary acl reconstruction: A systematic review with meta-analysis. *Orthop. J. Sports Med.* **2021**, *9*, 23259671211023099. [PubMed]

12. Musahl, V.; Engler, I.D.; Nazzal, E.M.; Dalton, J.F.; Lucidi, G.A.; Hughes, J.D.; Zaffagnini, S.; Della Villa, F.; Irrgang, J.J.; Fu, F.H.; et al. Current trends in the anterior cruciate ligament part ii: Evaluation, surgical technique, prevention, and rehabilitation. *Knee Surg. Sports Traumatol. Arthrosc.* **2022**, *30*, 34–51. [PubMed]
13. Mouarbes, D.; Menetrey, J.; Marot, V.; Courtot, L.; Berard, E.; Cavaignac, E. Anterior cruciate ligament reconstruction: A systematic review and meta-analysis of outcomes for quadriceps tendon autograft versus bone-patellar tendon-bone and hamstring-tendon autografts. *Am. J. Sports Med.* **2019**, *47*, 3531–3540.
14. Lee, D.W.; Ro, D.H.; Lee, M.C.; Han, H.S. Rectangular-tunnel anterior cruciate ligament reconstruction using quadriceps tendon-patellar bone autograft can reduce early donor site morbidity while maintaining comparable short-term clinical outcomes. *Clin. Orthop. Surg.* **2024**, *16*, 49–56.
15. Bottoni, C.R.; Smith, E.L.; Shaha, J.; Shaha, S.S.; Raybin, S.G.; Tokish, J.M.; Rowles, D.J. Autograft versus allograft anterior cruciate ligament reconstruction: A prospective, randomized clinical study with a minimum 10-year follow-up. *Am. J. Sports Med.* **2015**, *43*, 2501–2509.
16. Cruz, A.I., Jr.; Beck, J.J.; Ellington, M.D.; Mayer, S.W.; Pennock, A.T.; Stinson, Z.S.; VandenBerg, C.D.; Barrow, B.; Gao, B.; Ellis, H.B., Jr. Failure rates of autograft and allograft acl reconstruction in patients 19 years of age and younger: A systematic review and meta-analysis. *JBJS Open Access* **2020**, *5*, e20.00106.
17. Runer, A.; Keeling, L.; Wagala, N.; Nugraha, H.; Özbek, E.A.; Hughes, J.D.; Musahl, V. Current trends in graft choice for primary anterior cruciate ligament reconstruction—Part II: In-vivo kinematics, patient reported outcomes, re-rupture rates, strength recovery, return to sports and complications. *J. Exp. Orthop.* **2023**, *10*, 40.
18. Liau, Z.Q.G.; Ng, M.S.P.; Low, S.S.E.; Chin, B.Z.; Hui, J.H.P.; Kagda, F.H.Y. A novel practical method to predict anterior cruciate ligament hamstring graft size using preoperative mri. *Knee Surg. Relat. Res.* **2024**, *36*, 17.
19. Boksh, K.; Sheikh, N.; Chong, H.H.; Ghosh, A.; Aujla, R. The role of anterolateral ligament reconstruction or lateral extra-articular tenodesis for revision anterior cruciate ligament reconstruction: A systematic review and meta-analysis of comparative clinical studies. *Am. J. Sports Med.* **2024**, *52*, 269–285.
20. Bosco, F.; Giustra, F.; Masoni, V.; Capella, M.; Sciannameo, V.; Camarda, L.; Massè, A.; LaPrade, R.F. Combining an anterolateral complex procedure with anterior cruciate ligament reconstruction reduces the graft reinjury rate and improves clinical outcomes: A systematic review and meta-analysis of randomized controlled trials. *Am. J. Sports Med.* **2024**, *52*, 2129–2147.
21. Sterne, J.A.C.; Savović, J.; Page, M.J.; Elbers, R.G.; Blencowe, N.S.; Boutron, I.; Cates, C.J.; Cheng, H.Y.; Corbett, M.S.; Eldridge, S.M.; et al. Rob 2: A revised tool for assessing risk of bias in randomised trials. *BMJ* **2019**, *366*, l4898. [PubMed]
22. Slim, K.; Nini, E.; Forestier, D.; Kwiatkowski, F.; Panis, Y.; Chipponi, J. Methodological index for non-randomized studies (minors): Development and validation of a new instrument. *ANZ J. Surg.* **2003**, *73*, 712–716.
23. Furukawa, T.A.; Barbui, C.; Cipriani, A.; Brambilla, P.; Watanabe, N. Imputing missing standard deviations in meta-analyses can provide accurate results. *J. Clin. Epidemiol.* **2006**, *59*, 7–10.
24. Gheibi, S.; Mahmoodzadeh, A.; Kashfi, K.; Jeddi, S.; Ghasemi, A. Data extraction from graphs using adobe photoshop: Applications for meta-analyses. *Int. J. Endocrinol. Metab.* **2019**, *17*, e95216.
25. Yang, H.Y.; Cheon, J.H.; Choi, J.H.; Song, E.K.; Seon, J.K. Combined anterior cruciate ligament and anterolateral ligament reconstruction decreases passive anterior tibial subluxation compared with isolated anterior cruciate ligament reconstruction despite similar rotational stability and clinical outcomes. *Arthroscopy* **2023**, *39*, 2513–2524.e2. [CrossRef]
26. Lee, D.W.; Lee, D.H.; Cho, S.I.; Yang, S.J.; Kim, W.J.; Lee, J.K.; Kim, J.G. Comparison of acl and anterolateral ligament reconstruction with isolated acl reconstruction using hamstring autograft: Outcomes in young female patients with high-grade pivot shift. *Orthop. J. Sports Med.* **2023**, *11*, 23259671231178048.
27. Gonnachon, A.; Labattut, L.; Abdoul Carime, N.; Orta, C.; Baulot, E.; Martz, P. Does combined anterior cruciate ligament and anterolateral ligament reconstruction improve return to sport? *Eur. J. Orthop. Surg. Traumatol.* **2023**, *34*, 981–987. [CrossRef]
28. Pioger, C.; Gousopoulos, L.; Hopper, G.P.; Vieira, T.D.; Campos, J.P.; El Helou, A.; Philippe, C.; Saithna, A.; Sonnery-Cottet, B. Clinical outcomes after combined acl and anterolateral ligament reconstruction versus isolated acl reconstruction with bone-patellar tendon-bone grafts: A matched-pair analysis of 2018 patients from the santi study group. *Am. J. Sports Med.* **2022**, *50*, 3493–3501.
29. Laboudie, P.; Douiri, A.; Bouguennec, N.; Biset, A.; Graveleau, N. Combined acl and all reconstruction reduces the rate of reoperation for graft failure or secondary meniscal lesions in young athletes. *Knee Surg. Sports Traumatol. Arthrosc.* **2022**, *30*, 3488–3498.
30. Hamido, F.; Habiba, A.A.; Marwan, Y.; Soliman, A.S.I.; Elkhadrawe, T.A.; Morsi, M.G.; Shoaeb, W.; Nagi, A. Anterolateral ligament reconstruction improves the clinical and functional outcomes of anterior cruciate ligament reconstruction in athletes. *Knee Surg. Sports Traumatol. Arthrosc.* **2021**, *29*, 1173–1180.
31. Goncharov, E.N.; Koval, O.A.; Dubrov, V.E.; Bezuglov, E.N.; Filimonova, A.M.; Goncharov, N.G. Clinical experience with combined reconstruction of the anterior cruciate and anterolateral ligaments of the knee in sportsmen. *Int. Orthop.* **2019**, *43*, 2781–2788. [PubMed]

32. Helito, C.P.; Camargo, D.B.; Sobrado, M.F.; Bonadio, M.B.; Giglio, P.N.; Pécora, J.R.; Camanho, G.L.; Demange, M.K. Combined reconstruction of the anterolateral ligament in chronic acl injuries leads to better clinical outcomes than isolated acl reconstruction. *Knee Surg. Sports Traumatol. Arthrosc.* **2018**, *26*, 3652–3659.
33. Torkaman, A.; Hosseinzadeh, M.; Mohammadyahya, E.; Torkaman, P.; Bahaeddini, M.R.; Aminian, A.; Tayyebi, H. All-inside anterior cruciate ligament reconstruction with and without anterolateral ligament reconstruction: A prospective study. *BMC Musculoskelet. Disord.* **2024**, *25*, 16.
34. Tavlo, M.; Eljaja, S.; Jensen, J.T.; Siersma, V.D.; Krogsgaard, M.R. The role of the anterolateral ligament in acl insufficient and reconstructed knees on rotatory stability: A biomechanical study on human cadavers. *Scand. J. Med. Sci. Sports* **2016**, *26*, 960–966.
35. Maletis, G.B.; Chen, J.; Inacio, M.C.S.; Love, R.M.; Funahashi, T.T. Increased risk of revision after anterior cruciate ligament reconstruction with bone-patellar tendon-bone allografts compared with autografts. *Am. J. Sports Med.* **2017**, *45*, 1333–1340.
36. Zeng, C.; Gao, S.G.; Li, H.; Yang, T.; Luo, W.; Li, Y.S.; Lei, G.H. Autograft versus allograft in anterior cruciate ligament reconstruction: A meta-analysis of randomized controlled trials and systematic review of overlapping systematic reviews. *Arthroscopy* **2016**, *32*, 153–163.e18.
37. Dai, W.; Leng, X.; Wang, J.; Cheng, J.; Hu, X.; Ao, Y. Quadriceps tendon autograft versus bone-patellar tendon-bone and hamstring tendon autografts for anterior cruciate ligament reconstruction: A systematic review and meta-analysis. *Am. J. Sports Med.* **2022**, *50*, 3425–3439.
38. He, X.; Yang, X.G.; Feng, J.T.; Wang, F.; Huang, H.C.; He, J.Q.; Hu, Y.C. Clinical outcomes of the central third patellar tendon versus four-strand hamstring tendon autograft used for anterior cruciate ligament reconstruction: A systematic review and subgroup meta-analysis of randomized controlled trials. *Injury* **2020**, *51*, 1714–1725.
39. Mohtadi, N.G.; Chan, D.S.; Dainty, K.N.; Whelan, D.B. Patellar tendon versus hamstring tendon autograft for anterior cruciate ligament rupture in adults. *Cochrane Database Syst. Rev.* **2011**, *2011*, Cd005960.
40. Chalidis, B.; Pitsilos, C.; Kitridis, D.; Givissis, P. Graft choices for anterolateral ligament knee reconstruction surgery: Current concepts. *World J. Clin. Cases* **2022**, *10*, 8463–8473.
41. Wytrykowski, K.; Swider, P.; Reina, N.; Murgier, J.; Laffosse, J.M.; Chiron, P.; Cavaignac, E. Cadaveric study comparing the biomechanical properties of grafts used for knee anterolateral ligament reconstruction. *Arthroscopy* **2016**, *32*, 2288–2294. [PubMed]
42. Pailhé, R.; Cavaignac, E.; Murgier, J.; Laffosse, J.M.; Swider, P. Biomechanical study of acl reconstruction grafts. *J. Orthop. Res.* **2015**, *33*, 1188–1196. [PubMed]
43. Almqvist, K.F.; Jan, H.; Vercruysse, C.; Verbeeck, R.; Verdonk, R. The tibialis tendon as a valuable anterior cruciate ligament allograft substitute: Biomechanical properties. *Knee Surg. Sports Traumatol. Arthrosc.* **2007**, *15*, 1326–1330. [PubMed]
44. Nazari, G.; Barton, K.I.; Bryant, D.; Getgood, A.; Brown, C.H., Jr. Five- and six-strand hamstring grafts consistently produce appropriate graft diameters for anterior cruciate ligament reconstruction. *Knee Surg. Sports Traumatol. Arthrosc.* **2021**, *29*, 2940–2947.
45. Itoh, M.; Itou, J.; Okazaki, K.; Iwasaki, K. Estimation failure risk by 0.5-mm differences in autologous hamstring graft diameter in anterior cruciate ligament reconstruction: A meta-analysis. *Am. J. Sports Med.* **2024**, *52*, 535–543.
46. Zhao, D.; Pan, J.K.; Lin, F.Z.; Luo, M.H.; Liang, G.H.; Zeng, L.F.; Huang, H.T.; Han, Y.H.; Xu, N.J.; Yang, W.Y.; et al. Risk factors for revision or rerupture after anterior cruciate ligament reconstruction: A systematic review and meta-analysis. *Am. J. Sports Med.* **2023**, *51*, 3053–3075.
47. Guglielmetti, L.G.B.; Shimba, L.G.; do Santos, L.C.; Severino, F.R.; Severino, N.R.; de Moraes Barros Fucs, P.M.; de Paula Leite Cury, R. The influence of femoral tunnel length on graft rupture after anterior cruciate ligament reconstruction. *J. Orthop. Traumatol.* **2017**, *18*, 243–250. [CrossRef]
48. Moon, H.S.; Choi, C.H.; Yoo, J.H.; Jung, M.; Lee, T.H.; Choi, K.H.; Kim, S.H. The graft insertion length in the femoral tunnel during anterior cruciate ligament reconstruction with suspensory fixation and tibialis anterior allograft does not affect surgical outcomes but is negatively correlated with tunnel widening. *Arthroscopy* **2021**, *37*, 2903–2914.e1.
49. Mistry, H.; Metcalfe, A.; Colquitt, J.; Loveman, E.; Smith, N.A.; Royle, P.; Waugh, N. Autograft or allograft for reconstruction of anterior cruciate ligament: A health economics perspective. *Knee Surg. Sports Traumatol. Arthrosc.* **2019**, *27*, 1782–1790.
50. Lee, J.K.; Seo, Y.J.; Jeong, S.Y.; Yang, J.H. Biomechanical function of the anterolateral ligament of the knee: A systematic review. *Knee Surg. Relat. Res.* **2020**, *32*, 6.

Journal of
Clinical Medicine

MDPI

Article

The Risk of Secondary Knee Procedures After Anterior Cruciate Ligament Reconstruction—A Nationwide Retrospective Cohort Study

Han-Kook Yoon [1], Chang-Min Lee [1], Hyun-Cheol Oh [1], Taemi Youk [2] and Sang-Hoon Park [1,*]

[1] Department of Orthopaedic Surgery, National Health Insurance Service Ilsan Hospital, Goyang 10444, Republic of Korea; hangugy@nhimc.or.kr (H.-K.Y.); changmini713@naver.com (C.-M.L.); hyuncoh@nhimc.or.kr (H.-C.O.)

[2] Research Institute, National Health Insurance Service Ilsan Hospital, Goyang 10444, Republic of Korea; tmyouk@nhimc.or.kr

* Correspondence: almania@nhimc.or.kr; Tel.: +82-31-900-0540; Fax: +82-31-900-0343

Abstract: Objectives: Some following up patients have poor clinical outcomes when they experience anterior cruciate ligament reconstruction. The patient will undergo progression of knee joint osteoarthritis or several secondary knee procedures such as high tibial osteotomy, total knee arthroplasty, menisectomy, meniscus repair, or meniscus transplantation on their knees after anterior cruciate ligament reconstruction. This may be related to the remaining instability of the knee joint, changes in the knee joint biomechanics, and progression of osteoarthritis. This study aims to determine which secondary knee procedures are performed over time after anterior cruciate ligament reconstruction. **Methods:** The National Health Insurance Service-Health Screening database analyzed 146,122 patients who underwent ACL reconstruction surgery between 1 January 2002 and 31 December 2021. Secondary knee procedures were investigated by categorizing them into revisional reconstruction, high tibial osteotomy, total knee arthroplasty, menisectomy, meniscus repair, and meniscus transplantation, respectively. Multivariable Cox Proportional Hazard model analysis was used. The significant predictors for complications ($p < 0.05$) were as follows. **Results:** Among a total of 146,122 patients with anterior cruciate ligament reconstruction, 1073 (0.7%) patients underwent HTO, 908 (0.6%) patients underwent TKA, 15,218 (10.4%) patients underwent meniscectomy, 7169 (4.9%) patients underwent meniscus repair, and 938 (0.6%) patients underwent meniscus transplantation. The hazard ratio differed according to graft type, gender, and age group. **Conclusions:** Patients who undergo ACL reconstruction may experience poor clinical outcomes, such as progression of osteoarthritis and undergoing secondary knee procedures several years after ACL reconstruction. It is important for decision-making, ongoing monitoring, and follow-up care for patients undergoing ACL reconstruction.

Keywords: anterior cruciate ligament; big data; knee

1. Introduction

The anterior cruciate ligament is the most frequently injured ligament in the knee that needs surgical treatment [1,2]. There are studies about the incidence of ACL injury and reconstruction surgery worldwide. For example, in the United States, studies reported that the annual incidence of ACL tears was 68.6 per 100,000 people, between the years of 1990 and 2010. The rate of ACL reconstruction increased significantly over time in all age groups [3]. Additionally, in Italy, the incidence rate of ACL reconstruction was 21.70

https://doi.org/10.3390/jcm14113823

to 33.60 per 100,000 people, between the years of 2001 and 2015. The number of ACL reconstruction procedures increased annually [4]. Additionally, a study on South Korean populations reported that the incidence of ACL reconstruction was 36.4 per 100,000 people in 2008 and increased to 46.4 per 100,000 people in 2016 [5].

However, to our knowledge, there has been no report on secondary knee procedures after anterior cruciate ligament reconstruction. As the number of people performing anterior cruciate ligament reconstruction increases, understanding the natural course of the patient and management after surgery also increases. Some patients undergoing ACL reconstruction undergo several secondary knee procedures, such as revisional reconstruction, high tibial osteotomy, total knee arthroplasty, meniscectomy, meniscus repair, or meniscus transplantation over time.

Analysis of National Health Insurance (NHI) data can provide optimal information on epidemiological patterns of such procedures.

This study aims to determine which secondary knee procedures are performed over time after anterior cruciate ligament reconstruction.

2. Methods

This study is a retrospective observational cohort study using extensive nationwide data provided by the National Health Insurance Service (National Health Insurance Service-HealthScreening; NHIS-HealS) with the approval of the institutional review committee of the Ethics Committee of Ilsan Hospital.

Among the patients who were diagnosed with ACL injury (diagnostic codes: S83.50, S83.52, M23.53, M23.63, M23.83, M23.93, M23.01, M23.11, M23.21, M23.31, M23.41, S83.7), patients who underwent ACL reconstruction (N0880, N0881) from 1 January 2003 to 31 December 2021 were included in the study. Additionally, after ACL reconstruction, secondary knee procedures were categorized to revision (N0880, N0881), high tibial osteotomy (N0304), total knee arthroplasty (N2072, N2077), menisectomy (N0821, N0826, N0822, N0827), meniscus repair (N0823, N0828, N0824, N0829) and meniscus transplantation (N0825, N0820).

We also evaluated and compared the hazard ratio (HR) of secondary knee procedures by graft type of reconstruction (autograft vs. allograft), gender (male vs. female), and age (<20, 20–39, 40–49, 50–59, ≥60).

SAS 9.4 (SAS Inc., Cary, NC, USA) was used for all analyses. Multivariable Cox Proportional Hazard model analysis was used for eight independent variables of postoperative complications. In the case of complications and hospital-related variables, there were no missing data due to the nature of the claim data. Cases in which patient-related variables were missing due to information errors were extremely rare, and these were excluded. HR and 95% confidence interval (CI) are presented. The level of significance was maintained with a p value of < 0.05.

3. Results

From 2003 to 2021, a total of 146,122 patients who underwent ACL reconstruction were found. Table 1 shows the total number of ACL reconstruction cases and the graft used.

Table 1. Total number of ACL reconstruction cases and the demographic factors.

Total 146,122		Allograft		Autograft		*p*-Value *
		N	%	N	%	
Sex	Male	94,935	78.4%	21,086	84.40%	<0.001
	Female	26,213	21.6%	3888	15.60%	

Table 1. *Cont.*

Total 146,122		Allograft N	Allograft %	Autograft N	Autograft %	p-Value *
Age	under 20	15,006	12.4%	3715	14.90%	<0.001
	20–39	60,901	50.3%	14,775	59.20%	
	40–49	24,911	20.6%	4430	17.70%	
	50–59	15,786	13.0%	1773	7.10%	
	over 60	4544	3.8%	284	1.10%	
Revision ACLR		11,102	9.2%	2171	8.7%	0.018

* The level of significance was maintained with a p value of < 0.05.

Table 2 shows which secondary knee procedure was done after ACL reconstruction. The results show that 1073 (0.7%) patients underwent HTO, 908 (0.6%) patients underwent TKA, 15,218 (10.4%) patients underwent menisectomy, 7169 (4.9%) patients underwent meniscus repair, and 938 (0.6%) patients underwent meniscus transplantation, respectively.

Table 2. The secondary knee procedures data after ACL reconstruction.

		Total	HTO After ACLR			TKA After ACLR			Meniscus After ACLR			Meniscus Repair After ACLR			Meniscus Transplantation After ACLR		
			N	(%)	p-Value *	N	(%)	p-Value *	N	(%)	p-Value *	N	(%)	p-Value *	N	(%)	p-Value *
Sex	Male	116,021	638	0.5%	<0.0001	360	0.3%	<0.0001	11,577	10.0%	<0.0001	5958	5.1%	<0.0001	797	0.7%	<0.0001
	Female	30,101	435	1.4%		548	1.8%		3641	12.1%		1211	4.0%		141	0.5%	
Age	under 20	18,718	18	0.1%	<0.0001	-	0.0%	<0.0001	2225	11.9%	<0.0001	1806	9.6%	<0.0001	121	0.6%	<0.0001
	20–39	75,676	300	0.4%		15	0.0%		7212	9.5%		4130	5.5%		608	0.8%	
	40–49	29,341	379	1.3%		162	0.6%		3190	10.9%		838	2.9%		182	0.6%	
	50–59	17,559	330	1.9%		446	2.5%		2190	12.5%		336	1.9%		26	0.1%	
	over 60	4828	46	1.0%		285	5.9%		401	8.3%		59	1.2%		1	0.0%	

* The level of significance was maintained with a p value of < 0.05.

Table 3 shows the hazard ratio of each secondary knee procedure according to type of graft, gender, and age. Due to the number of Autograft-used TKA cases being small, it does not show suitable results.

Table 3. Hazard ratio of reoperation after anterior cruciate ligament reconstruction due to risk factors.

Risk Factors		HTO After ACLR			Menisectomy After ACLR			Meniscus Repair After ACLR			Meniscus Transplantation After ACLR		
		HR *	95% C.I. Lower	Upper	HR *	95% C.I. Lower	Upper	HR *	95% C.I. Lower	Upper	HR *	95% C.I. Lower	Upper
Graft	Autograft	1.000			1.000			1.000			1.000		
	Allograft	1.581	1.304	1.916	1.223	1.171	1.279	1.192	1.121	1.267	0.951	0.811	1.115
Sex	Male	1.000			1.000			1.000			1.000		
	Female	2.081	1.834	2.361	1.232	1.185	1.280	0.927	0.871	0.987	0.857	0.715	1.028
Age	under 20	1.000			1.000			1.000			1.000		
	20–39	4.337	2.694	6.981	0.791	0.754	0.830	0.534	0.505	0.564	1.210	0.995	1.472
	40–49	11.795	7.351	18.927	0.838	0.794	0.884	0.261	0.241	0.284	0.919	0.730	1.157
	50–59	17.695	11.004	28.454	1.029	0.970	1.092	0.190	0.169	0.213	0.238	0.155	0.363
	over 60	10.802	6.259	18.644	0.768	0.690	0.854	0.143	0.110	0.185	0.038	0.005	0.271

* Compared the hazard ratio (HR) of secondary knee procedures by graft type of reconstruction (autograft vs. allograft), gender (male vs. female), and age (<20, 20–39, 40–49, 50–59, ≥60).

Table 4 shows the follow-up time. The index date was the first start date of medical treatment for anterior cruciate rupture or anterior cruciate ligament reconstruction, and the follow-up was conducted for up to 19 years from 2003 to 2021.

Table 4. Follow-up time: index date~31 December 2021 (or death date).

	N	Follow-Up Time (Years) Mean	s.d.	Q1 (p25)	Median	Q3 (p75)
Total	146,122	6.6	3.9	3.5	6.5	9.4
Autograft	24,974	7.4	4.1	4.2	7.5	10.3
Allograft	121,148	6.4	3.8	3.4	6.2	9.1

Table 5 shows the survival time. Survival time means from the start date of the first medical treatment related to the anterior cruciate ligament to the date of secondary surgical treatment. Tables 4 and 5 in this study provided median and quartile follow-up times.

Table 5. Survival time (years): index date~outcome to occur.

	N	HTO				Menisectomy				Meniscus Repair				Meniscus Transplantation			
		N	Median	Mean	s.d.	N	Median	Mean	s.d.	N	Median	Mean	s.d.	N	Median	Mean	s.d.
Total	146,122	1073	4.3	5.1	3.9	15,218	2.1	3.3	3.1	7169	2.9	3.7	3.0	938	1.6	2.9	3.1
Autograft	24,974	119	6.1	6.0	4.1	2368	2.7	3.8	3.3	1255	3.2	4.2	3.2	192	1.6	3.2	3.6
Allograft	121,148	954	4.1	5.0	3.9	12,850	2.0	3.2	3.0	5914	2.9	3.6	3.0	746	1.6	2.9	3.0

At first, we examined the difference according to the difference in the graft. Autograft shows lower HR than Allograft for all secondary knee procedures except meniscus transplantation. Each HR was 0.633 (range 0.522–0.767, 95% C.I.) in HTO, 0.817 (range 0.782–0.854, 95% C.I.) in menisectomy, 0.839 (range 0.789–0.892, 95% C.I.) in meniscus repair, and 1.051 (range 0.897–1.233, 95% C.I.) in meniscus transplantation. As seen from the result, meniscus transplantation did not have significant results.

Next, in terms of gender, females show a higher HR of HTO—2.081 (range 1.834–2.361, 95% C.I.); menisectomy—1.232 (range 1.185–1.280, 95% C.I.); a lower HR of meniscus repair—0.927 (range 0.871–0.987, 95% C.I.); and meniscus transplantation also did not have a significant result—0.857 (range 0.715–1.028, 95% C.I.).

Finally, comparing the HR according to age based on those under 20 s, HTO shows higher HR in all age groups (20–39, 40–49, 50–59, >=60). Meniscectomy shows lower HR in all age groups except 50–59, 1.029 (range 0.970–1.092, 95% C.I.), meniscus repair shows lower HR in all age groups, and meniscus transplantation shows lower HR in 50–59, >=60 groups.

4. Discussion

The current study provides valuable insights into the incidence and risk factors for secondary knee procedures after ACL reconstruction. Through this study, we found that the risk of secondary knee surgery increases after ACL reconstruction. Considering each risk, it was found that additional knee damage occurred or arthritis progressed.

ACL reconstruction does not entirely restore the functional level of the knee before damage. Remained instability is one of the most crucial complications after ACL reconstruction. Emily et al. reported that an average increase in anterior laxity of 2.7 ± 2.3 mm between the day of surgery and 7 years was significant ($p < 0.001$) [6]. Scott Tashman et al. reported that ACL reconstructed knees were more externally rotated on average by 3.8 +/− 2.3 degrees across all subjects and time points ($p = 0.0011$) [7].

Also, changes in natural knee biomechanism and progression of osteoarthritis may occur after ACL injury and reconstruction. Burak Akesen et al. showed elevated TNF-alpha, collagenase, and TIMP-1 levels due to a ruptured ACL [8]. Timothy W. Tourville et al. reported that ACL-injured patients with abnormal tibiofemoral joint space width had diminished quality of life, increased pain, and increased type II collagen urine CTX-II/serum CPII ratios compared with healthy controls [9]. Urine CTX-II concentrations were significantly higher in ACL reconstruction than the normal control group 16 weeks post-operative, and a high urine CTX-II level was related to knee pain and altered knee function [10].

Our study mainly focuses on the biomechanical explanation of the second procedure after ACL reconstruction. It is thought that this reason can be found in the recently reported ligament biology, especially in the recent development of epithelial membrane theory [11]. Based on our study, epithelial membrane tissue has a role in healing and joint degeneration after injury, and based on this, it provides insight into the cellular and extracellular matrix response of the epithelium after new ACL injury for ligament healing and remodeling—not later big data studies—and it is thought that specific studies on whether it affects joint instability and osteoarthritis progression after reconstruction are needed.

Short- and medium-term clinical outcomes after anterior cruciate ligament reconstruction are usually found to be good. Studies have shown that approximately 80–100% of patients reported normal or near-normal outcomes after surgery [12–15]. In particular, in the functional evaluation, the Lysholm score improved from 64 before surgery to an average of 92 after surgery, showing normal and similar functional recovery results. However, there are subtle differences when compared to normal knees. In the evaluation of the anterior stability of the joint, the measurement using KT-2000 showed a slight increase in the mean anterior potential at a short follow-up of 2.1 $\pm$ 1.4 mm, and 2.8 $\pm$ 1.8 mm at a medium follow-up, but it was still acceptable [12]. However, these figures indicate a complete difference from normal knees.

In a study comparing the clinical outcomes of reconstruction following acute and chronic anterior cruciate ligament injury, there were no significant differences between the two groups in mean quadriceps atrophy, Tegner activity score, Lachman test, IKDC score, etc. This suggests that the time between the time of injury and the time of surgery may not have a significant impact on clinical outcomes [6,7,12].

It is known that arthritis is likely to occur in the long term after ACLR [15]. Long-term follow-up revealed that ACL reconstruction does not completely change the natural course of post-traumatic arthritis (PTOA). At 14 years after ACL reconstruction, approximately 57% of patients developed knee osteoarthritis, whereas only 18% of the opposite normal knee developed arthritis. In addition, the prevalence of radiological knee osteoarthritis after ACL reconstruction tends to increase over time, with 11.3% at 5 years after surgery, 20.6% at 10 years, and 51.6% at 20 years [15]. However, compared to patients who underwent reconstruction but did not undergo reconstruction, the relative risk of developing arthritis (RR) in patients who underwent reconstruction was as low as 3.62 (RR in patients who did not undergo reconstruction was 4.98). This suggests that reconstruction does not completely prevent the development of arthritis but has the effect of delaying it to some extent [15].

Post-traumatic OA is the other most crucial complication after ACL injury and reconstruction. May Arna Risberg et al. reported that the prevalence of radiographic tibiofemoral and patellofemoral OA at the 20-year follow-up was 42% and 21%, respectively [16].

Up to 80% of the patients showed radiographic markers of knee OA, such as joint space narrowing and osteophyte formation, after ACL reconstruction within 15 years. Almost up to 50% of those patients with radiographic markers of OA also have symptoms such as stiffness, swelling, and pain [17–21].

These problems lead some patients to undergo secondary knee procedures. Among the secondary knee procedures, the frequency of the procedure was particularly high for the meniscus injury. There can be some contributing factors, such as abnormal loading on knee joints because of altered knee biomechanisms [10,16], there could be pre-existing meniscus injury [22], or improper surgical techniques.

These findings suggest that patients and clinicians should know the potential need for additional knee procedures and consider the risk factors in their decision-making process. For example, older patients or those with high BMI may need more cautious follow-up and rehabilitation—such as reduced body weight—after ACL reconstruction to prevent or delay the need for HTO or TKA [14,23,24]. In addition, there are studies that show differences in the possibility of reoperation of the anterior cruciate ligament according to the graft choice in reconstruction of the anterior cruciate ligament, but few studies have investigated the possibility of secondary surgery other than reoperation [13]. So, the choice of graft type and surgical technique may also affect the risk of secondary knee procedures, and further research is needed to investigate these factors.

Next, for hazard ratio, autograft reveals lower HR for all secondary knee procedures. This may be related to the autograft having a lower failure rate and incidence of complications than the allograft [25,26].

For gender, females reveal higher HR for HTO and menisectomy; however, males reveal higher HR for meniscus repair. We need more research and investigation to obtain this result.

For age, the younger age group (under 20) reveals higher HR for menisectomy and meniscus repair and lower HR for HTO than the older age group.

It may relate to younger individuals being more active than older individuals, which could increase their risk for knee injuries. Also, the biomechanics of the knee joint may differ between younger and older individuals, which could affect the likelihood of developing specific knee injuries. For example, younger individuals may be more prone to ACL tears due to factors such as ligament laxity or muscle recovery after surgery [27,28].

On the other hand, HTO is related to the degeneration of knee cartilage and joints; it can be explained that the older age group reveals a much higher HR of HTO than the younger age group.

Since this study was based on the claimed code data of the National Health Insurance Service (National Health Insurance Service-HealthScreening; NHIS-HealS), it was estimated that a lot of data or codes may be missing in the processing of each hospital. Due to the nature of big data research, the details of each patient cannot be grasped at all, and there is a problem that can only be viewed through a registered code.

There are a number of risk factors that can affect the results of this study, but this study shows that it is shown as a variable by graft type, gender, and age.

The patient's data include those who underwent surgery between 2003 and 2021, so the follow-up period is not constant. Therefore, some procedures' hazard ratios were inaccurate, and the trend was only checked. Furthermore, there is a lack of studies comparing regular patients who did not undergo primary ACL reconstruction.

There could be remaining instability or changes in the previous knee joint biomechanisms that can occur after ACL reconstruction. The accelerating progression of osteoarthritis may also occur. The results of our study show that after anterior cruciate ligament reconstruction, several secondary knee procedures such as HTO, TKA, menisectomy, meniscus repair, and meniscus transplantation will be necessary for the knee joint. The incidence of the procedures can be shown as a variable by graft type, gender, and age.

Another limitation of this study was that no mention is made of the possible consequences of opting for conservative management in cases where ACL reconstruction is clinically indicated. Since it is classified by the billing code, it is possible to classify more accurately when it comes to parts related to surgery, but it is difficult to distinguish between the type, duration, posterior tibial slope, and rehabilitation of conservative treatment. Therefore, it seems difficult to add content related to conservative treatment in the current study.

The study results also have important implications for both patients and healthcare providers. Patients considering ACL reconstruction should be informed about the potential risks of secondary knee procedures, and healthcare providers should consider the risk of secondary knee procedures when deciding whether to recommend ACL reconstruction as a treatment option.

The study also highlights the importance of ongoing monitoring and follow-up care for patients undergoing ACL reconstruction. Regular check-ups and monitoring of knee function can help identify potential problems early on, which may reduce the need for secondary knee procedures.

5. Conclusions

This study provides valuable information about the risks of secondary knee procedures after ACL reconstruction. Patients who undergo ACL reconstruction may experience poor clinical outcomes, such as progression of osteoarthritis and undergoing secondary knee procedures several years after ACL reconstruction. The findings underscore the importance of informed decision-making and ongoing monitoring and follow-up care for patients undergoing ACL reconstruction.

Author Contributions: Conceptualization, T.Y. and S.-H.P.; methodology, T.Y.; software, T.Y. and C.-M.L.; validation, H.-C.O., H.-K.Y. and S.-H.P.; formal analysis, T.Y. and C.-M.L.; investigation, S.-H.P.; data curation, T.Y. and C.-M.L.; writing—original draft preparation, H.-K.Y., C.-M.L. and S.-H.P.; writing—review and editing, H.-K.Y. and S.-H.P.; visualization, H.-C.O., H.-K.Y. and S.-H.P.; supervision, S.-H.P.; project administration, H.-C.O., H.-K.Y. and S.-H.P.; funding acquisition, S.-H.P. All authors have read and agreed to the published version of the manuscript.

Funding: This work was supported by the National Health Insurance Ilsan Hospital grant. This study used NHIS-NSC data, made by National Health Insurance Service (NHIS). The authors alone are responsible for the content and writing of the paper.

Institutional Review Board Statement: This study is a retrospective observational cohort study using extensive nationwide data provided by the National Health Insurance Service (National Health Insurance Service-HealthScreening; NHIS-HealS) with the approval of the institutional review committee of the Ethics Committee of Ilsan Hospital(NHIMC 2023-03-026, approved on 16 March 2023).

Informed Consent Statement: This study used NHIS-NSC data made by National Health Insurance Service (NHIS). The Institutional Review Board of National Health Insurance Service Ilsan Hospital waived the informed consent from the participants, because this study was expected to present no or minimal risk of harm to the participants, and all the data used were anonymized.

Data Availability Statement: All data during this study are not publicly available because all data have been deposited in the National Health Insurance Service-HealthScreening (NHIS-HealS) Database. But all data during this study are included in this Article.

Conflicts of Interest: The authors declare no conflict of interest.

References

1. Gianotti, S.M.; Marshall, S.W.; Hume, P.A.; Bunt, L. Incidence of anterior cruciate ligament injury and other knee ligament injuries: A national population-based study. *J. Sci. Med. Sport* **2009**, *12*, 622–627. [CrossRef] [PubMed]
2. Janssen, K.W.; Orchard, J.W.; Driscoll, T.R.; van Mechelen, W. High incidence and costs for anterior cruciate ligament reconstructions performed in Australia from 2003–2004 to 2007–2008: Time for an anterior cruciate ligament register by Scandinavian model? *Scand. J. Med. Sci. Sports* **2012**, *22*, 495–501. [CrossRef] [PubMed]
3. Sanders, T.L.; Maradit Kremers, H.; Bryan, A.J.; Larson, D.R.; Dahm, D.L.; Levy, B.A.; Stuart, M.J.; Krych, A.J. Incidence of Anterior cruciate ligament tears and reconstruction: A 21-year population-Based study. *Am. J. Sports Med.* **2016**, *44*, 1502–1507. [CrossRef] [PubMed]
4. Longo, U.G.; Nagai, K.; Salvatore, G.; Cella, E.; Candela, V.; Cappelli, F.; Ciccozzi, M.; Denaro, V. Epidemiology of Anterior Cruciate Ligament Reconstruction Surgery in Italy: A 15-Year Nationwide Registry Study. *J. Clin. Med.* **2021**, *10*, 223. [CrossRef]
5. Chung, K.S.; Kim, J.H.; Kong, D.H.; Park, I.; Kim, J.G.; Ha, J.K. An Increasing Trend in the Number of Anterior Cruciate Ligament Reconstruction in Korea: A Nationwide Epidemiologic Study. *Clin. Orthop. Surg.* **2022**, *14*, 220–226. [CrossRef]
6. Meike, E.; Howell, S.M.; Hull, M.L. Anterior laxity and patient-reported outcomes 7 years after ACL reconstruction with a fresh-frozen tibialis allograft. *Knee Surg. Sports Traumatol. Arthroscop.* **2017**, *25*, 1500–1509. [CrossRef]
7. Tashman, S.; Collon, D.; Anderson, K.; Kolowich, P.; Anderst, W. Abnormal rotational knee motion during running after anterior cruciate ligament reconstruction. *Am. J. Sports Med.* **2004**, *32*, 975–983. [CrossRef]
8. Akesen, B.; Demirag, B.; Budak, F. Evaluation of intra-articular collagenase, TIMP-1, and TNF-alpha levels before and after anterior cruciate ligament reconstruction. *Acta Orthop. Traumatol. Turc.* **2009**, *43*, 214–218. [CrossRef]
9. Tourville, T.W.; Johnson, R.J.; Slauterbeck, J.R.; Naud, S.; Beynnon, B.D. Relationship between markers of type II collagen metabolism and tibiofemoral joint space width changes after ACL injury and reconstruction. *Am. J. Sports Med.* **2013**, *41*, 779–787. [CrossRef]

10. Chmielewski, T.L.; Trumble, T.N.; Joseph, A.M.; Shuster, J.; Indelicato, P.A.; Moser, M.W.; Cicuttini, F.; Leeuwenburgh, C. Urinary CTX-II concentrations are elevated and associated with knee pain and function in subjects with ACL reconstruction. *Osteoarthr. Cartil.* **2012**, *20*, 1294–1301. [CrossRef]
11. Georgiev, G.P.; Yordanov, Y.; Olewnik, K.; Tubbs, R.S.; LaPrade, R.F.; Ananiev, J.; Slavchev, S.A.; Dimitrova, I.N.; Gaydarski, L.; Landzhov, B. Do the Differences in the Epiligament of the Proximal and Distal Parts of the Anterior Cruciate Ligament Explain Their Different Healing Capacities? Quantitative and Immunohistochemical Analysis of CD34 and α-SMA Expression in Relation to the Epiligament Theor. *Biomedicines* **2024**, *12*, 156.
12. Jeon, Y.S.; Choi, S.W.; Park, J.H.; Yoon, J.S.; Shin, J.S.; Kim, M.K. Mid-term outcomes of anterior cruciate ligament reconstruction with far anteromedial portal technique. *Knee Surg. Relat. Res.* **2017**, *29*, 19–25. [CrossRef]
13. Min, J.H.; Yoon, H.K.; Oh, H.C.; Youk, T.; Ha, J.W.; Park, S.H. Graft choice to decrease the revision rate of anterior cruciate ligament reconstruction: A nationwide retrospective cohort study. *Sci. Rep.* **2024**, *14*, 20004. [CrossRef] [PubMed]
14. Byun, J.; Yoon, H.K.; Oh, H.C.; Youk, T.; Ha, J.W.; Park, S.H. Relationship between revision rate, osteoarthritis, and obesity for ACL reconstruction: A nationwide retrospective cohort study. *Orthop. J. Sports Med.* **2024**, *12*, 23259671241266597. [CrossRef]
15. Cheung, E.C.; DiLallo, M.; Feeley, B.T.; Lansdown, D.A. Osteoarthritis and ACL Reconstruction-Myths and Risks. *Curr. Rev. Musculoskelet. Med.* **2020**, *13*, 115–122. [CrossRef]
16. Risberg, M.A.; Oiestad, B.E.; Gunderson, R.; Aune, A.K.; Engebretsen, L.; Culvenor, A.; Holm, I. Changes in Knee Osteoarthritis, Symptoms, and Function After Anterior Cruciate Ligament Reconstruction: A 20-Year Prospective Follow-up Study. *Am. J. Sports Med.* **2016**, *44*, 1215–1224. [CrossRef]
17. Lohmander, L.S.; Ostenberg, A.; Englund, M.; Roos, H. High prevalence of knee osteoarthritis, pain, and functional limitations in female soccer players twelve years after anterior cruciate ligament injury. *Arthrit. Rheumat.* **2004**, *50*, 3145–3152. [CrossRef]
18. Kessler, M.A.; Behrend, H.; Henz, S.; Stutz, G.; Rukavina, A.; Kuster, M.S. Function, osteoarthritis and activity after ACL-rupture: 11 years follow-up results of conservative versus reconstructive treatment. *Knee Surg. Sports Traumatol. Arthroscop.* **2008**, *16*, 442–448. [CrossRef]
19. Hui, C.; Salmon, L.J.; Kok, A.; Maeno, S.; Linklater, J.; Pinczewski, L.A. Fifteen-year outcome of endoscopic anterior cruciate ligament reconstruction with patellar tendon autograft for "isolated" anterior cruciate ligament tear. *Am. J. Sports Med.* **2011**, *39*, 89–98. [CrossRef]
20. Oiestad, B.E.; Holm, I.; Aune, A.K.; Gunderson, R.; Myklebust, G.; Engebretsen, L.; Fosdahl, M.A.; Risberg, M.A. Knee function and prevalence of knee osteoarthritis after anterior cruciate ligament reconstruction: A prospective study with 10 to 15 years of follow-up. *Am. J. Sports Med.* **2010**, *38*, 2201–2210. [CrossRef]
21. Oiestad, B.E.; Holm, I.; Engebretsen, L.; Risberg, M.A. The association between radiographic knee osteoarthritis and knee symptoms, function and quality of life 10–15 years after anterior cruciate ligament reconstruction. *Br. J. Sports Med.* **2011**, *45*, 583–588. [CrossRef] [PubMed]
22. Cinque, M.E.; Chahla, J.; Mitchell, J.J.; Moatshe, G.; Pogorzelski, J.; Murphy, C.P.; Kennedy, N.I.; Godin, J.A.; LaPrade, R.F. Influence of Meniscal and Chondral Lesions on Patient-Reported Outcomes After Primary Anterior Cruciate Ligament Reconstruction at 2-Year Follow-up. *Orthop. J. Sports Med.* **2018**, *6*, 2325967117754189. [CrossRef] [PubMed]
23. Landsmeer, M.L.A.; Runhaar, J.; van Middelkoop, M.; Oei, E.H.G.; Schiphof, D.; Bindels, P.J.E.; Bierma-Zeinstra, S.M.A. Predicting Knee Pain and Knee Osteoarthritis Among Overweight Women. *J. Am. Board Fam. Med.* **2019**, *32*, 575–584. [CrossRef] [PubMed]
24. Messier, S.P.; Mihalko, S.L.; Legault, C.; Miller, G.D.; Nicklas, B.J.; Devita, P.; Beavers, D.P.; Hunter, D.J.; Lyles, M.F.; Eckstein, F. Effects of intensive diet and exercise on knee joint loads, inflammation, and clinical outcomes among overweight and obese adults with knee osteoarthritis: The IDEA randomized clinical trial. *JAMA* **2013**, *310*, 1263–1273. [CrossRef]
25. Prodromos, C.; Joyce, B.; Shi, K. A meta-analysis of stability of autografts compared to allografts after anterior cruciate ligament reconstruction. *Knee Surg. Sports Traumatol. Arthroscop.* **2007**, *15*, 851–856. [CrossRef]
26. Kraeutler, M.J.; Bravman, J.T.; McCarty, E.C. Bone-patellar tendon-bone autograft versus allograft in outcomes of anterior cruciate ligament reconstruction: A meta-analysis of 5182 patients. *Am. J. Sports Med.* **2013**, *41*, 2439–2448. [CrossRef]
27. Lutz, P.M.; Feucht, M.J.; Wechselberger, J.; Rasper, M.; Petersen, W.; Wörtler, K.; Imhoff, A.B.; Achtnich, A. Ultrasound-based examination of the medial ligament complex shows gender- and age-related differences in laxity. *Knee Surg. Sports Traumatol. Arthroscop.* **2021**, *29*, 1960–1967. [CrossRef]
28. Iriuchishima, T.; Shirakura, K.; Horaguchi, T.; Wada, N.; Sohmiya, M.; Tazawa, F.M.; Fu, F.H. Age as a predictor of residual muscle weakness after anterior cruciate ligament reconstruction. *Knee. Surg. Sports Traumatol. Arthroscop.* **2012**, *20*, 173–178. [CrossRef]

Journal of
Clinical Medicine

MDPI

Article

Propensity Score-Matched Comparison of Six-Strand All-Inside and Conventional Four-Strand Hamstring Autografts for ACL Reconstruction

Young Jin Seo *, Si Young Song and Dongju Kim

Department of Orthopedic Surgery, Dongtan Sacred Heart Hospital, Hallym University College of Medicine, 7, Keunjaebong-gil, Hwaseong-si 18450, Republic of Korea; dkmn123@naver.com (D.K.)
* Correspondence: yjseoos@gmail.com; Tel.: +82-31-8086-2410

Abstract

Background/Objectives: All-inside ACL reconstruction has emerged as a minimally invasive alternative to conventional techniques, with potential advantages in graft configuration and reduced surgical trauma. This study aimed to compare the clinical outcomes of all-inside and full tibial tunnel ACL reconstruction, focusing on graft diameter, postoperative stability, and functional recovery. We hypothesized that the all-inside technique would allow for thicker grafts and yield superior postoperative knee stability and functional outcomes, with postoperative anterior laxity as a major outcome of interest. **Methods:** This retrospective comparative study reviewed patients who underwent ACL reconstruction between January 2020 and February 2024. From January 2020 to September 2022, a four-strand hamstring autograft with full tibial tunnel technique (FT-4) was used, while from September 2022, a six-strand hamstring autograft with the all-inside technique (AI-6) was adopted to enable thicker grafts and optimize fixation. Among a total of 103 patients, 1:1 propensity score matching (PSM) was performed based on age, sex, BMI, laterality, ALL reconstruction, meniscal lesion, and preoperative anterior laxity (SSD). Graft diameter and clinical outcomes, including knee stability and functional scores, were compared between the matched groups. **Results:** After PSM, two comparable groups of 29 patients each were established. Graft diameter was significantly larger in the AI-6 group (9.5 $\pm$ 0.7 mm) compared to the FT-4 group (7.8 $\pm$ 0.8 mm, $p < 0.001$), while other baseline characteristics remained well balanced between the groups. At the final follow-up, both groups exhibited significant improvements in anterior laxity, functional scores, and pivot shift grades (all $p < 0.001$). The AI-6 group demonstrated superior outcomes with a significantly higher Lysholm score (82.2 $\pm$ 6.7 vs. 75.6 $\pm$ 8.9, $p = 0.002$), lower WOMAC score (8.0 $\pm$ 4.3 vs. 12.9 $\pm$ 10.5, $p = 0.023$), and reduced anterior laxity (1.6 $\pm$ 1.1 mm vs. 2.5 $\pm$ 1.4 mm, $p = 0.005$) compared to the FT-4 group, whereas no significant differences were observed in the IKDC, Tegner, Korean knee score, or pivot shift test results. A simple linear regression revealed a significant negative correlation between graft diameter and postoperative anterior laxity ($B = -0.398$, $p = 0.048$). **Conclusions:** The present study demonstrated that the use of a six-strand hamstring graft configuration in the AI-6 technique resulted in significantly thicker grafts and was associated with reduced postoperative anterior knee laxity compared to the FT-4 technique. While interpretation of these findings requires caution in light of MCID thresholds, the AI-6 group showed favorable outcomes in anterior laxity and selected functional scores, such as the Lysholm and WOMAC. This technique may offer practical clinical value, particularly in populations prone to smaller graft diameters, as it facilitates adequate graft thickness through multifold preparation, with the all-inside approach accommodating the inherent graft shortening.

Keywords: anterior cruciate ligament; all-inside; reconstruction; hamstring; autograft

1. Introduction

The conventional approaches for anatomical anterior cruciate ligament (ACL) reconstruction, including the modified transtibial, anteromedial portal, and outside-in techniques, have been widely accepted. Meanwhile, all-inside ACL reconstruction has emerged as an alternative technique characterized by tibial socket preparation and the potential for combination with various femoral tunnel methods, with the aim of improving clinical outcomes. Originally facilitated by the development of retrograde drilling systems in the early 2000s, the technique was later refined and popularized by Lubowitz, who emphasized its minimally invasive nature and the advantages of controlled intra-articular fixation [1–4]. The key differences between these approaches lie in the tibial tunnel drilling technique, graft preparation, and fixation strategies. These technical differences have sparked discussions regarding their potential impact on biomechanical and functional outcomes [5–8].

Traditional anatomical ACL reconstruction employs a full-length tibial tunnel, where a consistent diameter tunnel is drilled from the tibial cortex to the intra-articular exit. In contrast, all-inside ACL reconstruction utilizes a socket-based tunnel design, where only a short socket is created at the tibial insertion sites, precisely matching the diameter and length of the graft [9].

This technique features a distinct tibial-side fixation method compared to the standard approach. In traditional ACL reconstruction with the hamstring autograft, the graft that extends outside the tibial tunnel is additionally secured using a screw and washer or a spike. In contrast, the all-inside technique employs an adjustable loop cortical button on both the femoral and tibial sides, allowing for controlled graft tensioning within the sockets and minimizing metal irritation on the tibial side [9].

Another distinction between the two techniques is the preparation of the hamstring autograft. In traditional ACL reconstruction, the hamstring tendons are typically folded twice to create a sufficiently strong graft. However, in cases where the harvested tendons are relatively small or when only the semitendinosus is used, this configuration may result in a smaller graft diameter, which could potentially increase the risk of graft failure in high-demand athletes or individuals with larger physiques [10–14].

In contrast, 5- or six-strand graft configurations form thicker grafts and offer a reliable method to increase the diameter of relatively small hamstring autografts, helping to avoid failures related to undersized grafts [15]. The ability to prepare a thicker graft, which results in a shorter graft length due to increased folding, represents a potential advantage of the all-inside technique over conventional ACL reconstruction, as the shorter graft is well suited for socket-based tunnel preparation [16]. A recent meta-analysis reported that all-inside ACL reconstruction was superior to full tibial tunnel ACL reconstruction in terms of functional outcomes and tibial tunnel expansion, while postoperative anterior translation was comparable between the two techniques [3]. However, in most of the cited studies, a four-strand semitendinosus graft was used for the all-inside group, whereas the full tibial tunnel group utilized doubled gracilis and semitendinosus tendons. This differs from the present study, in which a six-strand hamstring autograft was used in the all-inside group, potentially influencing graft diameter outcomes.

Therefore, this study aims to compare the clinical effectiveness of all-inside ACL reconstruction with traditional anatomical ACL reconstruction, focusing on key outcome measures such as graft thickness, postoperative stability, functional recovery, and patient satisfaction. We hypothesize that ACL reconstruction utilizing the all-inside technique in combination with a six-strand hamstring autograft will yield a greater graft diameter, which in turn will be associated with reduced postoperative knee laxity and improved functional outcomes compared to the conventional anatomical reconstruction technique employing a four-strand configuration.

2. Materials and Methods

2.1. Demographics

This study was approved by our Institutional Review Board and Ethics Committee (File No. HDT 2025-01-009-001). A retrospective review was conducted on consecutive patients who underwent anterior cruciate ligament reconstruction between January 2020 and February 2024. During the initial period from January 2020 to September 2022, ACL reconstruction was performed using a 4-strand hamstring autograft with the standard full tibia technique (FT-4). From September 2022 to February 2024, the surgical technique was modified to a 6-strand hamstring autograft utilizing the all-inside approach (AI-6). This transition was made to accommodate a thicker graft configuration, which may offer greater mechanical strength and the potential for improved long-term graft integrity, while also optimizing fixation and minimizing bone loss.

Patients were included if they were between 18 and 49 years of age and had undergone primary ACL reconstruction using either the FT-4 or AI-6 technique. Only those with complete ACL tears, confirmed through clinical examination and MRI, and with a minimum follow-up of 12 months were eligible for the study. Patients were excluded if they had multi-ligament knee injuries requiring additional reconstruction, underwent revision ACL surgery, or had associated fractures or osteochondral injuries necessitating additional procedures. Other exclusion criteria included the presence of infection, inflammatory arthritis, or an incomplete follow-up. All the included cases were unilateral, and the analysis was therefore performed on a per-patient basis.

All surgeries were performed by a single experienced surgeon (YJS) using the respective technique based on the time period of intervention.

Clinical and functional outcomes were assessed preoperatively and at the last postoperative follow-up. Postoperative follow-up was conducted at 1 month, 3 months, 6 months, and 12 months, and subsequently at annual intervals.

Both groups followed the same standardized rehabilitation protocol. Postoperative rehabilitation included immediate range of motion exercises and partial weight-bearing with crutches as tolerated. Full weight-bearing was generally allowed by 4 weeks after surgery. Closed-chain exercises and proprioceptive training were initiated starting from 4 weeks postoperatively. Return to sports activities was typically permitted at 6 to 9 months, depending on individual progress.

Complications were defined as any postoperative adverse event requiring additional medical or surgical management beyond routine rehabilitation and follow-up care. Based on this definition, one patient in the FT-4 group developed a postoperative flexion contracture that required two arthroscopic adhesiolysis procedures. A residual contracture of 5° was observed at final follow-up. No other postoperative complications occurred in either group, and no perioperative complications were identified.

2.2. Surgical Technique

In both groups, the femoral tunnel was established using either the outside-in approach or the transportal technique, depending on intraoperative considerations. According to the senior surgeon's operative strategy, the outside-in technique was favored in cases where preservation of the femoral remnant was feasible, as it provided better control over tunnel placement while minimizing disruption of the remaining native ACL fibers. In contrast, when the femoral side was characterized by an empty wall or minimal residual tissue, the transportal technique was employed.

In the outside-in technique, the femoral tunnel was created under visualization through the posteromedial portal. After inserting the arthroscope via the posteromedial portal, partial septal resection was performed to allow detailed visualization of the inner wall of the lateral femoral condyle, facilitating accurate tunnel placement. The femoral tunnel was positioned precisely at the anatomic ACL femoral footprint, targeting the anteromedial (AM) bundle's direct fiber attachment site. Using a retrograde FlipCutter (Arthrex, Naples, FL, USA), the femoral socket was drilled approximately 7 mm shorter than the total measured length to prevent outer cortex breakage. Alternatively, the femoral tunnel was created using the transportal technique. Under direct visualization through the anteromedial (AM) portal, the femoral tunnel was drilled at the same position described earlier, with the knee hyperflexed to over 120 degrees. The reamer was introduced via the far anteromedial portal to achieve the desired tunnel placement.

In the all-inside ACL reconstruction technique (AI-6 group), the graft was prepared using a triple-folded 6-strand hamstring autograft technique. Both the semitendinosus and gracilis tendons were harvested and whipstitched at both ends. Using a harvested hamstring length of approximately 22–25 cm, the final graft length was adjusted to approximately 7.5 cm (Figure 1(A)).

An adjustable cortical suspensory device was secured at each end of the folded graft to ensure proper fixation [17]. On the tibial side, the tibial socket was created in the AM bundle orientation at the native ACL footprint using a FlipCutter (Arthrex, Naples, FL, USA). To ensure that the combined length of the femoral tunnel, tibial tunnel, and intra-articular segment exceeded the total graft length, the angle of the tibial tunnel guide was adjusted accordingly (Figure 1(B)).

Before graft passage, leading sutures were advanced through the femoral and tibial tunnels and retrieved via the anteromedial portal. The sutures connected to the adjustable cortical suspensory devices at each graft end were then linked to the corresponding leading sutures. The graft was first passed and secured on the femoral side, followed by tibial passage and fixation, ensuring proper tensioning and stabilization.

In the standard full tibia group (FT-4 group), a full-length tibial tunnel was drilled using the conventional technique, starting from the anteromedial cortex. The graft was prepared using a double-folded 4-strand hamstring autograft, utilizing both the semitendinosus and gracilis tendons (Figure 2(A)).

Fixation in the FT-4 group was achieved using an adjustable suspensory device on the femoral side. On the tibial side, an interference screw was used for primary fixation, with additional fixation performed using a screw and spike washer (Figure 2(B)).

For both the AI-6 and FT-4 groups, anterolateral ligament (ALL) reconstruction was performed in patients with a pivot shift grade 2 or higher, particularly those actively participating in sports. ALL reconstruction was performed using a 5 mm allogeneic tibialis tendon. The graft was fixed on the femoral side just posterior and proximal to the lateral femoral epicondyle using either a SwiveLock® anchor (Arthrex, Naples, FL, USA) or a 6 mm interference screw. Tibial fixation was performed with a 6 mm interference screw at a point 15 mm below the joint line, midway between Gerdy's tubercle and the fibular head, with the knee in 30° flexion and neutral rotation.

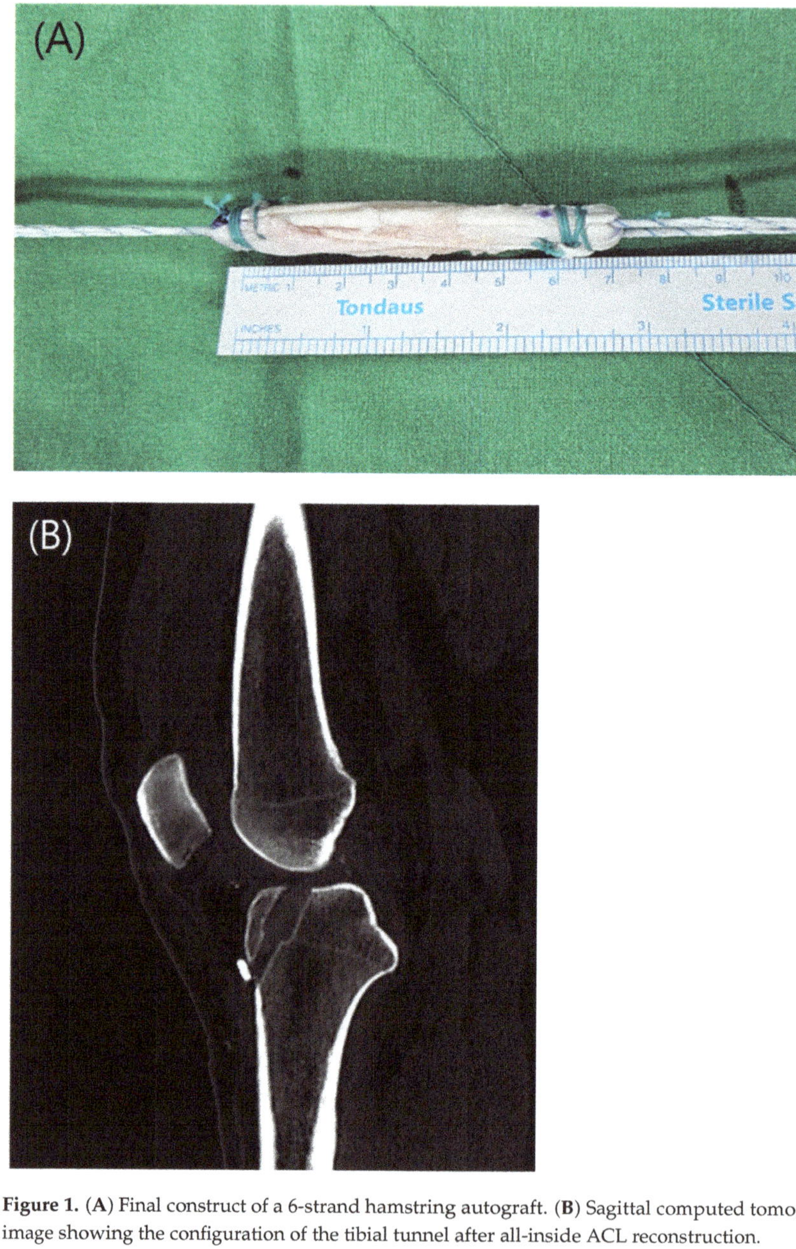

Figure 1. (**A**) Final construct of a 6-strand hamstring autograft. (**B**) Sagittal computed tomography image showing the configuration of the tibial tunnel after all-inside ACL reconstruction.

2.3. Outcome Measure

Graft diameter is recorded during surgery using a graft-sizing block (Arthrex, FL, USA) and defined as the largest diameter of the graft that could pass through the block. Meniscus injuries were documented based on their location (medial or lateral) and classified by type, including ramp lesions, root tears, longitudinal tears, horizontal tears, and others. Additionally, the treatment approach—whether repair or resection—was recorded for each case. The presence or absence of anterolateral ligament reconstruction was also documented.

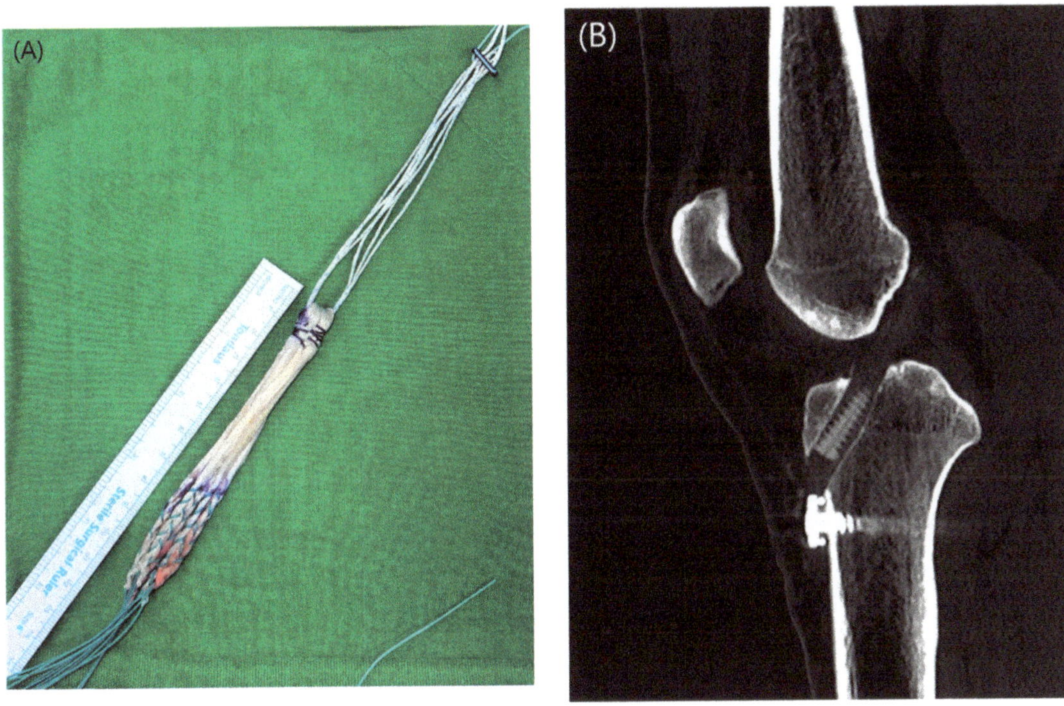

Figure 2. (**A**) Completed configuration of a four-strand hamstring autograft. (**B**) Sagittal computed tomography scan depicting the morphology of the full-length tibial tunnel after standard ACL reconstruction.

Anterior laxity is assessed using the Telos device (Telos GmbH, Hennigsdorf, Germany), which quantifies the side-to-side difference (SSD) in anterior tibial translation under a standardized force of 150 Newtons. The pivot shift test is graded on a scale from 0 to 3, and was performed by an experienced senior surgeon (YJS). Functional knee scores, including the International Knee Documentation Committee (IKDC) Subjective Knee Evaluation Form, Lysholm, Tegner, and Western Ontario and McMaster Universities Osteoarthritis Index (WOMAC), Korean knee score (KKS), were recorded. All the assessments were conducted preoperatively and at the final follow-up during outpatient visits. The WOMAC and KKS were only assessed at the final follow-up.

The score assessments were performed by a single evaluator who was blinded to the patient information.

2.4. Statistical Analysis

All statistical analyses were performed using SPSS for Windows (version 29.0, SPSS Inc, Chicago, IL, USA). The raw data was organized in an Excel (Microsoft, version 16.0) sheet and uploaded to SPSS for analysis. Descriptive statistics were used to summarize the demographic and clinical characteristics of the two groups. Continuous variables are expressed as means and standard deviations, while categorical variables are presented as frequencies and percentages.

For inter-group comparisons, normality of continuous variables was assessed using the Shapiro–Wilk test. Variables satisfying normality assumptions were analyzed using Student's t-test, while non-normally distributed variables were analyzed using the Mann–Whitney U test. Ordinal variables were also analyzed using the Mann–Whitney U test.

Nominal variables were compared using the chi-square test or Fisher's exact test, as appropriate. Statistical tests were selected based on distributional characteristics, and reanalysis was performed where necessary to ensure appropriate test application.

For intra-group comparisons, preoperative and postoperative data were analyzed using paired t-tests or the Wilcoxon signed-rank test. A significance level was set at $p < 0.05$.

To minimize selection bias and ensure comparability between the AI-6 and FT-4 groups, propensity score matching (PSM) was employed. The PSM method matched patients based on relevant baseline characteristics, including sex, age, BMI, laterality, concomitant anterolateral ligament (ALL) reconstruction, meniscal lesion, and preoperative anterior laxity (SSD).

The propensity scores were calculated using the PSM process embedded in SPSS, estimating the likelihood of receiving either the AI-6 or FT-4 technique based on these covariates. Patients were then matched 1:1 using the nearest neighbor matching algorithm with a caliper set to 0.1 to maintain balance across the variables in both groups. After matching, differences in clinical outcomes, such as knee stability and functional knee scores, were analyzed between the two groups.

Additionally, standardized mean differences (SMDs) were calculated to assess the balance between groups for variables used in PSM.

3. Results

A total of 121 cases were retrospectively reviewed, and 18 were excluded according to the predefined criteria. The remaining 103 patients were included in the analysis, comprising 30 patients in the AI-6 group and 73 in the FT-4 group. After PSM, 29 matched cases were selected for each group (Figure 3).

The mean follow-up duration was 27.1 ± 3.8 months (range, 20.3–35.1 months) in the AI-6 group and 29.6 ± 13.8 months (range, 12.1–57.3 months) in the FT-4 group. Preoperative characteristics of the matched cohorts are summarized in Table 1. Among the variables, graft diameter was significantly greater in the AI-6 group, whereas no significant differences were observed in other baseline characteristics. However, some SMDs exceeded the ideal cutoff of 0.1. Although an SMD below 0.1 is preferred, values up to 0.25 are sometimes considered acceptable. A few variables surpassed this threshold, likely due to small sample size and retrospective design, which should be acknowledged as an important limitation with the potential to affect the validity of the group comparisons.

3.1. Within-Group Analysis of Clinical Outcomes

At the final follow-up, analysis of clinical outcomes within each group revealed significant postoperative improvements. In the AI-6 group, postoperative anterior laxity (SSD), IKDC score, and Lysholm score improved to 1.58 ± 1.1 mm, 78.03 ± 7.0, and 82.2 ± 6.7, respectively (all $p < 0.001$). Similarly, the FT-4 group showed corresponding values of 2.5 ± 1.4 mm, 77.2 ± 8.4, and 75.6 ± 8.9 (all $p < 0.001$). Both groups showed significant gains in activity level, with Tegner scores increasing from a median [IQR] of 6 [1.5] in the AI-6 group and 5 [1.5] in the FT-4 group (all $p < 0.001$).

Postoperative pivot shift grades also improved significantly in both groups (all $p < 0.001$), with the AI-6 group showing 16 patients at grade 0, 12 at grade 1, and 1 at grade 2, while the FT-4 group had 16 at grade 0, 9 at grade 1, and 4 at grade 2.

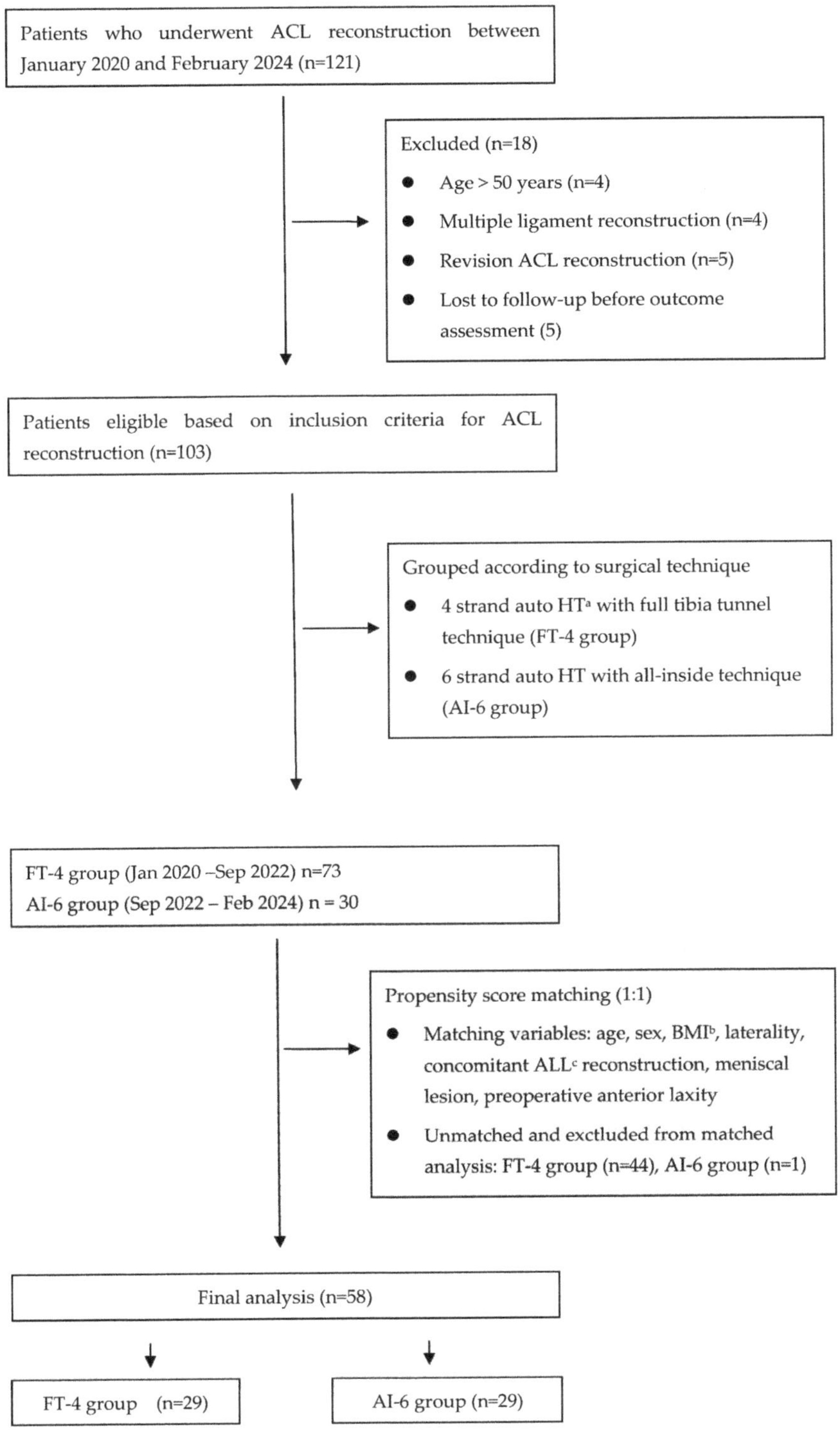

Figure 3. Flow diagram of patient selection and propensity score matching. [a] hamstring tendon, [b] body mass index, [c] anterolateral ligament.

Table 1. Comparison of patient characteristics after PSM.

Variables [a]	AI-6 (n = 29)	FT-4 (n = 29)	p-Value	SMD [h]
Age (year) *	27.7 ± 8.3	30.3 ± 12.2	0.629	0.249
Sex *				
Male (%)/Female (%)	18 (62.1)/11 (37.9)	19 (65.5)/10 (34.5)	1.0	0.072
Body mass index (kg/m^2) *	26.3 ± 3.5	26.5 ± 3.3	0.879	0.040
Side *				
Right (%)/Left (%)	18 (62.1)/11 (37.9)	21 (72.4)/8 (27.6)	0.401	0.221
Time from Injury to surgery (weeks)	3.9 ± 4.5	5.2 ± 5.0	0.249	
Time from surgery to final follow-up (months)	27.1 ± 3.8	29.6 ± 13.8	0.067	
Preop [b] anterior laxity (SSD [c], mm) *	6.0 ± 1.3	6.0 ± 1.6	0.972	0.009
Preop pivot shift grade under anesthesia (0/1/2/3) (%)	3 (10.3)/13 (44.8)/9 (31.0)/4 (13.8)	0 (0.0)/12 (41.4)/14 (48.3)/3 (10.3)	0.307	
Preop IKDC [d]	52.6 ± 5.1	49.7 ± 6.5	0.067	
Preop Lysholm	40.6 ± 8.7	43.8 ± 8.2	0.191	
Preop Tenger [e]	2 (2–3)	2 (2–3)	0.689	
Graft diameter (mm)	9.5 ± 0.7	7.8 ± 0.8	<0.001	
Femoral tunnel creation method (OI/TP) [f] (%)	20 (69.0)/9 (31.0)	15 (51.7)/14 (48.3)	0.283	
ALL reconstruction (%) *	20 (69.0)	23 (79.3)	0.368	0.237
Meniscus lesion *				
medial	15	13	0.793	0.138
Repair				
Ramp lesion	9	6		
Midbody-to Ph [g] longitudinal tear	4	2		
Ph radial tear	2	3		
Bucket handle tear		1		
Ph horizontal tear		1		
lateral	9	13	0.417	0.287
Repair				
Ph radial tear near root	6	4		
Ph radial tear		4		
Ph longitudinal tear	3	5		

[a] data are presented as the mean ± standard deviation or the number of patients. Depending on the characteristics of the variables, statistical analyses were conducted using Student's t-test, Mann–Whitney U test, Pearson chi-square test, or Fisher's exact test. [b] preoperative; [c] side-to-side difference; [d] International Knee Documentation Committee; [e] values are presented as median (range); [f] OI: outside-in; TP: transportal; [g] posterior horn; [h] standardized mean difference. * variables used for propensity score matching.

3.2. Between-Group Analysis of Clinical Outcomes

Inter-group comparisons of functional knee scores at the final follow-up demonstrated significantly superior outcomes in the AI-6 group for Lysholm and WOMAC scores, whereas no significant differences were observed in IKDC, Tegner, or KKS. A summary of the detailed data is shown in Table 2.

At the final outpatient follow-up, postoperative instability was compared between the two groups, revealing that the AI-6 group demonstrated significantly better results in anterior laxity (SSD), whereas no significant difference was observed between the groups in the pivot-shift test, as detailed in Table 3. The pivot-shift test was conducted in the outpatient clinic by a senior surgeon with extensive experience, ensuring adequate muscle relaxation to reduce the influence of voluntary guarding.

Table 2. Inter-group comparison of functional scores.

Variables [a]	Group	Mean ± SD	p-Value
Lysholm	AI-6 FT-4	82.2 ± 6.7 75.6 ± 8.9	0.003
IKDC [b]	AI-6 FT-4	78.0 ± 7.0 77.2 ± 8.4	0.684
Tegner [c]	AI-6 FT-4	6 [1.5] 5 [1.5]	0.289
WOMAC [d]	AI-6 FT-4	8.0 ± 4.3 12.9 ± 10.5	0.023
KKS [e]	AI-6 FT-4	83.5 ± 7.1 82.5 ± 7.2	0.528

[a] data are presented as the mean ± standard; [b] International Knee Documentation Committee; [c] Values are presented as median [interquatile range]; [d] Western Ontario and McMaster Universities Osteoarthritis Index; [e] Korean knee score.

Table 3. Inter-group comparison of postoperative instability.

Variables [a]	AI-6	FT-4	p-Value
Anterior laxity (SSD [b], mm)	1.6 ± 1.1	2.5 ± 1.4	0.005
pivot shift grade (0/1/2/3) (%)	16 (55.2)/12 (41.4)/1 (3.4)/0 (0.0)	16 (55.2)/9 (31.0)/4 (13.8)/0 (0.0)	0.732

[a] data are presented as the mean ± standard deviation or the number of patients. [b] side-to-side difference.

Given that key preoperative variables were balanced through propensity score matching, a simple linear regression was performed to assess the independent association between graft diameter and postoperative anterior laxity. The analysis revealed a significant negative relationship (B = −0.398, β = −0.287, p = 0.048; 95% CI: −0.791 to −0.005). Residual analysis showed no major violations of linearity, normality, or homoscedasticity. The residual sum of squares was 100.995 (df = 46) with a mean square error of 2.196. The model showed a modest fit (R = 0.287, R^2 = 0.083), indicating that a larger graft diameter was associated with reduced postoperative anterior laxity.

A post hoc power analysis was performed using G*Power 3.1 (Heinrich-Heine-University Düsseldorf, Germany), with postoperative anterior laxity selected as the main outcome variable for this analysis due to its clinical relevance. Based on the observed group difference (1.6 ± 1.1 mm in the AI-6 group vs. 2.5 ± 1.4 mm in the FT-4 group), the analysis yielded a Cohen's d of 0.71 and an estimated statistical power of 85.2% (one-tailed, α = 0.05), indicating that the sample size of 29 patients per group was sufficient to detect a clinically meaningful difference with adequate statistical rigor.

4. Discussion

The most important findings of this study were that the six-strand configuration used in the all-inside technique yielded significantly thicker grafts, which resulted in reduced postoperative anterior knee laxity compared to the full tibial tunnel technique. Although some functional outcomes, such as the IKDC, Tegner, and KKS, showed no significant differences between groups, the all-inside group demonstrated superior results in the Lysholm and WOMAC scores. These findings lend partial support to our hypothesis, given that the AI-6 group showed superior anterior knee stability and outperformed the FT-4 group in selected functional assessments.

Previous studies have yielded inconsistent findings regarding the relationship between graft diameter and postoperative knee outcomes, particularly in the context of autograft hamstring reconstruction. Although a direct comparison is limited due to differences in graft configurations, the findings of the current study align with the general trend reported in a recent network meta-analysis, which demonstrated that graft constructs with a greater number of strands, such as four-strands graft with augmentation, were associated with reduced anterior knee laxity compared to lower-strand configurations [18]. These findings suggest that the improved outcomes in the AI-6 group may be partially explained by the increased graft diameter inherent to the six-strand technique, which has been reported as a contributing factor to enhanced postoperative stability [18]. In contrast, a recent meta-analysis of Level I–II studies comparing five-strand and four-strand hamstring autografts demonstrated significantly larger graft diameters in the five-strand group (mean difference of 0.93 mm; 8.5–9.1 mm vs. 7.5–8.1 mm) and found no significant differences in anterior laxity based on the Lachman test [19]. Conversely, our study employing six-strand hamstring autografts revealed significant differences in instrumented anterior laxity. This discrepancy may be explained by both differences in anterior laxity evaluation methods and the distinct graft configurations utilized. Furthermore, this meta-analysis demonstrated that, although some PROMs, such as KOOS ADL and Lysholm scores, favored the five-strand group, the pivot shift test outcomes were similar across both groups, consistent with the findings of our study [19]. It is noteworthy that none of the mean differences in the aforementioned PROMs that favored the five-strand group surpassed the minimal clinically important difference (MCID) thresholds, suggesting comparable overall clinical outcomes [19]. Interestingly, one of the studies included in the aforementioned meta-analysis, by Wan KM et al., reported transitioning to the all-inside technique to accommodate shorter graft lengths, a method similar to the one employed in the present study [16]. They also described that a substantial proportion of Asian patients fail to achieve a graft diameter of 8.5 mm using a conventional four-strand hamstring technique [20–23].

Consequently, the five-strand technique has been considered particularly beneficial for Asian populations, where smaller graft diameters are more commonly encountered, and can be effectively applied in all-inside ACL reconstruction procedures.

In this context, the all-inside technique has garnered attention as a potential alternative to the traditional full tibia technique. Several recent meta-analyses comparing the two techniques have demonstrated comparable outcomes in terms of postoperative knee function, graft failure, and overall stability [3], while the all-inside technique has shown superior results regarding reduced postoperative pain, improved flexion strength, larger graft diameters, and decreased tunnel widening [1,2]. Upon closer examination focusing specifically on anterior laxity, however, a recent meta-analysis by Zhu et al. reported greater anterior laxity in the all-inside group compared to the full tibia group, which, somewhat surprisingly, contrasts with the findings of our study [24]. Although Zhu et al. speculated that factors such as adjustable loop elongation and the earlier initiation of rehabilitation protocols might contribute to this difference, the true cause remains uncertain. Notably, a detailed review of the three randomized controlled trials included in their analysis revealed that all three studies consistently utilized only the semitendinosus tendon in the all-inside group and both the gracilis and semitendinosus tendons in the full tibia group, resulting in similar graft diameters of approximately 8 mm without statistically significant differences [5,7,8]. Given that our study used a significantly thicker graft in the all-inside group, it is plausible that graft diameter, rather than the surgical technique alone, plays a key role in the differences observed in postoperative anterior laxity. However, further studies are warranted to confirm this notion.

Furthermore, upon closer inspection, two of these studies were conducted at the same institution and merely reported outcomes at different follow-up periods, and did not demonstrate statistically significant differences in anterior laxity [5,8]. Only one study reported a statistically significant difference in anterior laxity between the groups. However, despite the statistical significance, the mean SSD was 2.9 mm in the all-inside group and 2.3 mm in the full tibial tunnel group, which raises questions about the clinical relevance of this difference [7]. This critical discrepancy in graft configuration, sample size, and outcome reporting may account for the opposing findings, as our study demonstrated superior postoperative anterior laxity in the all-inside group, likely attributable to the larger graft diameters achieved in our cohort.

As previously discussed, most studies on the all-inside technique have reported results using only the semitendinosus to construct the graft, a method associated with several advantages, such as reduced soft tissue damage and improved flexor power, owing to gracilis sparing. Given these advantages, the all-inside approach also offers a notable technical merit in its ability to accommodate a graft that is relatively thick despite its short length. Although harvesting the semitendinosus alone may suffice in certain cases, it does not always yield a sufficiently thick graft, particularly when a more robust construct is desired. In our study, combining the semitendinosus and gracilis tendons to create a six-strand graft within the all-inside technique provided a practical and effective solution to achieve adequate graft diameter [10,19,25,26].

A key strength of this study is the direct comparison of two distinct graft constructions using propensity score-matched cohorts, providing practical insight into graft preparation strategies. This highlights the clinical relevance of the six-strand hamstring graft configuration, which enables the use of thicker grafts associated with improved postoperative anterior knee stability and select functional outcomes. Given the higher prevalence of smaller graft diameters among Asian populations, this approach may offer particular value in such cohorts by facilitating adequate graft thickness through multifold techniques. Additionally, the all-inside technique offers a practical solution to accommodate the shorter length inherent to six-strand grafts. However, this approach may introduce technical challenges during graft passage, as both femoral and tibial tunnel insertions must be accessed sequentially through the same portal.

Nevertheless, the purported advantages of the all-inside technique reported in this study should be interpreted with caution, considering the following limitations. First, graft failure was not included as a clinical endpoint in the analysis. Given that several previous studies have indicated a potential association between increased graft diameter and reduced failure rates, omission of this outcome may have limited the comprehensiveness of the findings [10–13]. Eggeling et al. reported that clinical failure following ACL reconstruction can be defined as postoperative anterior laxity (SSD) greater than 6 mm [27]. From this perspective, although graft failure was not included in the primary outcome analysis of the present study, one patient in the FT-4 group demonstrated postoperative anterior laxity (SSD) exceeding this threshold, thereby meeting the criteria for clinical failure. In contrast, no such cases were observed in the AI-6 group. While this finding was not statistically analyzed due to the limited sample size, it may suggest a potential difference in failure risk between graft configurations, warranting further investigation in future studies with larger cohorts and longer-term follow-up.

Second, when interpreted in light of the MCID, the clinical relevance of the observed inter-group differences warrants careful consideration. Although the AI-6 group showed statistically superior outcomes, the clinical magnitude of these differences varied across outcome measures. Specifically, the Lysholm score showed a mean difference of 6.6 points, exceeding the MCID range reported in prior studies (typically 4–10 points) with a corresponding effect size (Cohen's d) of 0.85, indicating a large effect [28]. In contrast, the WOMAC score demonstrated a mean difference of 4.9 points, which did not reach the commonly cited MCID threshold of 6–12 points, with an effect size of 0.58, corresponding to a medium effect [29,30]. Regarding anterior laxity, the SSD was 0.9 mm, with an effect size of 0.72. Although statistically significant, this difference may not be clinically perceptible, as MCID values for anterior translation are generally considered to be ≥2 mm [31]. These findings highlight the importance of considering both statistical and clinical relevance when interpreting postoperative outcomes.

Third, while the sample size in this study remains relatively small, the use of propensity score matching helps mitigate potential confounding factors and strengthens the validity of our findings. By matching participants on key baseline characteristics, this approach enhances the comparability between the AI-6 and FT-4 groups, providing a more reliable estimate of the treatment effects despite the limited sample size. Additionally, given the retrospective nature of the study, a formal primary endpoint was not prospectively designated. However, a post hoc power analysis was performed based on the observed difference in postoperative anterior laxity, which yielded a statistical power of 85.2%, supporting the reliability of this outcome measure in our analysis.

Fourth, this study's retrospective design inherently carries risks of selection bias and potential inconsistencies in data collection. Residual confounding from unmeasured variables cannot be entirely excluded. Additionally, the relatively short-term follow-up limits the assessment of long-term outcomes and graft durability. Therefore, further prospective studies with extended follow-up are warranted to validate and expand upon these findings.

5. Conclusions

The present study demonstrated that the use of a six-strand hamstring graft configuration in the AI-6 technique resulted in significantly thicker grafts and was associated with reduced postoperative anterior knee laxity compared to the FT-4 technique. While interpretation of these findings requires caution in light of MCID thresholds, the AI-6 group showed favorable outcomes in anterior laxity and selected functional scores, such as the Lysholm and WOMAC. This technique may offer practical clinical value, particularly in populations prone to smaller graft diameters, as it facilitates adequate graft thickness through multifold preparation, with the all-inside approach accommodating the inherent graft shortening.

Author Contributions: Conceptualization, Y.J.S.; Methodology, Y.J.S.; Software, Y.J.S.; Validation, Y.J.S.; Formal analysis, Y.J.S.; Investigation, Y.J.S. and D.K.; Resources, Y.J.S.; Data curation, Y.J.S. and S.Y.S.; Writing—original draft, Y.J.S.; Writing—review & editing, Y.J.S., S.Y.S. and D.K.; Visualization, Y.J.S.; Supervision, Y.J.S.; Project administration, Y.J.S. All authors have read and agreed to the published version of the manuscript.

Funding: This research received no external funding.

Institutional Review Board Statement: The study was conducted in accordance with the Declaration of Helsinki and approved by the Institutional Review Board of Dongtan Sacred Heart Hospital (protocol No: 2025-01-009-001, date of approval: 24 March 2025).

Informed Consent Statement: Patient consent was waived due to REASON (the study was retrospective in nature, posed no more than minimal risk to the subjects, and involved the use of existing clinical data that were de-identified, and the waiver was not expected to adversely affect the rights and welfare of the participants).

Data Availability Statement: The original contributions presented in this study are included in the article. Further inquiries can be directed to the corresponding author.

Acknowledgments: Our sincere thanks go to Jang Jun-Yeong for his help in compiling and organizing the data in Excel.

Conflicts of Interest: The authors declare no conflicts of interest.

References

1. Bhimani, R.; Shahriarirad, R.; Ranjbar, K.; Erfani, A.; Ashkani-Esfahani, S. Transportal versus all-inside techniques of anterior cruciate ligament reconstruction: A systematic review. *J. Orthop. Surg. Res.* **2021**, *16*, 734. [CrossRef]
2. Fu, C.W.; Chen, W.C.; Lu, Y.C. Is all-inside with suspensory cortical button fixation a superior technique for anterior cruciate ligament reconstruction surgery? A systematic review and meta-analysis. *BMC Musculoskelet. Disord.* **2020**, *21*, 445. [CrossRef]
3. Lv, X.; Wang, M.; Zhao, T.; Wang, L.; Dong, S.; Tan, H. All-inside versus complete tibial tunnel techniques in anterior cruciate ligament reconstruction: A systematic review and meta-analysis of randomized controlled trials. *J. Orthop. Surg. Res.* **2023**, *18*, 127. [CrossRef]
4. James, L.; Christopher, A.; Kyle, A. All-inside anterior cruciate ligament graft link technique: Second-generation, no incision anterior cruciate ligament reconstruction. *Arthroscopy* **2011**, *27*, 717–727. [CrossRef]
5. Eichinger, M.; Ploner, M.; Degenhart, G.; Rudisch, A.; Smekal, V.; Attal, R.; Mayr, R. Tunnel widening after ACL reconstruction with different fixation techniques: Aperture fixation with biodegradable interference screws versus all-inside technique with suspensory cortical buttons. 5-year data from a prospective randomized trial. *Arch. Orthop. Trauma. Surg.* **2023**, *143*, 6707–6718. [CrossRef] [PubMed]
6. Graf-Alexiou, L.; Karpyshyn, J.; Baptiste, J.J.; Hui, C.; Sommerfeldt, M.; Westover, L. Biomechanical Strength of All-Inside ACL Reconstruction Grafts Using Side-to-Side and Backup Fixation. *Orthop. J. Sports Med.* **2021**, *9*, 23259671211006521. [CrossRef]
7. Lin, R.; Zhong, Q.; Wu, X.; Cui, L.; Huang, R.; Deng, Q.; Zuo, J.; Jiang, C.; Li, W. Randomized controlled trial of all-inside and standard single-bundle anterior cruciate ligament reconstruction with functional, MRI-based graft maturity and patient-reported outcome measures. *BMC Musculoskelet. Disord.* **2022**, *23*, 289. [CrossRef]
8. Mayr, R.; Smekal, V.; Koidl, C.; Coppola, C.; Eichinger, M.; Rudisch, A.; Kranewitter, C.; Attal, R. ACL reconstruction with adjustable-length loop cortical button fixation results in less tibial tunnel widening compared with interference screw fixation. *Knee Surg. Sports Traumatol. Arthrosc.* **2020**, *28*, 1036–1044. [CrossRef] [PubMed]
9. Bosco, F.; Giustra, F.; Ghirri, A.; Cacciola, G.; Massè, A.; Capella, M. All-Inside Anterior Cruciate Ligament Reconstruction Technique: Tips and Tricks. *J. Clin. Med.* **2023**, *12*, 5793. [CrossRef]
10. Alomar, A.Z.; Nasser, A.S.B.; Kumar, A.; Kumar, M.; Das, S.; Mittal, S. Hamstring graft diameter above 7 mm has a lower risk of failure following anterior cruciate ligament reconstruction. *Knee Surg. Sports Traumatol. Arthrosc.* **2022**, *30*, 288–297. [CrossRef]
11. Mirzayan, R.; Chang, R.N.; Royse, K.E.; Reyes, C.E.; Prentice, H.A.; Maletis, G.B. Is There a Hamstring Autograft Diameter Threshold for Anterior Cruciate Ligament Reconstruction? *Orthop. J. Sports Med.* **2025**, *13*, 23259671241305427. [CrossRef] [PubMed]
12. Spragg, L.; Chen, J.; Mirzayan, R.; Love, R.; Maletis, G. The Effect of Autologous Hamstring Graft Diameter on the Likelihood for Revision of Anterior Cruciate Ligament Reconstruction. *Am. J. Sports Med.* **2016**, *44*, 1475–1481. [CrossRef]
13. Zhao, D.; Pan, J.K.; Lin, F.Z.; Luo, M.H.; Liang, G.H.; Zeng, L.F.; Huang, H.T.; Han, Y.H.; Xu, N.J.; Yang, W.Y.; et al. Risk Factors for Revision or Rerupture After Anterior Cruciate Ligament Reconstruction: A Systematic Review and Meta-analysis. *Am. J. Sports Med.* **2023**, *51*, 3053–3075. [CrossRef]
14. Masafumi, I.; Junya, I.; Ken, O.; Kiyotaka, I. Estimation failure risk by 0.5-mm differences in autologous hamstring graft diameter in anterior cruciate ligament reconstruction: A meta-analysis. *Am. J. Sports Med.* **2024**, *52*, 535–543. [CrossRef]
15. Attia, A.K.; Nasef, H.; ElSweify, K.H.; Adam, M.A.; AbuShaaban, F.; Arun, K. Failure Rates of 5-Strand and 6-Strand vs Quadrupled Hamstring Autograft ACL Reconstruction: A Comparative Study of 413 Patients With a Minimum 2-Year Follow-up. *Orthop. J. Sports Med.* **2020**, *8*, 2325967120946326. [CrossRef]
16. Wan, K.H.; Lai, C.Y.; Tang, S.P.; Ng, E.P.; Moy, R.L.; Chan, W.L.; Lee, R.H.; Wong, K.K. The Use of Five-Strand Hamstring Autograft to Increase the Graft Size in Anterior Cruciate Ligament Reconstruction-A Prospective Cohort Study With Satisfactory Early Clinical Results. *Arthrosc. Sports Med. Rehabil.* **2022**, *4*, e1923–e1931. [CrossRef]
17. Tanpowpong, T.; Kuptniratsaikul, S.; Itthipanichpong, T.; Limskul, D.; Thamrongskulsiri, N.; Supaluxmetha, S.; Rungsaksangmanee, P. Maximizing Graft Diameter: Unleashing the Power of Triple-fold Hamstring Autografts for Anterior Cruciate Ligament Reconstruction. *Arthrosc. Tech.* **2024**, *13*, 103131. [CrossRef]
18. Malesa, K.; Trams, E.; Kulinski, K.; Kaminski, R. The effectiveness of quadrupled semitendinosus graft technique in anterior cruciate ligament reconstruction: A network meta-analysis assessing various graft preparation techniques. *Knee Surg. Sports Traumatol. Arthrosc.* **2025**, *33*, 907–925. [CrossRef]
19. Vivekanantha, P.; Nedaie, S.; Grzela, P.; Cohen, D.; Hoshino, Y.; Nagai, K.; Kay, J.; de Sa, D. Though five-strand hamstring autografts demonstrate greater graft diameter, postoperative outcomes are equivocal to four-strand hamstring autograft preparations: A systematic review and meta-analysis of level I and II studies. *Knee Surg. Sports Traumatol. Arthrosc.* **2023**, *31*, 4437–4447. [CrossRef] [PubMed]
20. Ho, S.W.; Tan, T.J.; Lee, K.T. Role of anthropometric data in the prediction of 4-stranded hamstring graft size in anterior cruciate ligament reconstruction. *Acta Orthop. Belg.* **2016**, *82*, 72–77.

21. Liau, Z.Q.G.; Ng, M.S.P.; Low, S.S.E.; Chin, B.Z.; Hui, J.H.P.; Kagda, F.H.Y. A novel practical method to predict anterior cruciate ligament hamstring graft size using preoperative MRI. *Knee Surg. Relat. Res.* **2024**, *36*, 17. [CrossRef]
22. Tang, S.P.; Wan, K.H.; Lee, R.H.; Wong, K.K.; Wong, K.K. Influence of hamstring autograft diameter on graft failure rate in Chinese population after anterior cruciate ligament reconstruction. *Asia Pac. J. Sports Med. Arthrosc. Rehabil. Technol.* **2020**, *22*, 45–48. [CrossRef]
23. Xie, G.; Huangfu, X.; Zhao, J. Prediction of the graft size of 4-stranded semitendinosus tendon and 4-stranded gracilis tendon for anterior cruciate ligament reconstruction: A Chinese Han patient study. *Am. J. Sports Med.* **2012**, *40*, 1161–1166. [CrossRef]
24. Zhu, S.; Li, R. All-Inside Anterior Cruciate Ligament Reconstruction Had Clinical Outcome Similar to the Transtibial Technique Except for Improved Side-to-Side Difference and Tegner Activity Scale: A Systematic Review and Meta-analysis. *Arthroscopy* **2024**, *40*, 2276–2288. [CrossRef] [PubMed]
25. Marchand, J.B.; Ruiz, N.; Coupry, A.; Bowen, M.; Robert, H. Do graft diameter or patient age influence the results of ACL reconstruction? *Knee Surg. Sports Traumatol. Arthrosc.* **2016**, *24*, 2998–3004. [CrossRef] [PubMed]
26. Sarakatsianos, V.; Cristiani, R.; Edman, G.; Stalman, A. Diameter of Quadrupled Semitendinosus Autograft in Primary Anterior Cruciate Ligament Reconstruction Did Not Impact Early Revision Rate or Functional Outcome in a Large Cohort of Patients. *Arthroscopy* **2025**, *41*, 239–245. [CrossRef] [PubMed]
27. Eggeling, L.; Drenck, T.C.; Breer, S.; Frosch, K.H.; Akoto, R. Association of Remaining Anterior Knee Laxity With Inferior Outcomes After Revision ACL Reconstruction. *Orthop. J. Sports Med.* **2024**, *12*, 23259671231219695. [CrossRef]
28. Migliorini, F.; Maffulli, N.; Jeyaraman, M.; Schafer, L.; Rath, B.; Huber, T. Minimal clinically important difference (MCID), patient-acceptable symptom state (PASS), and substantial clinical benefit (SCB) following surgical knee ligament reconstruction: A systematic review. *Eur. J. Trauma. Emerg. Surg.* **2025**, *51*, 32. [CrossRef]
29. Kim, M.S.; Koh, I.J.; Choi, K.Y.; Sung, Y.G.; Park, D.C.; Lee, H.J.; In, Y. The Minimal Clinically Important Difference (MCID) for the WOMAC and Factors Related to Achievement of the MCID After Medial Opening Wedge High Tibial Osteotomy for Knee Osteoarthritis. *Am. J. Sports Med.* **2021**, *49*, 2406–2415. [CrossRef]
30. Maredupaka, S.; Meshram, P.; Chatte, M.; Kim, W.H.; Kim, T.K. Minimal clinically important difference of commonly used patient-reported outcome measures in total knee arthroplasty: Review of terminologies, methods and proposed values. *Knee Surg. Relat. Res.* **2020**, *32*, 19. [CrossRef]
31. Grassi, A.; Di Paolo, S.; Dal Fabbro, G.; Eroglu, O.N.; Macchiarola, L.; Lucidi, G.A.; Zaffagnini, S. Objective laxity and subjective outcomes are more influenced by meniscal treatment than anterior cruciate ligament reconstruction technique at minimum2 years of follow-up. *J. Isakos* **2022**, *7*, 54–59. [CrossRef] [PubMed]

Journal of
Clinical Medicine

MDPI

Article

Early Open Kinetic Chain Hamstring Exercise After ACL Reconstruction: A Retrospective Safety and Efficacy Study

Roberto Ricupito [1,*], Rosalba Castellucci [2], Filippo Maselli [3,4], Marco Bravi [5], Fabio Santacaterina [5], Riccardo Guarise [6] and Florian Forelli [7,8,9]

1 Restart Physiotherapy, Via Felice Grossi Gondi 35, 00162 Rome, Italy
2 Castellucci Private Clinic, Via Maiella, 75023 Montalbano Jonico, Italy; castellucci.ross@gmail.com
3 Sovrintendenza Sanitaria Regionale Puglia, INAIL, 70126 Bari, Italy; masellifilippo76@gmail.com
4 Department of Human Neurosciences, Sapienza University of Rome, 00185 Rome, Italy
5 Fondazione Policlinico Universitario Campus Bio-Medico, Via Alvaro del Portillo 200, 00128 Rome, Italy; m.bravi@policlinicocampus.it (M.B.); f.santacaterina@policlinicocampus.it (F.S.)
6 Physiotherapy Unit, CF Research Centre, Azienda Ospedaliera Universitaria Integrata di Verona (University Hospital of Verona), 37126 Verona, Italy
7 Haute-École Arc Santé, HES-SO University of Applied Sciences and Arts Western Switzerland, 2800 Delémont, Switzerland; florian.forelli@he-arc.ch
8 Orthopaedic Surgery Department, Clinic of Domont, Ramsay Health Care, OrthoLab, 95330 Domont, France
9 Société Française des Masseurs-Kinésithérapeutes du Sport (SFMKS) Lab, 93380 Pierrefitte-sur-Seine, France
* Correspondence: robertoricupito90@gmail.com; Tel.: +39-329-094-6509

Abstract

Background: Hamstring tendon autografts are frequently used for anterior cruciate ligament reconstruction (ACLR), but they are associated with persistent hamstring strength deficits and delayed functional recovery. Current rehabilitation guidelines often delay open kinetic chain (OKC) hamstring exercises due to safety concerns, despite the limited supporting evidence. This uncontrolled, underpowered, and exploratory study aimed to evaluate the safety and effectiveness of introducing OKC hamstring strengthening exercises as early as three weeks after ACLR. **Methods:** An exploratory retrospective observational study was conducted at a single physiotherapy center on 13 patients (aged 18–35) who underwent primary ACLR with semitendinosus–gracilis grafts. Participants followed a standardized rehabilitation program including isometric leg curls at 60° and 90° knee flexion and long-lever glute bridges twice weekly, starting from postoperative week 3. Safety was assessed through predefined "safety flags" (pain > 4/10, hematoma, clinical hamstring strain). Strength outcomes, including isometric knee flexion strength at 60° and 90°, limb symmetry index (LSI), and endurance tests, were assessed at 6 and 12 weeks. **Results:** All participants completed the program without major adverse events. Pain remained consistently low (median 2.5/10), with only one transient episode exceeding the threshold. No other complications were recorded. Isometric knee flexion strength significantly improved between week 6 and week 12 at both 60° ($p = 0.018$) and 90° ($p = 0.003$), with large effect sizes. LSI at 90° also increased significantly ($p = 0.006$), whereas improvements at 60° did not reach significance. Endurance testing showed functional gains as early as 6 weeks. **Conclusions:** The early introduction of OKC hamstring strengthening exercises three weeks after ACLR with hamstring autografts appears safe and promotes clinically meaningful improvements in strength and endurance. These findings, while from a small uncontrolled study, challenge conservative rehabilitation protocols and support the reconsideration of early hamstring loading. Given the retrospective, uncontrolled, and underpowered design, these findings are hypothesis-generating and not generalizable beyond young adults with hamstring autografts; larger randomized trials are required.

J. Clin. Med. **2025**, *14*, 6871 https://doi.org/10.3390/jcm14196871

Keywords: anterior cruciate ligament reconstruction; hamstrings; open kinetic chain

1. Introduction

Anterior cruciate ligament (ACL) injuries are prevalent in athletes and are frequently associated with persistent functional limitations, sub-optimal return to previous performance levels, elevated reinjury risk, and, in some cases, shorter athletic careers [1–3]. In soccer, pooled data indicate that 72–90% of players resume competitive play; however, only 53–80% recover their pre-injury standard of performance [4–6]. The careers of soccer players after ACL injury last on average 3–8 years and are typically 1–2 years shorter than those of their uninjured peers [4–6]. Such persistent deficits after ACL injury may contribute to the growing reliance on surgical reconstruction (ACLR), whose incidence in the United States increased from 40.9 to 47.8 procedures per 10,000 individuals between 2004 and 2009 [7–9].

ACLR is mainly performed using either autografts, where tissue is harvested from the patient's own body (commonly the hamstrings or patellar tendon), or allografts, where tissue is obtained from a donor. One of the key aspects after ACLR with hamstring tendon (HT) autograft is the harvesting procedure, which leads to persistent hamstring strength deficits commonly associated with loss of medial rotation, knee flexion, and varus strength [10]. The evidence for what kind of graft reduces the risk of re-rupture is not clear, but some authors suggest a slight increase in the risk for HT [11,12]. These findings underscore the necessity of incorporating adjunctive external stabilization techniques, such as lateral extra-articular tenodesis [13,14]. We can only hypothesize that the reported rise in graft re-rupture is linked to altered kinetic variables—such as a loss of knee-flexion range—but, although the current evidence does not support a definitive correlation, the impact of graft-harvesting techniques on the rotational stability and varus-moment control of the knee remains largely unexplored [15].

Hamstrings are crucial for dynamic knee stability and ACL protection [16,17]. In fact, hamstrings play an important role in knee joint stability by preventing medial femoral condyle lift-off, valgus opening, anterior tibial translation, and external rotation [16,18]. At mid- to long-term follow-up (1–2 years and beyond), a significant proportion of patients continue to experience measurable hamstring strength deficits compared to their uninjured limb or healthy controls [19–22]. Girdwood et al. [23] reported that knee flexor strength deficits of 5–7% compared to the contralateral limb are typical at 1 year, with little further improvement up to 5 years after ACLR. These deficits are even larger when compared to uninjured controls instead of the contralateral limb. Furthermore, a recent study reported limb symmetry index (LSI) values of 54%, 70%, and 76% for isometric knee flexor strength at 4, 8, and 12 weeks following ACLR using a hamstring graft [24]. These findings highlight the persistence of strength deficits in the early postoperative period after ACLR [24]. Moreover, hamstring weakness after ACLR tends to be more pronounced at deeper flexion angles (from >70° to max knee flexion) (i.e., shorter muscle lengths), during slower contraction speeds, and is especially evident when assessing rate of force development rather than peak strength alone [24]. After ACLR with HT, there is often a selective reduction in semitendinosus muscle thickness, with reported atrophy ranging from 10% to 28% [20]. After ACLR with hamstring graft, the semitendinosus often shows selective atrophy (10–28%), frequently accompanied by gracilis atrophy (~30%). If not compensated by hypertrophy of the semimembranosus or biceps femoris, this can lead to overall hamstring volume loss, reduced knee flexion strength, and imbalances between medial and lateral hamstrings that may impair transverse plane knee stability [21,25–27].

In addition to maximal strength, hamstring endurance is another clinically relevant aspect that may influence the postoperative recovery [28]. Endurance, defined as the ability to sustain repeated submaximal contractions over time, is crucial for functional knee stability during prolonged physical activity [29,30]. Importantly, endurance deficits may persist even when peak strength partially recovers, suggesting that monitoring endurance could provide complementary insights into muscle function after ACLR [31].

While rehabilitation protocols have evolved towards accelerated approaches [32,33] (which involve early unrestricted movement, immediate weight-bearing within limits, removal of immobilization braces, and a patient-centered goal of returning to high-level physical activity or sports within 6 months post-surgery), current guidelines often maintain a cautious approach to the early introduction of hamstring strengthening exercises, particularly open kinetic chain (OKC) leg curls, due to concerns about harvest site healing. Most research suggests waiting 6–8 weeks before starting to load the knee flexion [34–36].

However, this cautious approach is largely based on expert consensus [37] rather than high-level evidence [9]. At the same time, it is well established that early muscle activation is fundamental to counteract neural inhibition and muscle atrophy [38]. Given the persistence of hamstring strength deficits observed after ACLR with HT and the absence of robust data on the effects of early introduction of specific OKC exercises such as leg curls and bridges [20,37], there is a compelling need to reconsider the timing of their introduction. To date, no studies have specifically evaluated the safety and effectiveness of early OKC exercises on hamstring strength after ACLR. Seeking to address this gap in the literature, the present study aims to evaluate the potential for hamstring strength recovery associated with early OKC exercise implementation and analyze the incidence of potential adverse effects. We hypothesize that the early introduction of OKC exercises may facilitate faster recovery without increasing the risk of complications.

2. Materials and Methods

2.1. Study Design and Participants

An exploratory retrospective observational study was conducted in accordance with the Strengthening the Reporting of Observational Studies in Epidemiology (STROBE) guidelines [39].

This was a retrospective observational study conducted at a single outpatient physiotherapy center. The study followed the ethical principles outlined in the Declaration of Helsinki and its subsequent amendments. Ethical approval was obtained from the Institutional Review Board (Ethics Committee) of the Conseil d'Orientation Scientifique—GCS Ramsay Santé pour l'Enseignement et la Recherche (IORG0009085; IRB00010835; protocol code COS-RGDS-2025-06-002-FORELLI-F; approval date 11 June 2023), and all participants provided written informed consent for the use of their anonymized data.

We reviewed the records of 25 patients who underwent primary ACLR with autologous semitendinosus–gracilis grafts between December 2023 and December 2024 (all procedures were performed by the same surgical team). The inclusion criteria of an age range of 18–35 years and a Tegner Activity Scale score of ≥5 were chosen to focus on a population of physically active adults and athletes. This specific cohort is highly represented in ACL injuries and shares common rehabilitation goals, such as a high-level return to sport. Excluding pediatric and older adult patients helped to mitigate potential confounding factors related to age-dependent variations in muscle development, strength, and recovery rates.

The inclusion criteria were as follows:

- Age 18–35 years;
- Tegner Activity Scale ≥ 5;

- Isolated ACLR or combined with partial meniscectomy or lateral extra-articular tenodesis;
- Baseline knee range of motion $\geq 90°$ [40];
- Resting knee pain $\leq 3/10$ on the Numeric Pain Rating Scale (NPRS);
- Absence of clinical signs of effusion or acute inflammatory flare (joint swelling < Trace on Stroke test compared to contralateral side, no redness or local heat or any other warning signs) [41].

The exclusion criteria were as follows

- Meniscal repair;
- Concomitant Posterior Cruciate Ligament or posterolateral corner injuries;
- Use of grafts other than hamstring tendons;
- ACL revision surgery;
- Additional ligament injuries requiring protection beyond standard ACLR rehab;
- Cartilage procedures requiring protected loading (e.g., microfracture);
- Clinically relevant postoperative complications before week 3 (e.g., infection, arthrofibrosis).

Of the 25 patient records reviewed, 12 were excluded due to concomitant procedures or alternative graft types, leaving 13 eligible records included in the final analysis (Figure 1). The same 13 participants were assessed at all timepoints, ensuring valid paired comparisons.

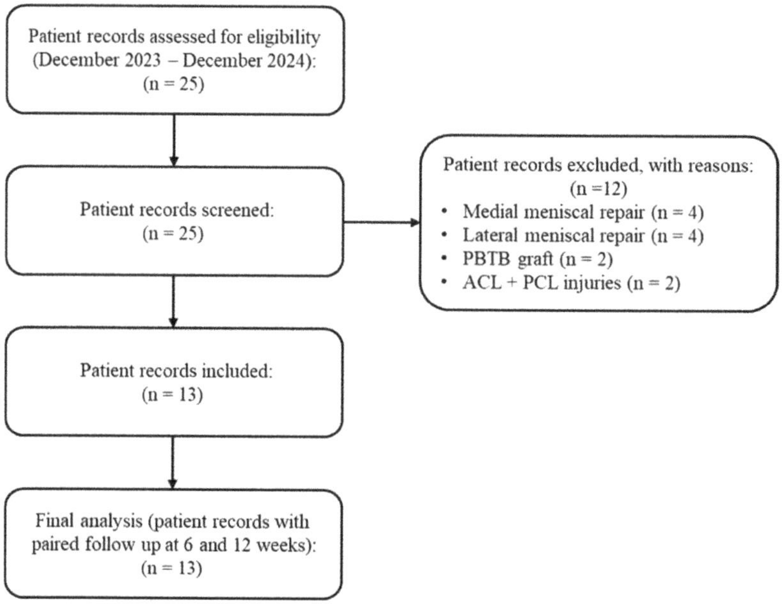

Figure 1. Flowchart of the retrospective selection process.

2.2. Rehabilitation Protocol

All participants began a hamstring strengthening protocol at 3 weeks after ACLR, two times per week. The protocol included 2 open kinetic chain exercises (leg curl) and 1 closed kinetic chain exercise (long lever glute bridge). During this period, no other isolated hamstring exercises were performed. Every patient followed a 3 times per week (every 48 h) strict rehabilitation protocol focusing on quadriceps, calf, core, hip, and balance and two hamstring exercises completed 2 times per week every 96 h (Table 1).

Table 1. Structure of the rehabilitation program weeks 3–6.

Day 1	Day 2	Day 3
10′ bike	10′ bike	10′ bike
Seated hamstring isometric curl at 90°	Horizontal single leg press	Seated hamstring isometric curl at 90°
Seated hamstring isometric curl at 60°		Seated hamstring isometric curl at 60°
Isometric long lever glute bridge	Seated leg isometric leg extensions	Isometric long lever glute bridge
Horizontal single leg press	Standing calf raise	Horizontal single leg press
Seated leg isometric leg extensions	Bent knee calf raise	Seated leg isometric leg extensions
Standing calf raise	Lateral walk with mini band	Standing calf raise
Bent knee calf raise	Adductor plank	Bent knee calf raise
Lateral walk with mini band	Single leg balance exercise with eyes closed	Lateral walk with mini band
Adductor plank		Adductor plank
Single leg balance exercise with eyes closed		Single leg balance exercise with eyes closed

After 10′ of bike as warm-up, the intervention was structured in two primary phases: initially, OKC exercises were performed, followed by closed kinetic chain (CKC) exercises.

The first exercise was an isometric seated single leg curl on a leg curl machine at 90°, the second was an isometric seated leg curl on a leg curl machine at 60°, and the third was long lever glute bridges (patients lie supine with the knee flexed at 30°, foot in contact with the ground, and arms on the chest. For the seated leg curl machine, the range of motion (ROM) was standardized using the built-in lateral adjustment device, which allows the movement to be fixed at predefined joint angles (Seated Leg Curl R.O.M. machine, Technogym®, Cesena, Italy); for the glute bridge, we standardized the knee joint angle using a goniometer to ensure consistent ROM across participants. These exercises were completed at the beginning of each rehabilitation session.

Following the two hamstring primary exercises, participants completed a standardized protocol consisting of the following:

- Two quadriceps-focused exercises (leg extension and leg press),
- Two calf exercises (bent-knee and straight-knee calf raises),
- Two core stabilization exercises (plank and side plank),
- Two hip-focused exercises targeting the adductors and abductors (Copenhagen plank and lateral walk with a mini-band positioned at the ankles),
- One single leg balance exercise with eye closed.

From postoperative week 3 to week 6, every patient entered a three-week strengthening program consisting of three supervised sessions per week (nine sessions in total). All work was overseen and logged—sets × repetitions × external load or time-under-tension (TUT), plus any symptoms (including pain and/or burning sensation in harvest site or cramping in the posterior/medial side of the thigh), by the same physiotherapist, who has more than ten years' experience in ACLR rehabilitation.

Each session began with quadriceps-dominant and multi-joint lower-limb exercises (e.g., leg extension, leg press). These drills followed a linear periodization scheme [42]: the earliest sessions used high repetitions with low external resistance, and subsequent sessions progressively reduced the repetition count while increasing the load, but only when the patient maintained full movement control throughout the range of motion.

Hamstring strengthening was scheduled twice per week. During those two sessions, patients performed three unilateral exercises: (i) an isometric leg curl hold at 90° of knee flexion, (ii) an isometric leg curl hold at 60° of knee flexion, and (iii) a long lever glute bridge. The initial prescription for each hamstring drill was five sets of forty-five-second holds, with thirty seconds of rest between sets; the injured limb was always trained first, followed by the uninjured side to avoid contralateral detraining. Starting loads were chosen to provoke neither pain with an NPRS less than 3 out 10 nor compensatory patterns like anterior pelvic tilt or feeling fatigue from the calf muscle. Quality was deemed acceptable when no anterior pelvic tilt (no lumbar lift-off from the backrest) appeared during the leg-curl holds and when the hip height remained stable during the glute bridge, with no height drop from the position reached at the beginning of the set. Whenever all sets met these criteria, with a numeric rating pain scale < 3, the next session's external load was increased by ten per cent, and the TUT for each set was shortened by five seconds [43]. If a patient could not yet stabilize a single-leg glute bridge for the full TUT, the exercise began in the double-leg position and progressed to unilateral execution once a forty-five-second hold was achieved without loss of hip height.

The third weekly session omitted hamstring exercises but retained the same quadriceps and multi-joint progression, ensuring adequate recovery for the flexor muscles while maintaining overall lower-limb loading throughout the three-week block.

After 6 weeks, patients started a progressive isotonic slow resistance training with 0–90° range of motion in seated leg curl and full hip range of motion with knees at 30° of flexion on single leg long lever glutes bridge (Table 2).

Table 2. Structure of the rehabilitation program weeks 6–12.

Day 1	Day 2	Day 3
10′ bike	10′ bike	10′ bike
Seated isotonic leg curl	Horizontal single leg press	Seated isotonic leg curl
Isotonic long lever glute bridge	Seated leg isometric leg extensions	Isotonic long lever glute bridge
Horizontal single leg press	Standing calf raise	Horizontal single leg press
Seated leg isometric leg extensions	Bent knee calf raise	Seated leg isometric leg extensions
Standing calf raise	Lateral walk with mini band	Standing calf raise
Bent knee calf raise	Adductor plank	Bent knee calf raise
Lateral walk with mini band	Single leg balance exercise with eyes closed	Lateral walk with mini band
Adductor plank		Adductor plank
Single leg balance exercise with eyes closed		Single leg balance exercise with eyes closed

For the isotonic seated leg curl and long lever glutes bridge, the strength progression was based on a linear periodization.

The initial load was 4 sets of 15 repetitions (with 2 repetitions in reverse) at a slow controlled tempo, and progression of the load was increased by 5–10%, depending on the pain tolerance (maximum NPRS score less than 3 out 10). With each load increase, repetitions were decreased by two (i.e., 15 → 12 → 10 → 8 → 6), while maintaining 4 sets and a 2 min rest between them. Once the patient reached 6 repetitions per set, the volume (sets and reps) was held constant, and only the external load was progressively increased.

2.3. Outcome Measures

The primary outcome is the safety and tolerability of the early introduction of OKC exercises. For each physiotherapy session, we searched the notes for three predefined "safety flags" recorded during the workout or within the following 24 h:

1. Pain rated > 4/10 on the NPRS.
2. Hematoma in the posterior thigh or at the graft-harvest site, described on inspection or palpation and, when necessary, confirmed by musculoskeletal ultrasound.
3. Clinical signs of hamstring-muscle strain, identified by acute localized pain in the posterior thigh or tendon, pain exacerbated by stretching or palpation, and, when suspected, confirmed by magnetic-resonance imaging [44].

Whenever one or more of these events appeared in the chart, the treating therapist halted the OCK component of the program. OKC work was restarted only after the patient was completely pain-free and never earlier than postoperative week 8, in line with our physiotherapy center guidelines.

The secondary outcome was the recovery of the hamstring muscle strength and endurance. Hamstring strength values recorded at postoperative week 3 served as the baseline, while measurements at weeks 6 and 12 were used to evaluate the progression of muscle strength over time. Before the test, patients underwent a standardized warm-up regimen, which consisted of 10 min on a stationary bike, followed by ten submaximal repetitions at 50% and 75%, and then one to two repetitions at 90% of their maximum voluntary contraction in the testing device [45,46].

At 6 weeks, the isometric strength of the hamstring muscles was tested at 90° and 60° of knee flexion using a fixed dynamometer with 1000 Hz frequency (K-push, Kinvent, France). The dynamometer force arm was calibrated according to the manufacturer's guidelines before each testing session. The non-testing thigh was secured to the test bench with a strap at its mid-thigh level.

The force arm of the dynamometer was secured 2 cm proximal to the lateral malleolus to ensure a consistent lever arm across all participants. We calculated the lever arm for each participant by measuring the distance in meters between the lateral femoral condyle and the point where the dynamometer was placed on the lower leg, which was 2 cm proximal to the lateral malleolus. Patients were asked to push as hard and fast as they could for 5 s trying to avoid countermovement prior the start. In order to have a more detailed picture of the recovery, we also calculated the hamstring-to-quadriceps strength ratio. Quadriceps strength was assessed in a sitting position with the knee at 60° of flexion, in order to avoid stress on the graft [47]. The isometric test consisted of three 3 s maximal voluntary contractions with a 30 s rest interval [44,48]. The average of the three trials was calculated and used to compute the LSI.

We calculated the torque as the force, expressed in Newton normalized to the body weight, expressed in kilograms (N/kg) [49].

The endurance was tested through the glute bridge endurance test [31]: patients performed as many single-leg repetitions as possible in a supine position with the hip flexed at 45° and the knee at 90°, maintaining dorsiflexion [31]. Before starting the test, a target height was determined based on the patient's maximal hip extension during a preliminary trial. The test was performed to the rhythm of 60 beats per minute. The test was stopped when the patient could no longer reach the target height or failed to maintain the rhythm. This test was chosen to assess both maximal and endurance strength of the posterior chain at the 6-week timepoint.

At the 12-week follow-up, all the same isometric strength tests were repeated, with the exception of the glute bridge endurance test, which was replaced by a 90°–90° isometric hamstring test (with both the hip and knee flexed at 90°) [44,48]. For both strength assessments test, the uninjured limb was tested first. Each isometric test consisted of three 3 s maximal voluntary contractions with a 30 s rest interval [44,48]. The average of the three trials was calculated and used to compute the LSI.

The LSI was computed through the following formula:

$$\text{LSI} = (\text{Injured limb strength}/\text{Healthy limb strength}) \times 100. \quad (1)$$

2.4. Statistical Analysis

All statistical analyses were conducted using JASP (Version 0.95.1; JASP Team, Amsterdam, The Netherlands). A descriptive analysis was performed for anthropometric and clinical characteristics. Normality tests were conducted for all variables with Shapiro–Wilk test and inspection of Q–Q plots. Given the small sample size (n = 13) and the limited power of normality testing, non-parametric methods were adopted regardless of the distributional results. When reported, safety outcomes (pain > 4/10, hematoma, clinical signs of strain) were summarized as counts and percentages. Continuous variables were reported as the median and interquartile range (IQR). A comparison analysis of differences in the hamstring isometric strength (60° and 90° knee flexion), quadriceps strength, hamstring-to-quadriceps ratio, and limb symmetry index (LSI) between week 6 and week 12 was performed using the Wilcoxon signed-rank test. The glute bridge endurance test was only descriptively reported (median [IQR]), as it was only performed at week 6. Effect sizes for paired non-parametric tests were expressed as the rank–biserial correlation (r), with 95% confidence intervals (CI). All statistical tests were two-tailed, with the significance level set at $\alpha = 0.05$. No adjustment for multiple comparisons was applied, given the exploratory nature of the study. No a priori sample size calculation was performed; therefore, the analyses are underpowered, and the potential for type II error must be acknowledged when interpreting non-significant findings.

3. Results

3.1. Safety

All 13 participants (descriptive characteristics in Table 3) completed the rehabilitation protocol without interruption.

Table 3. Demographic data.

Characteristics	ACL Patients (n = 13)
Age [1]	27 (25–30)
Gender	
Male, n (%)	9 (69.2)
Female, n (%)	4 (30.8)
Weight (Kg) [1]	71 (68–79)
Height (cm) [1]	178 (172–183)
Graft type	
R HT/G, n (%)	6
L HT/G, n (%)	7
Time from surgery (weeks)	21 (19–22)

[1] Data are reported as median (IQR). Yr = years; HT = hamstring tendons, Kg = kilograms.

Pain diaries documented consistently low discomfort levels throughout the 18 supervised sessions (234 observations in total). The median pain intensity recorded across all sessions was 2.5 (range 1.2–4.4). Inter-session values showed no clinically relevant differences, with most ratings remaining stably below the threshold of 4. Across the

234 monitored sessions, only one patient (7.7%) reported pain exceeding the clinical threshold (NPRS 4.4 at session 12). This was an isolated episode and did not require protocol interruption. No posterior thigh hematomas, graft site complications, or clinical signs of hamstring strain were observed. The distribution of pain scores across sessions and patients is illustrated in Figure 2.

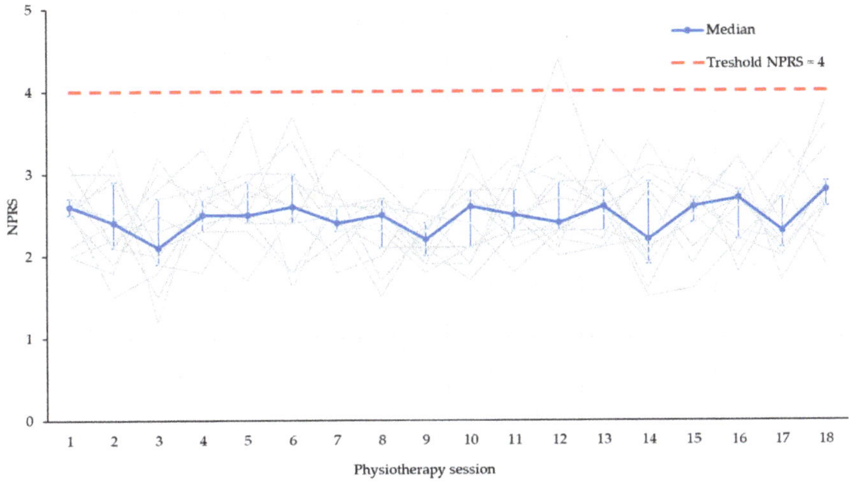

Figure 2. Individual pain trajectories (NPRS) recorded across the 18 supervised rehabilitation sessions. Thin grey lines represent single-patient values, while the blue line depicts the session-by-session median with interquartile range error bars. The dashed red line indicates the clinical threshold of 4 points.

3.2. Strength Recovery

At 6 weeks, the isometric knee flexion strength of the operated limb was 0.25 N/kg (range 0.14–0.36) at 60° and 0.19 N/kg (range 0.04–0.27) at 90°. At 12 weeks, the strength increased to 0.28 N/kg (range 0.12–0.42) at 60° and 0.26 N/kg (range 0.10–0.34) at 90°. Paired comparisons between 6 and 12 weeks showed a significant improvement in isometric strength at both 60° ($Z = -2.40$, $p = 0.018$) and 90° ($Z = -3.04$, $p = 0.003$). The effect size, expressed as rank-biserial correlation suggested a large improvement both at 60° ($r = -0.82$, 95% CI −0.95 to −0.45) and 90° ($r = -0.96$, 95% CI −0.99 to −0.86). These results are illustrated in Figure 3.

The median LSI for isometric knee flexion tested at 60° was 70.4% (IQR: 42.9–93.4%) at 6 weeks, increasing to 82.4% (IQR: 54.2–96.3%) at 12 weeks. This difference was not statistically significant ($p = 0.108$). The effect size, expressed as the rank–biserial correlation, suggested a moderate improvement ($r = -0.52$, 95% CI: −0.83 to 0.05). The median LSI for isometric knee flexion tested at 90° was 65% (IQR: 36.4–29.2%) at 6 weeks, increasing to 82.7% (IQR: 67.9–126%) at 12 weeks. The Wilcoxon signed-rank test revealed a significant improvement in the LSI at 90° from 6 to 12 weeks ($p = 0.006$), with a large effect size ($r = -0.82$, 95% CI −0.95 to −0.50). Detailed descriptive and inferential statistics are reported in Table 4 and illustrated in Figure 3.

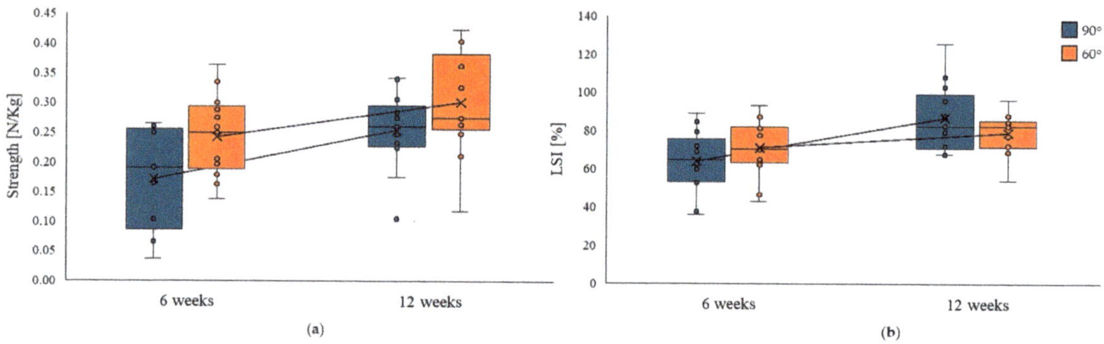

Figure 3. Distribution of quadriceps isometric strength measured at 90° (blue box plots) and 60° (orange box plots) of knee flexion in the ACLR limb at 6 and 12 weeks postoperatively. Box plots display the median, interquartile range, and individual data points; connecting lines represent individual trajectories between timepoints. An overall improvement in strength is observed in the operated limb, particularly at 90°, with inter-individual variability. The strength asymmetry between limbs appears to decrease over time. (**a**) show improvement in strength, (**b**) improvement in the limb symmetry index (LSI).

Table 4. Limb symmetry index at 6 and 12 weeks post-ACLR. Hamstring strength tests performed in a seated position at 60° and 90° of knee flexion.

Isometric Hamstring Muscle Test	LSI at 6 Weeks Median [IQR]	LSI at 12 Weeks Median [IQR]	Δ LSI	*Z*	*p*-Value	r	95% Confidence Interval
Knee flexion = 60°	70.4% [42.9–93.4]	82.4% [54.2–96.3]	+9.5%	−1.64	0.108	−0.52	−0.83 to 0.05
Knee flexion = 90°	65% [36.4–89.2]	82.7% [67.9–126]	+19.5%	−2.62	0.006	−0.82	−0.95 to −0.50

Note: IQR = interquartile range; Δ LSI = change in limb symmetry index between 6 and 12 weeks. Wilcoxon signed-rank test was used. r = effect size calculated using rank–biserial correlation.

At 6 weeks, participants performed a median of 25 (IQR: 14–57) repetitions with the uninjured limb and 25 (IQR: 12–55) with the injured limb. The difference was statistically significant ($Z = -2.43$, $p = 0.016$), with a large effect size ($r = -0.80$, 95% CI −0.94 to −0.42). The corresponding LSI was 95.45%.

4. Discussion

The aims of this study were to evaluate the hamstring strength recovery and the safety of introducing both OKC and CKC hamstring exercises as early as three weeks after ACLR using a hamstring graft. The findings indicate that early implementation of these exercises appears to be safe and may promote improvements in hamstring strength and endurance, but these results should be interpreted with caution given the sample size and study design.

A previous study initiated hamstring-loading protocols at four weeks following ACLR with hamstring tendon autografts and documented progressive improvements in hamstring strength at 8 and 12 weeks, with an LSI of 69% and 75% at 60° of knee flexion, respectively; however, no significant gains were noted at 90° [47]. Greater deficits in knee flexion strength have been reported at deeper flexion angles (>70°), particularly in patients who underwent harvest of both semitendinosus and gracilis tendons, with residual weakness ranging from 3% to 27% even at 32 months after ACL [50]. Persistent weakness has also been observed at 18 months after ACLR, with LSIs as low as 60% at 90° and 70% at 70° of knee flexion in a prone position in the semitendinosus–gracilis group [51]. Moreover, one study documented reduced active knee flexion range of motion one year after surgery, suggesting ongoing deficits in muscular function and neuromuscular control [52]. Our results support the hypothesis that early introduction of both OKC and CKC hamstring exercises may counteract such long-term deficits [53]. No adverse events occurred during the intervention period. Patients reported only mild discomfort (median NPRS: 2.5) during or following training sessions, and no cases of hematoma, donor site complications, or hamstring strain were observed. These findings challenge the traditionally conservative approach of delaying OKC hamstring exercises after ACLR, a strategy primarily based on theoretical concerns rather than empirical evidence. Instead, our data suggest that earlier loading may be both safe and beneficial for optimizing the early recovery of hamstring strength and endurance.

4.1. Clinical Implications

The preliminary findings of this retrospective study suggest that early voluntary isometric and isotonic exercises, introduced at three weeks after ACLR in patients with isolated reconstructions and no meniscal repair, may be feasible and safe. While such early loading could potentially help counteract neural inhibition and support recovery of functional strength [54–56], these observations are based on a small sample and should be interpreted with caution. We cannot state whether natural healing, general exercise, or familiarizations could be plausible alternative explanations. Larger controlled studies are required before drawing firm conclusions about clinical implications [57].

4.2. Limitations

This study has several methodological and analytical limitations that must be acknowledged. First, given the small sample size, the study had limited statistical power. As such, non-significant findings cannot be interpreted as evidence of no effect, but rather as inconclusive results that require confirmation in larger cohorts. Second, the testing procedures were not fully consistent across time points, as different strength assessments were used, potentially affecting the comparability of the results over time. We decided to address endurance strength only at 6 weeks, because it is not considered a clinical milestone for 12 weeks assessment; so, we do not know whether the result achieved is consistent over time. Third, the chosen effect size metric may not have been the most appropriate for the type of data analyzed, which could lead to an over- or underestimation of the true magnitude of change. Fourth, some outcome measures were either insufficiently described or lacked clear operational definitions, reducing the transparency and reproducibility. In addition, safety outcomes were reported narratively rather than through systematic collection and quantification of adverse events, which limits the robustness of our safety claims. It is important to note that the small sample size and the narrative nature of the safety data collection limit the robustness of these findings. While the completion of 234 sessions with only one pain episode is a reassuring preliminary signal, this study is not powered to detect rare or uncommon adverse events; furthermore, because pain is subjective, and the source data were routine clinical records, outcome misclassification is possible. Rare adverse events cannot be excluded in a cohort of this size. Therefore, our safety claims should be interpreted as hypothesis-generating, with a need for larger prospective studies to systematically quantify and confirm the safety profile of this intervention. We also cannot address the effect on graft laxity due to the absence of the laxity test, but this was not an objective of the study. Another important limitation concerns the reliance on the LSI as the primary marker of recovery: while useful, LSI does not capture absolute strength values and may therefore introduce bias, especially if the contralateral limb is also affected by deconditioning. Moreover, the retrospective design without a control group, the small sample size (n = 13), single surgical team, single rehabilitation center, and standardized treatment by the same therapist limit the internal validity. Selection and reporting biases are possible, and causal inference is not warranted. The external validity is restricted to young physically active adults (18–35 years) who underwent primary ACLR with hamstring autografts without meniscal repair. Finally, the absence of a control group prevents any causal inferences regarding the superiority of early hamstring loading over standard rehabilitation protocols and limits the generalizability of the findings. Collectively, these limitations highlight the preliminary nature of our results and underscore the need for future prospective randomized controlled trials with larger sample sizes, standardized outcome measures, systematic safety reporting, and long-term follow-up to confirm and expand upon these observations.

4.3. Future Directions

Future studies should build on the present findings by prospectively testing whether the early introduction of voluntary isometric and isotonic hamstring exercises at three weeks post-ACLR leads to superior recovery of hamstring strength compared with standard protocols. Randomized controlled trials with adequately powered sample sizes are warranted to evaluate not only the LSI but also the absolute strength values, functional performance measures, and long-term return-to-sport and re-injury outcomes. Methodological refinements should include the use of consistent strength assessments across time points, systematic collection of adverse events to better characterize safety, and appropriate effect size metrics to capture the magnitude of change. Additionally, future research should explore whether the timing and intensity of early strengthening differentially affect patients with various graft types or concomitant procedures and whether targeted interventions can mitigate the atherogenic muscle inhibition observed in this population.

5. Conclusions

Introducing open-kinetic-chain hamstring strengthening from week 3 post-ACLR with a hamstring autograft appeared feasible and was associated with short-term improvements in inter-limb strength symmetry and endurance. No adverse events were observed, and meaningful improvements in inter-limb strength symmetry and endurance were obtained. These findings challenge the traditionally conservative approach and provide a rationale for reconsidering early hamstring loading in postoperative rehabilitation protocols. These preliminary observations should be interpreted with caution and require confirmation in adequately powered randomized controlled trials with standardized safety monitoring and longer follow-up.

Author Contributions: CRediT author statement: Conceptualization, R.R. and F.F.; methodology, R.R. and F.M.; software, M.B.; validation, R.R., R.C. and R.G.; formal analysis, F.F.; investigation, R.R., M.B. and F.S.; resources, R.C. and R.G.; data curation, M.B. and F.S.; writing—original draft preparation, R.R. and F.F.; writing—review and editing, R.C., F.M., M.B., F.S. and R.G.; visualization, F.M.; supervision, F.F.; project administration, R.R. All authors have read and agreed to the published version of the manuscript.

Funding: This research received no external funding.

Institutional Review Board Statement: The study was conducted in accordance with the Declaration of Helsinki and approved by the Institutional Review Board (Ethics Committee) of the Conseil d'Orientation Scientifique—GCS Ramsay Santé pour l'Enseignement et la Recherche (IORG0009085; IRB00010835; protocol code COS-RGDS-2025-06-002-FORELLI-F; approval date 11 June 2023).

Informed Consent Statement: Informed consent was obtained from all subjects involved in the study. Written informed consent has been obtained from the patient(s) to publish this paper.

Data Availability Statement: The data supporting the findings of this study are available from the authors upon request.

Conflicts of Interest: The authors declare no conflicts of interest.

References

1. Farinelli, L.; Abermann, E.; Meena, A.; Ueblacker, P.; Hahne, J.; Fink, C. Return to Play and Pattern of Injury After ACL Rupture in a Consecutive Series of Elite UEFA Soccer Players. *Orthop. J. Sports Med.* **2023**, *11*, 23259671231153629. [CrossRef]
2. Manojlovic, M.; Ninkovic, S.; Matic, R.; Versic, S.; Modric, T.; Sekulic, D.; Drid, P. Return to Play and Performance After Anterior Cruciate Ligament Reconstruction in Soccer Players: A Systematic Review of Recent Evidence. *Sports Med.* **2024**, *54*, 2097–2108. [CrossRef] [PubMed]
3. Niederer, D.; Engeroff, T.; Wilke, J.; Vogt, L.; Banzer, W. Return to Play, Performance, and Career Duration after Anterior Cruciate Ligament Rupture: A Case-Control Study in the Five Biggest Football Nations in Europe. *Scand. J. Med. Sci. Sports* **2018**, *28*, 2226–2233. [CrossRef] [PubMed]
4. Lai, C.C.H.; Ardern, C.L.; Feller, J.A.; Webster, K.E. Eighty-Three per Cent of Elite Athletes Return to Preinjury Sport after Anterior Cruciate Ligament Reconstruction: A Systematic Review with Meta-Analysis of Return to Sport Rates, Graft Rupture Rates and Performance Outcomes. *Br. J. Sports Med.* **2018**, *52*, 128–138. [CrossRef] [PubMed]
5. Longstaffe, R.; Leiter, J.; Gurney-Dunlop, T.; McCormack, R.; MacDonald, P. Return to Play and Career Length After Anterior Cruciate Ligament Reconstruction Among Canadian Professional Football Players. *Am. J. Sports Med.* **2020**, *48*, 1682–1688. [CrossRef]
6. Van Melick, N.; Van Cingel, R.E.H.; Brooijmans, F.; Neeter, C.; Van Tienen, T.; Hullegie, W.; Nijhuis-Van Der Sanden, M.W.G. Evidence-Based Clinical Practice Update: Practice Guidelines for Anterior Cruciate Ligament Rehabilitation Based on a Systematic Review and Multidisciplinary Consensus. *Br. J. Sports Med.* **2016**, *50*, 1506–1515. [CrossRef]
7. Leathers, M.P.; Merz, A.; Wong, J.; Scott, T.; Wang, J.C.; Hame, S.L. Trends and Demographics in Anterior Cruciate Ligament Reconstruction in the United States. *J. Knee Surg.* **2015**, *28*, 390–394. [CrossRef]
8. Pinheiro, V.H.; Borque, K.A.; Laughlin, M.S.; Jones, M.; Balendra, G.; Kent, M.R.; Ajgaonkar, R.; Williams, A. Determinants of Performance in Professional Soccer Players at 2 and 5 Years After ACL Reconstruction. *Am. J. Sports Med.* **2023**, *51*, 3649–3657. [CrossRef]
9. Ricupito, R.; Grassi, A.; Mourad, F.; Di Filippo, L.; Gobbo, M.; Maselli, F. Anterior Cruciate Ligament Return to Play: "A Framework for Decision Making". *J. Clin. Med.* **2025**, *14*, 2146. [CrossRef]
10. Briem, K.; Zebis, M.K.; Haraldsson, B.Þ.; Bencke, J.; Fernandes, L. Rehabilitation Guidelines after Autograft Anterior Cruciate Ligament Reconstruction Need More Graft-Specific Exercise Recommendations—A Scoping Review. *Knee Surg. Sports Traumatol. Arthrosc.* **2025**. [CrossRef]
11. Persson, A.; Fjeldsgaard, K.; Gjertsen, J.E.; Kjellsen, A.B.; Engebretsen, L.; Hole, R.M.; Fevang, J.M. Increased Risk of Revision with Hamstring Tendon Grafts Compared with Patellar Tendon Grafts after Anterior Cruciate Ligament Reconstruction: A Study of 12,643 Patients from the Norwegian Cruciate Ligament Registry, 2004–2012. *Am. J. Sports Med.* **2014**, *42*, 285–291. [CrossRef]
12. Yang, J.S.; Prentice, H.A.; Reyes, C.E.; Lehman, C.R.; Maletis, G.B. Risk of Revision and Reoperation After Quadriceps Tendon Autograft ACL Reconstruction Compared with Patellar Tendon and Hamstring Autografts in a US Cohort of 21,973 Patients. *Am. J. Sports Med.* **2024**, *52*, 670–681. [CrossRef]
13. Sonnery-Cottet, B.; Carrozzo, A.; Saithna, A.; Monaco, E.; Vieira, T.D.; Musahl, V.; Getgood, A.; Helito, C.P.; Bedi, A.; Bryant, D.; et al. Surgical Treatment and Complications of Lateral Extra-Articular Procedures in the ACL Reconstructed Knee: Part II of An International Consensus Statement. *Arthrosc. J. Arthrosc. Relat. Surg.* **2025**, *41*, 3313–3321. [CrossRef]
14. Sonnery-Cottet, B.; Carrozzo, A.; Saithna, A.; Monaco, E.; Vieira, T.D.; Musahl, V.; Getgood, A.; Helito, C.P.; Bedi, A.; Bryant, D.; et al. Indications for Lateral Extra-Articular Procedures in the ACL Reconstructed Knee: Part I of An International Consensus Statement. *Arthrosc. J. Arthrosc. Relat. Surg.* **2025**, *41*, 3303–3312. [CrossRef]
15. Sundberg, A.; Senorski, R.H.; Högberg, J.; Piussi, R.; Samuelsson, K.; Thomeé, R.; Senorski, E.H. Persistent Isokinetic Knee Flexion Strength Deficits at the Time of Return to Sport Are Not Associated with a Second ACL Injury. *Knee Surg. Sports Traumatol. Arthrosc.* **2025**, *333*, 2971–2983. [CrossRef]
16. Draganich, L.F.; Vahey, J.W. An in Vitro Study of Anterior Cruciate Ligament Strain Induced by Quadriceps and Hamstrings Forces. *J. Orthop. Res.* **1990**, *8*, 57–63. [CrossRef] [PubMed]
17. More, R.C.; Karras, B.T.; Neiman, R.; Fritschy, D.; Woo, S.L.Y.; Daniel, D.M. Hamstrings—An Anterior Cruciate Ligament Protagonist: An in Vitro Study. *Am. J. Sports Med.* **1993**, *21*, 231–237. [CrossRef]
18. Scanlan, S.F.; Chaudhari, A.M.W.; Dyrby, C.O.; Andriacchi, T.P. Differences in Tibial Rotation during Walking in ACL Reconstructed and Healthy Contralateral Knees. *J. Biomech.* **2010**, *43*, 1817–1822. [CrossRef] [PubMed]

19. Verrall, G.M.; Slavotinek, J.P.; Barnes, P.G.; Fon, G.T.; Spriggins, A.J. Clinical Risk Factors for Hamstring Muscle Strain Injury: A Prospective Study with Correlation of Injury by Magnetic Resonance Imaging. *Br. J. Sports Med.* **2001**, *35*, 435–439. [CrossRef] [PubMed]
20. Bourne, M.N.; Bruder, A.M.; Mentiplay, B.F.; Carey, D.L.; Patterson, B.E.; Crossley, K.M. Eccentric Knee Flexor Weakness in Elite Female Footballers 1–10 Years Following Anterior Cruciate Ligament Reconstruction. *Phys. Ther. Sport* **2019**, *37*, 144–149. [CrossRef]
21. Messer, D.J.; Shield, A.J.; Williams, M.D.; Timmins, R.G.; Bourne, M.N. Hamstring Muscle Activation and Morphology Are Significantly Altered 1–6 Years after Anterior Cruciate Ligament Reconstruction with Semitendinosus Graft. *Knee Surg. Sports Traumatol. Arthrosc.* **2020**, *28*, 733–741. [CrossRef]
22. Bouzekraoui Alaoui, I.; Moiroux-Sahraoui, A.; Mazeas, J.; Kakavas, G.; Biały, M.; Douryang, M.; Forelli, F. Impact of Hamstring Graft on Hamstring Peak Torque and Maximum Effective Angle After Anterior Cruciate Ligament Reconstruction: An Exploratory and Preliminary Study. *Bioengineering* **2025**, *12*, 465. [CrossRef]
23. Girdwood, M.; Culvenor, A.G.; Rio, E.K.; Patterson, B.E.; Haberfield, M.; Couch, J.; Mentiplay, B.; Hedger, M.; Crossley, K.M. Tale of Quadriceps and Hamstring Muscle Strength after ACL Reconstruction: A Systematic Review with Longitudinal and Multivariate Meta-Analysis. *Br. J. Sports Med.* **2025**, *59*, 423–434. [CrossRef] [PubMed]
24. Baumgart, C.; Welling, W.; Hoppe, M.W.; Freiwald, J.; Gokeler, A. Angle-Specific Analysis of Isokinetic Quadriceps and Hamstring Torques and Ratios in Patients after ACL-Reconstruction. *BMC Sports Sci. Med. Rehabil.* **2018**, *10*, 23. [CrossRef]
25. Williams, G.N.; Snyder-Mackler, L.; Barrance, P.J.; Axe, M.J.; Buchanan, T.S. Muscle and Tendon Morphology after Reconstruction of the Anterior Cruciate Ligament with Autologous Semitendinosus-Gracilis Graft. *J. Bone Jt. Surg.* **2004**, *86*, 1936–1946. [CrossRef]
26. Irie, K.; Tomatsu, T. Atrophy of Semitendinosus and Gracilis and Flexor Mechanism Function after Hamstring Tendon Harvest for Anterior Cruciate Ligament Reconstruction. *Orthopedics* **2002**, *25*, 491–495. [CrossRef] [PubMed]
27. Snow, B.J.; Wilcox, J.J.; Burks, R.T.; Greis, P.E. Evaluation of Muscle Size and Fatty Infiltration with MRI Nine to Eleven Years Following Hamstring Harvest for ACL Reconstruction. *J. Bone Jt. Surg.* **2012**, *94*, 1274–1282. [CrossRef] [PubMed]
28. Biały, M.; Wilczyński, B.; Forelli, F.; Hewett, T.E.; Gnat, R. Functional Deficits in Non-Elite Soccer (Football) Players: A Strength, Balance, and Movement Quality Assessment After Anterior Cruciate Lig Ament Reconstruction. *Cureus* **2024**, *16*, e75846. [CrossRef]
29. Stergiou, M.; Calvo, A.L.; Forelli, F. Effectiveness of Neuromuscular Training in Preventing Lower Limb Soccer Injuries: A Systematic Review and Meta-Analysis. *J. Clin. Med.* **2025**, *14*, 1714. [CrossRef]
30. Forelli, F.; Traulle, M.; Bechaud, N.; Sansonnet, C.; Marine, P.; Vandebrouck, A.; Duffiet, P.; Mazeas, J. Predict Anterior Cruciate Ligament Injury in Elite Male Soccer Players? Focus On the Five Factors Maximum Model. *Int. J. Physiother.* **2021**, *8*, 211–216. [CrossRef]
31. Buckthorpe, M.; Della Villa, F. Optimising the 'Mid-Stage' Training and Testing Process After ACL Reconstruction. *Sports Med.* **2020**, *50*, 657–678. [CrossRef]
32. Saketh, A.S.P.V.S.; Subramanyam, K. Anterior Cruciate Ligament Rehabilitation Dilemma: Finding the Optimal Path between Conservative and Accelerated Methods. *J. Telangana Orthop. Surg. Assoc.* **2023**, *1*, 25. [CrossRef]
33. Hiranyakumar, S.; Karthik, M.N. Functional Outcome of Accelerated Rehabilitation in Arthroscopic Anterior Cruciate Ligament Reconstruction with Semitendinosis and Gracilis Graft. *Int. J. Sci. Study* **2015**, *3*, 40–44. [CrossRef]
34. Carofino, B.; Fulkerson, J. Medial Hamstring Tendon Regeneration Following Harvest for Anterior Cruciate Ligament Reconstruction: Fact, Myth, and Clinical Implication. *Arthrosc. J. Arthrosc. Relat. Surg.* **2005**, *21*, 1257–1265. [CrossRef]
35. Escamilla, R.F.; MacLeod, T.D.; Wilk, K.E.; Paulos, L.; Andrews, J.R. Anterior Cruciate Ligament Strain and Tensile Forces for Weight-Bearing and Non-Weight-Bearing Exercises: A Guide to Exercise Selectiona. *J. Orthop. Sports Phys. Ther.* **2012**, *42*, 208–220. [CrossRef] [PubMed]
36. Ristanis, S.; Tsepis, E.; Giotis, D.; Stergiou, N.; Cerulli, G.; Georgoulis, A.D. Electromechanical Delay of the Knee Flexor Muscles Is Impaired after Harvesting Hamstring Tendons for Anterior Cruciate Ligament Reconstruction. *Am. J. Sports Med.* **2009**, *37*, 2179–2186. [CrossRef] [PubMed]
37. Buckthorpe, M.; Danelon, F.; La Rosa, G.; Nanni, G.; Stride, M.; Della Villa, F. Recommendations for Hamstring Function Recovery After ACL Reconstruction. *Sports Med.* **2021**, *51*, 607–624. [CrossRef]
38. Hasegawa, S.; Kobayashi, M.; Arai, R.; Tamaki, A.; Nakamura, T.; Moritani, T. Effect of Early Implementation of Electrical Muscle Stimulation to Prevent Muscle Atrophy and Weakness in Patients after Anterior Cruciate Ligament Reconstruction. *J. Electromyogr. Kinesiol.* **2011**, *21*, 622–630. [CrossRef]
39. von Elm, E.; Altman, D.G.; Egger, M.; Pocock, S.J.; Gøtzsche, P.C.; Vandenbroucke, J.P. The Strengthening the Reporting of Observational Studies in Epidemiology (STROBE) Statement: Guidelines for Reporting Observational Studies. *J. Clin. Epidemiol.* **2008**, *61*, 344–349. [CrossRef]

40. Forelli, F.; Mazeas, J.; Korakakis, V.; Ramtoola, H.; Vandebrouck, A.; Duffiet, P.; Ratte, L.; Kakavas, G.; Bouzekaroui Alaoui, I.; Douryang, M.; et al. Criteria-Based Decision Making for Introducing Open Kinetic Chain Exercise after-ACL Reconstruction: A Scoping Review. *Sports Med. Open* **2025**, *11*, 37. [CrossRef] [PubMed]
41. Sturgill, L.P.; Snyder-Mackler, L.; Manal, T.J.; Axe, M.J. Interrater Reliability of a Clinical Scale to Assess Knee Joint Effusion. *J. Orthop. Sports Phys. Ther.* **2009**, *39*, 845–849. [CrossRef]
42. Medeiros, D.M.; de Quadros Robaina, B.; Rigotti, V.V.W.; Baroni, B.M. Resistance Training with Linear Periodization Is Superior to the '3 × 10 Reps Protocol' after Anterior Cruciate Ligament Reconstruction: A Randomized Controlled Trial. *Phys. Ther. Sport* **2025**, *74*, 75–82. [CrossRef]
43. American College of Sports Medicine. American College of Sports Medicine Position Stand. Progression Models in Resistance Training for Healthy Adults. *Med. Sci. Sports Exerc.* **2009**, *41*, 687–708. [CrossRef]
44. Martin, R.R.L.; Cibulka, M.T.; Bolgla, L.A.; Koc, T.A.; Loudon, J.K.; Manske, R.C.; Weiss, L.; Christoforetti, J.J.; Heiderscheit, B.C. Hamstring Strain Injury in Athletes. *J. Orthop. Sports Phys. Ther.* **2022**, *52*, CPG1–CPG44. [CrossRef]
45. Högberg, J.; Piussi, R.; Simonsson, R.; Wernbom, M.; Samuelsson, K.; Thomeé, R.; Hamrin Senorski, E. The NordBord Test Reveals Persistent Knee Flexor Strength Asymmetry When Assessed Two and Five Years after ACL Reconstruction with Hamstring Tendon Autograft. *Phys. Ther. Sport* **2024**, *66*, 53–60. [CrossRef]
46. Manchado, I.; Motta, L.M.; Blanco, G.; González, J.; Garcés, G.L. Isometric Knee Muscle Strength and Patient-Reported Measures Five Years after Anterior Cruciate Ligament Reconstruction: Comparison of Single versus Dual Autograft Hamstring Tendon Harvesting. *J. Clin. Med.* **2022**, *11*, 5682. [CrossRef]
47. Harput, G.; Erkan Kilinc, H.; Ozer, H.; Baltaci, G.; Mattacola, C.G. Quadriceps and Hamstring Strength Recovery during Early Neuromuscular Rehabilitation after ACL Hamstring-Tendon Autograft Reconstruction. *J. Sport Rehabil.* **2015**, *24*, 398–404. [CrossRef] [PubMed]
48. van Melick, N.; van der Weegen, W.; van der Horst, N. Quadriceps and Hamstrings Strength Reference Values for Athletes With and Without Anterior Cruciate Ligament Reconstruction Who Play Popular Pivoting Sports, Including Soccer, Basketball, and Handball: A Scoping Review. *J. Orthop. Sports Phys. Ther.* **2022**, *52*, 142–155. [CrossRef] [PubMed]
49. Lesnak, J.; Anderson, D.; Farmer, B.; Katsavelis, D.; Grindstaff, T.L. Validity of Hand-Held Dynamometry in Measuring Quadriceps Strength and Rate of Torque Development. *Int. J. Sports Phys. Ther.* **2019**, *14*, 180–187. [CrossRef]
50. Ardern, C.L.; Webster, K.E.; Taylor, N.F.; Feller, J.A. Hamstring Strength Recovery After Hamstring Tendon Harvest for Anterior Cruciate Ligament Reconstruction: A Comparison Between Graft Types. *Arthrosc. J. Arthrosc. Relat. Surg.* **2010**, *26*, 462–469. [CrossRef] [PubMed]
51. Ardern, C.; Webster, K. Knee Flexor Strength Recovery Following Hamstring Tendon Harvest for Anterior Cruciate Ligament Reconstruction: A Systematic Review. *Orthop. Rev.* **2009**, *1*, e12. [CrossRef] [PubMed]
52. Adachi, N.; Ochi, M.; Uchio, Y.; Sakai, Y.; Kuriwaka, M.; Fujihara, A. Harvesting Hamstring Tendons for ACL Reconstruction Influences Postoperative Hamstring Muscle Performance. *Arch. Orthop. Trauma Surg.* **2003**, *123*, 460–465. [CrossRef] [PubMed]
53. Belloir, M.; Mazeas, J.; Traullé, M.; Vandebrouck, A.; Duffiet, P.; Ratte, L.; Forelli, F. Influence of the Open Kinetic Chain on the Distension of the Transplant After Anterior Cruciate Ligament Surgery with Hamstring Graft: Search for Risk Factors. *Int. J. Physiother.* **2020**, *7*. [CrossRef]
54. Moiroux-Sahraoui, A.; Forelli, F.; Mazeas, J.; Rambaud, A.J.; Bjerregaard, A.; Riera, J. Quadriceps Activation After Anterior Cruciate Ligament Reconstruction: The Early Bird Gets the Worm! *Int. J. Sports Phys. Ther.* **2024**, *19*, 1044. [CrossRef]
55. Moiroux-Sahraoui, A.; Mazeas, J.; Gold, M.; Kakavas, G.; Forelli, F. Neuromuscular Control Deficits After Anterior Cruciate Ligament Reconstruction: A Pilot Study Using Single-Leg Functional Tests and Electromyography. *J. Funct. Morphol. Kinesiol.* **2025**, *10*, 98. [CrossRef]
56. Forelli, F.; Moiroux-Sahraoui, A.; Mazeas, J.; Dugernier, J.; Cerrito, A. Rethinking the Assessment of Arthrogenic Muscle Inhibition After ACL Reconstruction: Implications for Return-to-Sport Decision-Making—A Narrative Review. *J. Clin. Med.* **2025**, *14*, 2633. [CrossRef] [PubMed]
57. Sonnery-Cottet, B.; Hopper, G.P.; Gousopoulos, L.; Vieira, T.D.; Thaunat, M.; Fayard, J.M.; Freychet, B.; Ouanezar, H.; Cavaignac, E.; Saithna, A. Arthrogenic Muscle Inhibition Following Knee Injury or Surgery: Pathophysiology, Classification, and Treatment. *Video J. Sports Med.* **2022**, *2*. [CrossRef]

Journal of
Clinical Medicine

MDPI

Review

Biologic Augmentation in Anterior Cruciate Ligament Reconstruction and Beyond: A Review of PRP and BMAC

Grant M. Pham

Regenerative Medicine, Arlington Regenerative Medicine Institute, Arlington, TX 76013, USA;
grantmpham@gmail.com

Abstract

This narrative review synthesizes PubMed- and Scopus-indexed studies from 2020 to 2025, including preclinical animal models, prospective cohort studies, and level I and II randomized trials, to compare two leading biologic augmentation strategies: platelet-rich plasma (PRP) and bone marrow aspirate concentrate (BMAC). The review examines underlying mechanisms of action, delivery techniques, imaging biomarkers of graft maturation, patient-reported and functional outcomes, safety profiles, cost-effectiveness, and regulatory frameworks. PRP provides early anti-inflammatory and proangiogenic signaling, while BMAC delivers a concentrated population of mesenchymal stem cells and growth factors to the tendon–bone interface. Both modalities consistently enhance MRI-defined graft maturation, yet evidence of long-term functional or biomechanical superiority remains inconclusive. Emerging therapies such as peptide hydrogels, adipose-derived stem cells, and exosome delivery offer promising avenues for future research. Standardized protocols and large multicenter trials are needed to clarify comparative efficacy and inform personalized rehabilitation strategies.

Keywords: anterior cruciate ligament reconstruction; platelet-rich plasma; platelet-rich fibrin; bone marrow aspirate concentrate; biologic augmentation; regenerative sports medicine

1. Introduction

Introduction and Background

Anterior cruciate ligament (ACL) injuries represent a major orthopedic and public health challenge, particularly among athletes. Annually, over 200,000 ACL injuries are diagnosed in the United States, resulting in a significant number of surgical reconstructions, many of which occur in individuals aged 15 to 35 [1,2]. The ramifications of these injuries extend beyond mechanical instability, often affecting athletic careers, daily mobility, and long-term joint health. Anterior cruciate ligament injury is also a known risk factor for post-traumatic osteoarthritis, especially when combined with meniscal or cartilage damage [3]. Thus, successful ACL reconstruction is essential for restoring joint kinematics and preventing degenerative changes.

Over the past two decades, surgical advancements such as anatomical tunnel placement using anteromedial and all-inside approaches, improved graft fixation technologies including cortical suspensory systems and interference screws, and the adoption of minimally invasive arthroscopic techniques have substantially enhanced the precision and reproducibility of ACL reconstruction [4]. However, achieving consistent biological integration of the graft remains a clinical challenge [2]. Issues at the tendon-to-bone interface, including inadequate fibrocartilage formation, excessive inflammation, and graft motion, continue to hinder the formation of a robust, native-like enthesis [5]. The restoration of the native enthesis, or tendon-to-bone interface, is vital for long-term graft survival. Healing at this interface is slow and often incomplete, limiting early functional recovery and increasing re-rupture rates in young, active populations.

The biologic remodeling of the tendon graft after ACL reconstruction proceeds through distinct stages, initial necrosis and inflammation, followed by vascular invasion, cellular repopulation, and extracellular matrix reorganization, culminating in graft maturation or ligamentization. Despite this orchestrated sequence, the process often remains incomplete, and the healed graft rarely matches the structural and mechanical profile of the native ACL [5–7]. Factors such as patient age, comorbidities, smoking status, and timing of surgery can further complicate biologic healing. Therefore, strategies that accelerate and improve graft incorporation have become a focus of modern regenerative and orthopedic medicine.

Biologic augmentation aims to enhance the local healing environment using autologous or engineered biologics to support graft integration. Platelet-rich plasma (PRP) and bone marrow aspirate concentrate (BMAC) are among the most studied in this field [8]. Platelet-rich plasma offers a concentrated source of growth factors, including vascular endothelial growth factor (VEGF) and transforming growth factor beta 1 (TGF-β1), that stimulate angiogenesis and tissue repair [9]. Bone marrow aspirate concentrate provides a heterogeneous mix of cells, including mesenchymal stem cells (MSCs), capable of differentiating into ligamentous tissue and modulating inflammation. Emerging preclinical evidence suggests that these biologics may reduce tunnel widening, promote fibrocartilage formation, and increase mechanical strength at the graft interface [10].

Foundational reviews have consolidated the mechanistic rationale for biologic therapies. Andriolo et al. (2020) and Dulic et al. (2025) underscored the potential for PRP and MSCs to influence healing outcomes, while Rodríguez-Merchán (2021) critically evaluated clinical evidence and called for standardized methodologies [11–13]. In parallel, novel delivery platforms, including bioresorbable scaffolds, growth factor-binding peptides, and hydrogel matrices, have been developed to prolong the residence time of biologics and optimize their spatial distribution at the tendon–bone junction.

Recent interest has also turned to combining biologics with rehabilitation protocols to synchronize mechanical loading with peak biologic activity. For example, early neuromuscular stimulation may enhance cell migration and improve matrix alignment in biologically augmented grafts. Imaging tools such as quantitative MRI and ultrasound elastography are also being explored to monitor biologic activity and guide return-to-sport decisions. Collectively, these approaches reflect a shift toward personalized ACL reconstruction that integrates surgical, biologic, and rehabilitative strategies. Therefore, the aim of this review is to synthesize current evidence on biologic augmentation strategies for ACL reconstruction, with a specific focus on their role in enhancing graft healing and integration at the critical tendon–bone interface. It will evaluate the mechanistic rationale, preclinical findings, and clinical outcomes of prominent biologics such as PRP and BMAC. Furthermore, this review will explore emerging trends, including novel delivery systems and the integration of biologic therapies with personalized rehabilitation protocols, to provide a comprehensive overview of the present and future of biologics in optimizing ACL reconstruction outcomes.

2. Methods

This review synthesizes data from 2020 to 2025 drawn from studies indexed in PubMed and Scopus, including preclinical animal models, prospective cohort studies, and randomized controlled trials at levels I and II, to compare platelet-rich plasma (PRP) and bone marrow aspirate concentrate (BMAC) in ACL reconstruction. A search of both databases identified records from January 2020 through July 2025; titles and abstracts were screened, and full texts were reviewed by the author. The exact combinations used were (anterior cruciate ligament OR ACL) AND (reconstruct* OR repair*) AND (platelet-rich plasma OR PRP OR platelet-rich fibrin OR PRF); (anterior cruciate ligament OR ACL) AND (reconstruct* OR repair*) AND (bone marrow aspirate concentrate OR BMAC OR bone marrow aspirate); (anterior cruciate ligament OR ACL) AND (reconstruct* OR repair*) AND (mesenchymal stem cell* OR mesenchymal stromal cell* OR MSC); and (anterior cruciate ligament OR ACL) AND (reconstruct* OR repair*) AND (biologic augmentation OR biological augmentation). The review explicitly lists preclinical studies, randomized trials, prospective and retrospective cohorts, meta-analyses, and prior reviews, with priority given to level I and II clinical evidence where available. It then focuses on mechanisms of action, delivery strategies, clinical outcomes, imaging markers, and synchronization with rehabilitation protocols, and evaluates safety, cost-effectiveness, and regulatory considerations while highlighting key gaps and future directions in regenerative sports medicine.

3. Discussion

3.1. Biologic Mechanisms of PRP and BMAC

Platelet-rich plasma (PRP) and its scaffold-forming derivative platelet-rich fibrin (PRF) are prepared from autologous whole blood using centrifugation protocols that isolate the platelet-rich component [14]. These platelets harbor a reservoir of bioactive molecules, including platelet-derived growth factor (PDGF), TGF-β, VEGF, insulin-like growth factor 1 (IGF-1), epidermal growth factor (EGF), and fibroblast growth factor (FGF), each of which plays a role in modulating inflammation, angiogenesis, and extracellular matrix (ECM) synthesis [15]. Upon activation, either through calcium chloride or mechanical stress, these platelets release their growth factors, initiating a cascade that promotes cellular chemotaxis and matrix deposition.

In ACL reconstruction, PRP can be applied by soaking grafts, injecting into bone tunnels, or layering around the graft–tunnel interface [16]. Platelet-rich fibrin forms a three-dimensional fibrin network that functions as a slow-release system, prolonging growth factor bioavailability and acting as a scaffold for progenitor cells [17]. The resulting biologic environment is enriched for regenerative signaling, though the magnitude and duration of these effects depend heavily on PRP formulation, particularly whether leukocytes are included. Leukocyte-rich PRP contains higher levels of white blood cells and pro-inflammatory cytokines, while leukocyte-poor PRP has minimal leukocyte content and promotes anti-inflammatory and anabolic responses. Other critical variables include platelet concentration and timing of delivery. Numerous analyses since 2020 have demonstrated that leukocyte-poor PRP yields less inflammation, reduces catabolic cytokine release, and better supports tissue healing than leukocyte-rich PRP [18].

Preclinical animal models support these findings. In rabbit ACL reconstruction models, PRP and PRF-treated grafts exhibited higher vascular density and collagen fiber organization at postoperative follow-up [19,20]. Canine studies have shown improved pull-out strength and histologic evidence of early fibrocartilage formation in PRP-augmented tunnels [21]. However, some studies have reported minimal differences in mechanical properties at longer follow-ups, highlighting the need for sustained biologic stimuli or combination therapies [22].

Bone marrow aspirate concentrate (BMAC) contains MSCs, endothelial progenitor cells, mononuclear cells, and a broad spectrum of cytokines [23]. Unlike PRP, BMAC provides both a cellular and humoral component, potentially offering a more sustained regenerative effect [10]. MSCs contribute to healing by differentiating into ligamentous fibroblasts and by secreting exosomes and paracrine factors that reduce inflammation and encourage ECM remodeling. Several mechanistic pathways have been proposed to explain BMAC's effects [23]. Stromal cell-derived factor 1 (SDF-1), secreted by local tissues, may attract circulating MSCs to the graft site, where they participate in tissue remodeling. Growth factors like basic fibroblast growth factor (bFGF) and hepatocyte growth factor (HGF) enhance angiogenesis and promote fibroblast proliferation. In vivo, BMAC-treated ACL grafts demonstrate increased mineralized tissue at the bone–tendon junction, reduced tunnel widening, and improved biomechanical properties. Optimization of BMAC preparation is critical. Studies have shown that factors such as volume of aspirate, centrifugation speed, and anticoagulant use influence cell viability and growth factor concentration. Moreover, combining BMAC with bioresorbable scaffolds or hydrogels has been shown to improve cell retention and distribution, enhancing its efficacy [23]. Newer approaches involve pre-conditioning BMAC with hypoxic environments or mechanical stimulation to prime cells before implantation.

3.2. Clinical Applications & Delivery Techniques

Clinically, PRP and PRF are widely utilized during ACL reconstruction for their regenerative potential [24]. Platelet-rich plasma is typically administered intraoperatively by soaking graft materials or injecting directly into femoral and tibial bone tunnels, with the aim of enhancing the biologic environment and supporting early-phase healing. Platelet-rich fibrin, by contrast, is prepared as a gel or membrane that can be applied around grafts or within tunnels, offering a dual role as both a biologic reservoir and a structural scaffold [25]. A randomized study by Anz et al. (2025) showed preoperative PRP injections in patients with acute ACL tears significantly reduced synovial inflammation and chondrodegenerative biomarkers, suggesting a protective intra-articular effect prior to reconstruction [9]. Postoperatively, adjunctive intra-articular injections of PRP are sometimes used at regular one-month intervals to sustain the healing cascade, particularly in the early phases of ligamentization [22,24]. Such practices are more common in high-performance athletes or in patients with slower initial recovery [14].

The methods used to prepare PRP and PRF, such as the choice of centrifugation speed, platelet concentration targets, and inclusion or exclusion of leukocytes, significantly impact the final product's composition and bioactivity [25]. Leukocyte-rich PRP may provoke a stronger inflammatory response, which could be beneficial or detrimental depending on timing and delivery site. Double-spin centrifugation typically produces higher concentrations of platelets but may reduce growth factor diversity (Table 1). Platelet-rich fibrin, with its fibrin mesh, offers slow-release kinetics and provides a more durable carrier for cellular and molecular components [17,25].

Table 1. A summary comparing the composition, mechanism of action, key benefits, and inherent limitations of PRP and BMAC to inform decision-making.

Biological Augmentation	Platelet-Rich Plasma (PRP)	Bone Marrow Aspirate Concentrate (BMAC)
Core Composition	Concentrate of autologous platelets, growth factors, and fibrinogen.	Heterogeneous concentrate of autologous cells including mesenchymal stem cells (MSCs), hematopoietic stem cells, platelets, and growth factors.
Primary Mechanism of Action	Delivery of a supraphysiologic dose of growth factors (e.g., VEGF, TGF-β, PDGF) to stimulate and accelerate native healing processes like angiogenesis, cell proliferation, and collagen synthesis.	Provides a cellular scaffold with osteogenic and chondrogenic potential. Stem cells can differentiate into target tissues, modulate the immune response, and secrete paracrine factors to orchestrate regeneration.

Table 1. *Cont.*

Biological Augmentation	Platelet-Rich Plasma (PRP)	Bone Marrow Aspirate Concentrate (BMAC)
Key Advantages	- Minimally invasive harvest (peripheral venipuncture). - Relatively low cost and quick preparation. - Excellent safety profile with minimal risk of immunogenic reaction. - Wide availability and extensive clinical experience. - Significant heterogeneity in preparation systems (leukocyte-rich vs. poor, single vs. double spin).	- Contains progenitor cells with true regenerative potential. - Higher concentration of MSCs and other nucleated cells. - Potentially more potent effect on bone tunnel healing and enthesis formation. - May have a stronger anti-inflammatory and immunomodulatory effect.
Key Limitations/Challenges	- Significant heterogeneity in preparation systems (leukocyte-rich vs. poor, single vs. double spin). - Growth factor concentration and release kinetics are short-lived. - Limited evidence for structural improvement in high-quality human trials.	- Invasive and painful harvest from the iliac crest. - Higher cost and more complex preparation requiring specialized kits. - Variable MSC yield depending on patient age, comorbidities, and technique.

Bone marrow aspirate concentrate (BMAC) is harvested intraoperatively, most often from the posterior or anterior iliac crest, and concentrated using centrifugation to isolate a nucleated cell-rich fraction. It is typically injected into the bone tunnels or applied directly to graft surfaces before fixation. In some advanced protocols, BMAC is incorporated with scaffolds such as collagen membranes or demineralized bone matrix to enhance retention and prolong cellular viability. The delivery strategy of BMAC often depends on the surgical technique and graft type. For example, in all-inside techniques using suspensory fixation, BMAC may be injected retrograde into the tunnel following graft insertion. In full tibial tunnel approaches, it can be combined with bone chips or soaked into the graft construct prior to passage. Emerging technologies like intraosseous injection systems and scaffold-assisted delivery platforms aim to improve spatial localization and integration of biologics [26]. Moreover, in select cases of partial ACL tears or chronic laxity where surgery is deferred, ultrasound-guided BMAC or PRP injections have been used as part of non-operative biologic management strategies. Early reports suggest these approaches may offer symptom relief and imaging-based evidence of healing, though randomized controlled trials are needed to substantiate efficacy [27].

Standardization of biologic delivery remains a key challenge. Variability in concentration, preparation technique, timing of application, and host factors all influence treatment response. Future directions may include point-of-care cell characterization, real-time biologic activity assays, and integration with personalized rehabilitation timelines to tailor delivery for maximal impact.

Taken together, PRP and BMAC represent complementary strategies for biologic augmentation. PRP acts quickly, providing a burst of growth factors during the early healing phase, while BMAC offers a more durable cellular response. PRP can transiently increase PDGF, TGF-β, VEGF, and downshift inflammatory markers [9]. Understanding how these agents influence the molecular and mechanical milieu of ACL grafts will be essential for developing next-generation biologic therapies, as depicted in Table 1. Further studies are needed to compare their efficacy directly, identify optimal dosing and delivery schedules, and assess their synergy with evolving rehabilitation paradigms.

3.3. Clinical Evidence and Comparative Outcomes

A meta-analysis by Lv et al. (2021) of 17 randomized controlled trials including 970 ACL reconstruction patients found that PRP significantly reduced early postoperative pain (mean VAS decrease of ~1.1 points) and improved short to mid-term IKDC and Lysholm scores, though long-term functional significance remained limited [28]. These findings highlight the potential value of PRP in facilitating early recovery and symptomatic relief. However, these benefits were not sustained at 12 months, and PRP did not improve tunnel widening or objective knee stability. Functional outcomes, such as return-to-sport readiness and re-injury rates, showed no significant difference compared to control groups in long-term follow-up. These results suggest that while PRP may support early-phase biological remodeling, its utility in driving long-term clinical success remains limited (Table 1). Additionally, the heterogeneity in PRP formulations, preparation techniques, and application timing further complicates the interpretation of existing data [29,30]. Compounding this, Kasl et al. (2022) evaluated Vivostat™, a platelet-rich fibrin prepared intraoperatively from autologous venous blood in a closed system (centrifugation and controlled polymerization yielding a sprayable fibrin matrix) [31]. The PRF was applied to the graft and tunnel apertures during ACLR. They found no significant differences in MRI ligamentization or patient-reported outcomes at 6 and 12 months versus controls, and recommended larger trials focused on the immediate postoperative window, where short-lived effects might be detected. In contrast, Milovanovic et al. (2024) used the same Vivostat PRF technique during bone patellar tendon–bone ACL reconstruction, with additional application to the patellar and tibial donor sites [32]. They reported reduced kneeling pain and faster narrowing of harvest site bone defects at 8 and 12 months, but no statistically significant differences immediately after surgery or at 4 months. Together, these studies suggest any PRF benefit may be time dependent and more evident in later structural remodeling than in early postoperative imaging or symptoms.

Bone marrow aspirate concentrate (BMAC) has shown promise in enhancing biological graft incorporation. Several small-scale trials and prospective studies have reported improved MRI-based parameters, including lower signal intensity and increased synovial coverage of the graft [33]. Enhanced bone tunnel integration and reduced tunnel widening were also noted in patients receiving BMAC augmentation. One particular study by Jordan et al. (2025) involving the application of BMAC with a collagen matrix in allograft ACL reconstruction demonstrated appeared safe and yielded favorable clinical outcomes at two-year follow-up [23]. Moreover, there is some emerging evidence that BMAC may influence the timeline for graft maturation, potentially enabling earlier initiation of dynamic rehabilitation [33]. Nonetheless, the magnitude of clinical improvement remains modest, and studies vary significantly in methodological quality.

Importantly, direct head-to-head comparisons between PRP and BMAC remain rare [29]. Existing trials often differ in inclusion criteria, graft type, outcome measures, and follow-up duration, making it difficult to draw definitive conclusions regarding superiority. Only a few comparative analyses have attempted to evaluate PRP versus BMAC within the same clinical protocol. These studies tend to suggest that BMAC may confer greater benefits in terms of imaging and tunnel morphology, whereas PRP provides more pronounced short-term symptomatic improvement [30]. There is currently insufficient evidence to determine whether one biologic is clearly superior across all outcome domains.

Moving forward, more robust randomized controlled trials are needed to clarify the comparative efficacy of these interventions. Ideally, future studies should employ standardized biologic preparation methods, consistent imaging modalities, and validated functional scoring systems. In addition, the integration of biomechanical testing, molecular biomarkers, and long-term outcome tracking will be critical to fully elucidate the therapeutic value of biologic augmentation in ACL reconstruction. Until such data are available, clinicians must continue to individualize biologic strategies based on patient-specific factors, graft selection, and surgical technique.

3.4. Safety, Cost, and Regulatory Issues

Platelet-rich plasma (PRP) enjoys a favorable safety profile and is generally well-tolerated by patients (Table 1). Minor adverse effects reported include localized swelling, mild discomfort at the injection site, or transient joint pain, all of which are typically self-limiting [34]. Due to its autologous nature, the risk of immunogenic reactions or transmission of infectious agents is negligible. The preparation and administration are straightforward, often performed in an outpatient setting, making it a viable option across a broad patient population [35]. Financially, PRP is relatively inexpensive, with single treatments costing between $300 and $700 depending on preparation protocols and clinical setting [30]. These costs are generally out-of-pocket expenses, as PRP is not consistently covered by insurance.

Conversely, BMAC involves additional procedural complexity and cost (Table 1). Harvesting BMAC requires an invasive aspiration procedure, most commonly from the iliac crest, which can result in donor site pain, hematoma, or, in rare cases, infection [36]. The need for sterile technique, surgical expertise, and specialized equipment makes BMAC significantly more expensive, ranging from $1500 to $2700 per treatment [36]. Despite these challenges, BMAC offers a cellular component that may provide sustained regenerative support, particularly in biologically compromised or revision ACL cases. While PRP and intraoperative BMAC are typically regulated under the U.S. Food and Drug Administration (FDA)'s 361 Human Cells, Tissues, and Cellular and Tissue-Based Products (HCT/P) designation as minimally manipulated autologous biologics, expanded or engineered MSCs fall under the stricter 351 pathway, which requires premarket approval through a Biologics License Application (BLA) due to their classification as more than minimally manipulated products [37].

A 2023 Markov decision analysis evaluated three strategies for isolated meniscal repair biologically analogous to ACL reconstruction, namely PRP augmentation, marrow venting procedure (MVP), and repair without biologic adjuncts. It found that both PRP and MVP yielded more quality-adjusted life years (QALYs) compared to standard repair. However, PRP came at a significantly higher cost, with an incremental cost-effectiveness ratio (ICER) of $161,742 per QALY, far above the standard $50,000 willingness-to-pay threshold. In contrast, the MVP approach produced similar QALY gains at a substantially lower cost, making it the more economically viable option [38].

Beyond direct costs, indirect factors such as faster return to work or reduced need for revision surgeries may further influence the economic appeal of biologic therapies. However, the literature remains limited in long-term cost–benefit analyses, particularly for BMAC [10]. Additionally, reimbursement policies vary widely, with most payers regarding these interventions as experimental. As biologic augmentation grows more common, health policies must adapt to address clinical evidence, real-world effectiveness, and equitable access. Ultimately, economic feasibility will determine how widely these therapies are adopted for routine ACLR.

3.5. Practical Implications and Rehabilitation Integration

Biologic augmentation techniques hold the potential to significantly influence rehabilitation timelines by enhancing graft healing and maturation. Improved MRI-defined graft signal intensity following biologic interventions, such as PRP or BMAC, has been correlated with tissue revascularization, collagen remodeling, and more organized ligamentization [39]. These biological improvements may enable clinicians to consider earlier initiation of progressive loading, weight-bearing protocols, and neuromuscular re-education. Such early mobilization strategies have been shown in general ACL rehabilitation literature to promote proprioceptive recovery and improve long-term function. Beyzadeoglu et al. (2020) conducted a cohort MRI study and found that applying PRF during ACL reconstruction was associated with improved graft maturation scores, suggesting a positive effect on early healing [17]. However, evidence directly linking biologically enhanced MRI outcomes to clinically validated return-to-sport (RTS) acceleration remains limited. Most studies to date use surrogate endpoints, such as graft signal intensity or patient-reported knee scores, rather than objective RTS metrics. Furthermore, differences in imaging protocols, interpretation criteria, and biologic product standardization complicate attempts to define universal RTS readiness thresholds based on imaging alone [39,40].

Despite these limitations, interest in biologic-enhanced rehabilitation continues to grow, particularly among high-performance athletes and motivated patients. These individuals are often eager to shorten recovery timeframes and reduce their risk of graft failure or contralateral injury, both of which are elevated during the vulnerable post-reconstruction period. Some centers have adopted integrated care models where MRI findings post-biologic augmentation are discussed collaboratively between radiologists, surgeons, sports physicians, and physical therapists to tailor rehabilitation progression [41]. Thus, a multidisciplinary team delivers care through a clinician-led, shared decision-making model. The medical lead (surgeon or sports physician) oversees surgical readiness and safety, while the rehabilitation lead (physical therapist) directs daily progress and testing. The extended team may include athletic training, strength coaching, and specialist support. Governance is clear: both leads must agree on advancement to high-level activities like running once the criteria are met. The return-to-sport decision is a consensus.

The integration of biologics into ACL reconstruction and rehabilitation introduces critical considerations around patient selection, response monitoring, and cost–benefit balance. Studies like Spierings et al. (2025) have demonstrated significant individual variability in graft-derived cytokine profiles, independent of age, suggesting the existence of biologic 'responders' who might benefit most from augmentation [42,43]. Similarly, reviews have highlighted how excessive inflammation and uneven tendon-to-bone healing can impair outcomes, reinforcing the rationale for stratifying patients based on inflammatory or regenerative markers to personalize therapy [5]. Additionally, as wearable technologies and digital health platforms advance, it may become possible to correlate biologic-enhanced healing markers with kinetic and kinematic movement patterns during rehabilitation [44]. Ultimately, a successful biologic-enhanced rehabilitation model will require multidisciplinary collaboration, real-time outcome feedback, and rigorous clinical validation to transition from a conceptual promise to the standard of care.

4. Conclusions

Future Directions and Research Gaps

Recent preclinical investigations have revealed a wide array of innovative biologic strategies aimed at improving tendon-to-bone healing in ACL reconstruction. Among these, peptide-based approaches, gene therapies, and exosome-enriched biologics are gaining traction due to their scalability and translational potential [8,45]. For example, in a murine ACL reconstruction model, a self-assembling KI24RGDS peptide hydrogel significantly improved zonal tendon-to-bone attachment, fibrocartilage formation, and early mechanical fixation strength [46]. This hydrogel mimics the extracellular matrix and supports endogenous cell recruitment and matrix deposition. Preclinical studies suggest that tissue-engineered ACL grafts enhanced with MSC affinity components can significantly improve tendon-to-bone integration. Building on this concept, Tang et al. (2021) developed a biomimetic biphasic electrospun scaffold in a rat ACL model, which supported MSC-based fibroblast differentiation in vitro and promoted ligament regeneration and joint stability in vivo, highlighting its potential to enhance tendon-to-bone healing [47]. Similarly, nanofiber-reinforced 3D acellular tendon scaffolds incorporating MSC-binding peptide motifs demonstrated enhanced tendon–bone attachment and structural regeneration in large animal models, as shown by Yu et al. (2024) [48].

Along with these peptide-based advances, adipose-derived stem cells (ADSCs) have also emerged as a compelling biologic adjunct for ACL repair [49,50]. In a rabbit ACL reconstruction model, Matsumoto et al. (2021) demonstrated that ADSC sheet application nearly doubled early graft failure load (~17 N → ~37 N at 2 weeks and ~29 N → ~47 N at 4 weeks), enhanced collagen fiber diameter and organization, and limited bone tunnel widening, despite diminishing differences beyond 8 weeks, suggesting an early mechanobiologic advantage of this technique [50]. However, these were animal models. Future studies must evaluate safety, optimal dosing, delivery vehicles such as cell sheets, extracellular vesicles, or scaffolds, and comparative efficacy versus existing biologics in human trials [51].

Recent preclinical work has also evaluated a variety of cell-free peptide-based strategies that offer innovative alternatives to conventional cell-based therapies. Additionally, tissue-engineered grafts incorporating MSC-affinity peptides have shown improved integration and biomechanical performance in large animal studies. These developments suggest that short, synthetic peptides could offer scalable, off-the-shelf biologic options that eliminate the need for cell harvesting or specialized processing.

Beyond peptides, other innovative strategies under investigation include gene therapy vectors, exosome-based therapies, and smart biomaterials that release growth factors in a temporally controlled fashion. Gene editing tools, such as CRISPR-Cas9, are being explored to locally upregulate anabolic signaling pathways, potentially enhancing ligament regeneration at the molecular level [52]. Similarly, exosomes derived from MSCs and other progenitor cells are under investigation for their ability to deliver signaling molecules such as microRNAs, growth factors, and cytokines that enhance angiogenesis, regulate macrophage polarization, and remodel extracellular matrix at the tendon–bone interface [53]. Although these technologies remain largely experimental, they represent potential directions for biologic augmentation in ACL repair.

The future of ACL biologic augmentation will also benefit from advances in biomaterials science. For example, biodegradable scaffolds loaded with peptide sequences or growth factors are being designed to mimic the native enthesis and to guide zonal tissue regeneration. Hybrid constructs combining multiple strategies such as scaffold + PRP + exosome or scaffold + BMAC + peptide are also being tested to optimize the healing microenvironment [8,26]. These combinatory approaches may hold the key to overcoming the limitations of single-modality therapies. A randomized control, double blind study involving PRP + BMAC in ACL reconstruction by Lin et al. (2024) showed improved tendon-femoral bone interface and increased laxity compared to the control (nonaugmented) group [54].

Before these promising therapies can be widely adopted, key challenges must be addressed. Their efficacy is so far limited to animal studies, and moving to human clinical use means carefully assessing dosage, delivery techniques, and long-term biocompatibility.

Ultimately, human trials for these peptide-based and hybrid solutions are needed to prove their safety and effectiveness. Furthermore, large-scale trials that directly compare PRP and BMAC using standardized methods are essential to determine which is more effective [22].

Moving forward, the integration of imaging biomarkers, functional outcome metrics, and personalized rehabilitation protocols will be vital for tailoring biologic treatments to individual patient profiles. Advances in MRI, such as UTE-T2* and T2* relaxation mapping and ultrasound elastography, now enable real-time, quantitative monitoring of graft maturation and biomechanical properties, potentially transforming how we assess biologic activity and guide safe return-to-sport timelines [55]. Combined with machine learning and wearable sensor data, these tools could facilitate precision medicine approaches in sports orthopedics [56]. Ultimately, the success of biologic ACL augmentation will depend on multidisciplinary collaboration, rigorous trial design, and the development of standardized clinical guidelines informed by both basic science and clinical evidence.

Funding: This research received no external funding.

Institutional Review Board Statement: Not applicable.

Informed Consent Statement: Not applicable.

Data Availability Statement: No new data were created or analyzed in this study.

Conflicts of Interest: The author declares no conflicts of interest.

Abbreviations

The following abbreviations are used in this manuscript:

ACL	Anterior Cruciate Ligament
PRP	Platelet-Rich Plasma
PRF	Platelet-Rich Fibrin
BMAC	Bone Marrow Aspirate Concentrate
MSC	Mesenchymal Stem Cell
EVs	Extracellular Vesicles
ADSCs	Adipose-Derived Stem Cells
ADRCs	Adipose-Derived Regenerative Cells
MRI	Magnetic Resonance Imaging
US	Ultrasound
UTE-T2*	Ultrashort Echo Time T2-star (advanced MRI mapping sequence)
T2*	T2-star relaxation time (MRI parameter sensitive to tissue microstructure and field inhomogeneity)
CRISPR-Cas9	Clustered Regularly Interspaced Short Palindromic Repeats/CRISPR-associated protein 9 (gene editing tool)
RCT	Randomized Controlled Trial
IKDC	International Knee Documentation Committee score
KOOS	Knee Injury and Osteoarthritis Outcome Score
Lysholm	Lysholm Knee Scoring Scale
PROs	Patient Reported Outcomes
DBM	Demineralized Bone Matrix
LP-PRP	Leukocyte-Poor Platelet Rich Plasma
LR-PRP	Leukocyte-Rich Platelet Rich Plasma
BLA	Biologics License Application
FDA	U.S. Food and Drug Administration
HCT/P	Human Cells, Tissues, and Cellular and Tissue-Based Products
VEGF	Vascular Endothelial Growth Factor
PDGF	Platelet-Derived Growth Factor
TGF-β	Transforming Growth Factor Beta

IL-1β	Interleukin-1 Beta
TNF-α	Tumor Necrosis Factor Alpha
MMPs	Matrix Metalloproteinases
TIMP-1	Tissue Inhibitor of Metalloproteinase-1

References

1. Silvers-Granelli, H. Why Female Athletes Injure Their ACL's More Frequently? What can we do to mitigate their risk? *Int. J. Sports Phys. Ther.* **2021**, *16*, 971–977. [CrossRef]
2. Looney, A.M.; Leider, J.D.; Horn, A.R.; Bodendorfer, B.M. Bioaugmentation in the surgical treatment of anterior cruciate ligament injuries: A review of current concepts and emerging techniques. *SAGE Open Med.* **2020**, *8*, 2050312120921057. [CrossRef] [PubMed]
3. Wang, L.J.; Zeng, N.; Yan, Z.P.; Li, J.T.; Ni, G.X. Post-traumatic osteoarthritis following ACL injury. *Arthritis Res. Ther.* **2020**, *22*, 57. [CrossRef] [PubMed]
4. Bosco, F.; Rovere, G.; Giustra, F.; Masoni, V.; Cassaro, S.; Capella, M.; Risitano, S.; Sabatini, L.; Lucenti, L.; Camarda, L. Advancements in Anterior Cruciate Ligament Repair—Current State of the Art. *Surgeries* **2024**, *5*, 234–247. [CrossRef]
5. Yao, S.; Yung, P.S.H.; Lui, P.P.Y. Tackling the Challenges of Graft Healing After Anterior Cruciate Ligament Reconstruction-Thinking from the Endpoint. *Front. Bioeng. Biotechnol.* **2021**, *9*, 756930. [CrossRef]
6. Moretti, L.; Bizzoca, D.; Cassano, G.D.; Caringella, N.; Delmedico, M.; Moretti, B. Graft Intra-Articular Remodeling and Bone Incorporation in ACL Reconstruction: The State of the Art and Clinical Implications. *J. Clin. Med.* **2022**, *11*, 6704. [CrossRef]
7. Boyd, E.; Endres, N.K.; Geeslin, A.G. Postoperative healing and complications based on anterior cruciate ligament reconstruction graft type. *Ann. Jt.* **2024**, *9*, 30. [CrossRef]
8. Goulian, A.J.; Goldstein, B.; Saad, M.A. Advancements in Regenerative Therapies for Orthopedics: A Comprehensive Review of Platelet-Rich Plasma, Mesenchymal Stem Cells, Peptide Therapies, and Biomimetic Applications. *J. Clin. Med.* **2025**, *14*, 2061. [CrossRef]
9. Anz, A.W.; Branch, E.A.; Jordan, S.E.; Ostrander, R.V.; Kindle, B.J.; Presley, J.C.; Hackel, J.G.; Maggi, E.; Plummer, H.A. Preoperative Platelet-Rich Plasma Injections Decrease Inflammatory and Chondrodegenerative Biomarkers in Patients with Acute Anterior Cruciate Ligament Tears: A Pilot Randomized Controlled Trial. *Orthop. J. Sports Med.* **2025**, *13*, 23259671241312754. [CrossRef]
10. Park, J.Y.; Ng Hing Cheung, J.A.; Todorov, D.; Park, S.J.; Lim, H.; Shin, E.; Yoon, A.; Ha, J. Biological augmentation of anterior cruciate ligament reconstruction with bone marrow aspirate concentrate: A systematic review and meta-analysis of randomised controlled trials. *Int. Orthop.* **2025**, *49*, 35–43. [CrossRef]
11. Andriolo, L.; Reale, D.; Di Martino, A.; De Fillippis, R.; Sessa, A.; Zaffagnini, S.; Filarddo, G. Long-term Results of Arthroscopic Matrix-Assisted Autologous Chondrocyte Transplantation: A Prospective Follow-up at 15 Years. *Am. J. Sports Med.* **2020**, *48*, 2994–3001. [CrossRef]
12. Rodriguez-Merchan, E.C. Anterior Cruciate Ligament Reconstruction: Is Biological Augmentation Beneficial? *Int. J. Mol. Sci.* **2021**, *22*, 12566. [CrossRef]
13. Dulic, O.; Abazovic, D.; Matijevic, S.; Rasovic, P.; Obradovic, M.; Bjelobrk, M.; Tosic, M.; Lalic, I.; Baljak, B.; Milinkov, M. Quality of life changes in patients suffering from knee osteoarthritis treated with bone marrow aspirate concentrate, platelet-rich plasma and hyaluronic acid injections. *Regen. Med.* **2025**, *20*, 87–96. [CrossRef]
14. El Zouhbi, A.; Yammine, J.; Hemdanieh, M.; Korbani, E.T.; Nassereddine, M. Utility of Platelet-Rich Plasma Therapy in the Management of Meniscus Injuries: A narrative review. *Orthop. Rev.* **2024**, *16*, 94240. [CrossRef]
15. Chalidis, B.; Givissis, P.; Papadopoulos, P.; Pitsilos, C. Molecular and biologic effects of platelet-rich plasma (PRP) in ligament and tendon healing and regeneration: A systematic review. *Int. J. Mol. Sci.* **2023**, *24*, 2744. [CrossRef] [PubMed]
16. Gill, S.S.; Cenci, G.; Falcinelli, S.; Marzano, F.; Carriero, B.; Filippi, N.; Pace, V. Platelet rich plasma and anterior cruciate ligament repair: A new frontier, or a short term adjunct. *World J. Orthop.* **2025**, *16*, 100693. [CrossRef] [PubMed]
17. Beyzadeoglu, T.; Pehlivanoglu, T.; Yildirim, K.; Buldu, H.; Tandogan, R.; Tuzun, U. Does the Application of Platelet-Rich Fibrin in Anterior Cruciate Ligament Reconstruction Enhance Graft Healing and Maturation? A Comparative MRI Study of 44 Cases. *Orthop. J. Sports Med.* **2020**, *8*, 2325967120902013. [CrossRef] [PubMed]
18. Zhao, D.; Han, Y.-H.; Pan, J.-K.; Yang, W.-Y.; Zeng, L.-F.; Liang, G.-H.; Liu, J. The clinical efficacy of leukocyte-poor platelet-rich plasma in arthroscopic rotator cuff repair: A meta-analysis of randomized controlled trials. *J. Shoulder Elb. Surg.* **2021**, *30*, 918–928. [CrossRef]
19. Weng, P.W.; Chen, C.H.; Lin, Y.C.; Chen, K.-H.; Yeh, Y.-Y.; Lai, J.-M.; Chiang, C.-J.; Wong, C.-C. Platelet-Rich Fibrin-Augmented Gap-Bridging Strategy in Rabbit Anterior Cruciate Ligament Repair. *Am. J. Sports Med.* **2023**, *51*, 642–655. [CrossRef]

20. Zhang, L.; Zhang, Q.; Cui, L.; Wu, L.; Gao, S. Kartogenin Combined Platelet-Rich Plasma (PRP) Promoted Tendon-Bone Healing for Anterior Cruciate Ligament (ACL) Reconstruction by Suppressing Inflammatory Response Via targeting AKT/PI3K/NF-kappaB. *Appl. Biochem. Biotechnol.* **2023**, *195*, 1284–1296. [CrossRef]
21. Sample, S.J.; Racette, M.A.; Hans, E.C.; Volstad, N.J.; Schaefer, S.L.; Bleedorn, J.A.; Little, J.P.; Waller, K.R., III; Hao, Z.; Block, W.F.; et al. Use of a platelet-rich plasma-collagen scaffold as a bioenhanced repair treatment for management of partial cruciate ligament rupture in dogs. *PLoS ONE* **2018**, *13*, e0197204. [CrossRef]
22. Ye, Z.; Chen, H.; Qiao, Y.; Wu, C.; Cho, E.; Wu, X.; Li, Z.; Wu, J.; Lu, S.; Xie, G.; et al. Intra-Articular Platelet-Rich Plasma Injection After Anterior Cruciate Ligament Reconstruction: A Randomized Clinical Trial. *JAMA Netw. Open* **2024**, *7*, e2410134. [CrossRef]
23. Jordan, S.E.; Anz, A.W.; Ostrander, R.V.; Branch, E.A.; Denney, T.S.; Cohen, A.; Truett, J.; Andrews, J.R. Augmenting an Allograft for ACL Reconstruction with a Collagen Matrix and BMAC Injection Appears Safe and Produces Favorable Clinical Outcomes at 2-year Follow Up. *Arthrosc. Sports Med. Rehabil.* **2025**, *in press*. [CrossRef]
24. Narayanaswamy, R.; Patro, B.P.; Jeyaraman, N.; Gangadaran, P.; Rajendran, R.L.; Nallakumarasamy, A.; Jeyaraman, M.; Ramani, P.; Ahn, B.-C. Evolution and Clinical Advances of Platelet-Rich Fibrin in Musculoskeletal Regeneration. *Bioengineering* **2023**, *10*, 58. [CrossRef] [PubMed]
25. Bai, M.-Y.; Vy, V.P.T.; Tang, S.-L.; Hung, T.N.K.; Wang, C.-W.; Liang, J.-Y.; Wong, C.-C.; Chan, W.P. Current Progress of Platelet-Rich Derivatives in Cartilage and Joint Repairs. *Int. J. Mol. Sci.* **2023**, *24*, 12608. [CrossRef] [PubMed]
26. Yang, C.; Teng, Y.; Geng, B.; Xiao, H.; Chen, C.; Chen, R.; Yang, F.; Xia, Y. Strategies for promoting tendon-bone healing: Current status and prospects. Review. *Front. Bioeng. Biotechnol.* **2023**, *11*, 1118468. [CrossRef] [PubMed]
27. Wasilczyk, C. Nanosurgical and Bioengineering Treatment of Human Anterior Cruciate Ligament Tears with Ultrasound-Guided Injection of Modified Platelet-Rich Plasma Using Human Cell Memory Based on Clinical, Ultrasound, MRI, and Nanoscope Analyses: A Double-Blind Randomized Trial. *J. Clin. Med.* **2024**, *13*, 2475. [CrossRef]
28. Lv, Z.-t.; Zhang, J.-M.; Pang, Z.-Y.; Wang, Z.; Huang, J.-M.; Zhu, W.-T. The efficacy of platelet rich plasma on anterior cruciate ligament reconstruction: A systematic review and meta-analysis. *Platelets* **2021**, *33*, 229–241. [CrossRef]
29. Zhang, Z.; Liu, P.; Xue, X.; Zhang, Z.; Wang, L.; Jiang, Y.; Zhang, C.; Zhou, H.; Lv, S.; Shen, W.; et al. The role of platelet-rich plasma in biomedicine: A comprehensive overview. *iScience* **2025**, *28*, 111705. [CrossRef]
30. Zhu, T.; Zhou, J.; Hwang, J.; Xu, X. Effects of Platelet-Rich Plasma on Clinical Outcomes After Anterior Cruciate Ligament Reconstruction: A Systematic Review and Meta-analysis. *Orthop. J. Sports Med.* **2022**, *10*, 23259671211061535. [CrossRef]
31. Kasl, J.; Zeman, P.; Pavelka, T.; Cibulková, J.; Pilný, J.; Matějka, J. Clinical Outcomes of the Application of Platelet-Rich Fibrin during Anatomic Anterior Cruciate Ligament Reconstruction: Results of Prospective Randomised Study. *Acta Chir. Orthop. Traumatol. Cechoslov.* **2022**, *89*, 279–285. [CrossRef] [PubMed]
32. Milovanovic, D.; Vukman, P.; Gavrilovic, D.; Begovic, N.; Stijak, L.; Sreckovic, S.; Kadija, M. The Influence of Platelet-Rich Fibrin on the Healing of Bone Defects after Harvesting Bone-Patellar Tendon-Bone Grafts. *Medicina* **2024**, *60*, 154. [CrossRef] [PubMed]
33. Forsythe, B.; Chahla, J.; Korrapati, A.; Lavoie-Gagne, O.; Forlenza, E.; Diaz, C.C.; Beletsky, A.; Chung, C.B.; Bae, W.C.; Bach, B.R.; et al. Bone Marrow Aspirate Concentrate Augmentation May Accelerate Allograft Ligamentization in Anterior Cruciate Ligament Reconstruction: A Double-Blinded Randomized Controlled Trial. *Arthroscopy* **2022**, *38*, 2255–2264. [CrossRef] [PubMed]
34. Glinkowski, W.M.; Gut, G.; Śladowski, D. Platelet-Rich Plasma for Knee Osteoarthritis: A Comprehensive Narrative Review of the Mechanisms, Preparation Protocols, and Clinical Evidence. *J. Clin. Med.* **2025**, *14*, 3983. [CrossRef] [PubMed]
35. Utrilla, G.S.; Degano, I.R.; D'Ambrosi, R. Efficacy of platelet-rich plasma in meniscal repair surgery: A systematic review of randomized controlled trials. *J. Orthop. Traumatol.* **2024**, *25*, 63. [CrossRef]
36. Lavender, C.D.; Schaver, A.L.; Taylor, S.; Peluso, R.; Berdis, G.; Singh, V.; Cipriani, K.; Lycans, D.; Jasko, J.; Hewett, T.E. Anterior Cruciate Ligament Reconstruction Augmentation With Bone Marrow Aspirate Concentrate, Demineralized Bone Matrix, and Suture Tape Shows No Difference in Outcomes-But Faster Functional Recovery-Versus Non-augmented Anterior Cruciate Ligament Reconstruction. *Arthroscopy.* **2025**, *41*, 1496–1508. [CrossRef]
37. U.S. Department of Health and Human Services. *Regulatory Considerations for Human Cells, Tissues, and Cellular and Tissue-Based Products: Minimal Manipulation and Homologous Use;* U.S. Department of Health and Human Services: Washington, DC, USA, 2020.
38. Oeding, J.F.; Berlinberg, E.J.; Lu, Y.; Marigi, E.M.; Okoroha, K.R.; Camp, C.L.; Barlow, J.D.; Krych, A.J. Platelet-Rich Plasma and Marrow Venting May Serve as Cost-Effective Augmentation Techniques for Isolated Meniscal Repair: A Decision-Analytical Markov Model-Based Analysis. *Arthroscopy* **2023**, *39*, 2058–2068. [CrossRef]
39. Zhou, T.; Xu, Y.; Zhang, A.; Zhang, X.; Deng, K.; Wu, H.; Xu, W. Association of Graft Maturity on MRI With Return to Sports at 9 Months After Primary Single-Bundle ACL Reconstruction with Autologous Hamstring Graft. *Orthop. J. Sports Med.* **2024**, *12*, 23259671241248202. [CrossRef]
40. Ricupito, R.; Grassi, A.; Mourad, F.; Di Filippo, L.; Gobbo, M.; Maselli, F. Anterior Cruciate Ligament Return to Play: "A Framework for Decision Making". *J. Clin. Med.* **2025**, *14*, 2146. [CrossRef]
41. D'Ambrosi, R.; Sconfienza, L.M.; Albano, D.; Meena, A.; Abermann, E.; Fink, C. Can MRI predict return to sport after anterior cruciate ligament reconstruction? A systematic review of the literature. *Radiol. Med.* **2025**, *130*, 638–649. [CrossRef]

42. Spierings, J.; van Doeselaar, M.; Buenen, M.; Abinzano, F.; van der Steen, M.; Janssen, R.; Ito, K.; Foolen, J. Inflammatory factors released by ACL reconstruction tendon grafts and their potential for macrophage polarization. *Sci. Rep.* **2025**, *15*, 19091. [CrossRef]
43. Sinkler, M.A.; Furdock, R.J.; McMellen, C.J.; Calcei, J.G.; Voos, J.E. Biologics, Stem Cells, Growth Factors, Platelet-Rich Plasma, Hemarthrosis, and Scaffolds May Enhance Anterior Cruciate Ligament Surgical Treatment. *Arthroscopy* **2023**, *39*, 166–175. [CrossRef]
44. Tan, T.; Gatti, A.A.; Fan, B.; Shea, K.G.; Sherman, S.L.; Uhlrich, S.D.; Hicks, J.L.; Delp, S.L.; Shull, P.B.; Chaudhari, A.S. A scoping review of portable sensing for out-of-lab anterior cruciate ligament injury prevention and rehabilitation. *npj Digit. Med.* **2023**, *6*, 46. [CrossRef] [PubMed]
45. Yu, X.; Hu, J.; Li, Y.; Wen, Y.; Li, B. ACL injury management: A comprehensive review of novel biotherapeutics. *Front. Bioeng. Biotechnol.* **2024**, *12*, 1455225. [CrossRef] [PubMed]
46. Fujino, K.; Yamamoto, N.; Yoshimura, Y.; Yokota, A.; Hirano, Y.; Neo, M. Repair potential of self-assembling peptide hydrogel in a mouse model of anterior cruciate ligament reconstruction. *J. Exp. Orthop.* **2024**, *11*, e12061. [CrossRef] [PubMed]
47. Tang, Y.; Tian, J.; Li, L.; Huang, L.; Shen, Q.; Guo, S.; Jiang, Y. Biomimetic Biphasic Electrospun Scaffold for Anterior Cruciate Ligament Tissue Engineering. *Tissue Eng. Regen. Med.* **2021**, *18*, 819–830. [CrossRef]
48. Yu, C.; Chen, R.; Chen, J.; Wang, T.; Wang, Y.; Zhang, X.; Wang, Y.; Wu, T.; Yu, T. Enhancing tendon-bone integration and healing with advanced multi-layer nanofiber-reinforced 3D scaffolds for acellular tendon complexes. *Mater. Today Bio.* **2024**, *26*, 101099. [CrossRef]
49. Wang, C.; Hu, Y.; Zhang, S.; Ruan, D.; Huang, Z.; He, P.; Cai, H.; Heng, B.C.; Chen, X.; Shen, W. Application of Stem Cell Therapy for ACL Graft Regeneration. *Stem Cells Int.* **2021**, *2021*, 6641818. [CrossRef]
50. Matsumoto, T.; Sato, Y.; Kobayashi, T.; Suzuki, K.; Kimura, A.; Soma, T.; Ito, E.; Kikuchi, T.; Kobayashi, S.; Harato, K.; et al. Adipose-Derived Stem Cell Sheets Improve Early Biomechanical Graft Strength in Rabbits After Anterior Cruciate Ligament Reconstruction. *Am. J. Sports Med.* **2021**, *49*, 3508–3518. [CrossRef]
51. Xu, Z.; Xu, W.; Zhang, T.; Luo, L. Mechanisms of tendon-bone interface healing: Biomechanics, cell mechanics, and tissue engineering approaches. *J. Orthop. Surg. Res.* **2024**, *19*, 817. [CrossRef]
52. Amini, M.; Venkatesan, J.K.; Liu, W.; Leroux, A.; Nguyen, T.N.; Madry, H.; Migonney, V.; Cucchiarini, M. Advanced Gene Therapy Strategies for the Repair of ACL Injuries. *Int. J. Mol. Sci.* **2022**, *23*, 14467. [CrossRef]
53. Zou, M.; Wang, J.; Shao, Z. Therapeutic Potential of Exosomes in Tendon and Tendon-Bone Healing: A Systematic Review of Preclinical Studies. *J. Funct. Biomater.* **2023**, *14*, 299. [CrossRef]
54. Lin, Y.C.; Chen, Y.J.; Fan, T.Y.; Chou, P.H.; Lu, C.C. Effect of bone marrow aspiration concentrate and platelet-rich plasma combination in anterior cruciate ligament reconstruction: A randomized, prospective, double-blinded study. *J. Orthop. Surg. Res.* **2024**, *19*, 4. [CrossRef]
55. Retzky, J.S.; Koff, M.F.; Nwawka, O.K.; Rodeo, S.A. Novel Noninvasive Imaging Techniques to Assess Structural, Functional, and Material Properties of Tendon, Ligament, and Cartilage: A Narrative Review of Current Concepts. *Orthop. J. Sports Med.* **2025**, *13*, 23259671251317223. [CrossRef]
56. Di Paolo, S.; Lopomo, N.F.; Della Villa, F.; Paolini, G.; Figari, G.; Bragonzoni, L.; Grassi, A.; Zaffagnini, S. Rehabilitation and Return to Sport Assessment after Anterior Cruciate Ligament Injury: Quantifying Joint Kinematics during Complex High-Speed Tasks through Wearable Sensors. *Sensors* **2021**, *21*, 2331. [CrossRef]

Journal of
Clinical Medicine

MDPI

Article

"Returning to Sport Is Not Just About the Knee": Physiotherapists' Experiences of the Management of Anterior Cruciate Ligament Injury: A Qualitative Study

Sultan A. Alanazi [1,*], Samia A. Alamrani [2], Sarah S. Bajuaifer [3], Layan Alhammad [1], Nouf Alotaibi [1], Naif Z. Alrashdi [1,4], Msaad Alzhrani [1], Ahmad D. Alanazi [1], Ahmed M. Almansour [1], Abdulmajeed Alfayyadh [5] and Aqeel M. Alenazi [6]

1 Department of Physical Therapy and Health Rehabilitation, College of Applied Medical Sciences, Majmaah University, Al-Majmaah 11952, Saudi Arabia; LayannDPT@gmail.com (L.A.); Noufenadalotaibi@gmail.com (N.A.); n.alrashedy@mu.edu.sa (N.Z.A.); m.alzhrani@mu.edu.sa (M.A.); aalanazi@mu.edu.sa (A.D.A.); ah.almansour@mu.edu.sa (A.M.A.)

2 Department of Health Rehabilitation Sciences, Faculty of Applied Medical Sciences, University of Tabuk, Tabuk 71491, Saudi Arabia; salamrani@ut.edu.sa

3 Department of Rehabilitation Sciences, College of Health and Rehabilitation Sciences, Princess Nourah Bint Abdulrahman University, P.O. Box 84428, Riyadh 11671, Saudi Arabia; ssbajuaifer@pnu.edu.sa

4 Health and Basic Sciences Research Center, Majmaah University, Al-Majmaah 11952, Saudi Arabia

5 Department of Physical Therapy and Health Rehabilitation, College of Applied Medical Sciences, Jouf University, Sakaka 72346, Saudi Arabia; abalfayyadh@ju.edu.sa

6 Department of Health and Rehabilitation Sciences, College of Applied Medical Sciences, Prince Sattam Bin Abdulaziz University, Al-Kharj 11942, Saudi Arabia; aqeel.alanazi@psau.edu.sa

* Correspondence: sa.alanazi@mu.edu.sa

Abstract

Objectives: To explore sport physiotherapists' perspectives and experiences on the management of anterior cruciate ligament (ACL) injuries in Saudi Arabia and to understand the key challenges that influence rehabilitation practice. **Methods:** A qualitative semi-structured interviews were conducted with sport physiotherapists recruited from different regions and clinical settings (Public, private and sport clubs) in Saudi Arabia. Eligibility criteria included $\geq$2 years' post-qualification experience in ACL injuries management. Interviews were audio-recorded, transcribed verbatim, and analyzed using reflexive thematic analysis. A total of twenty-six sport physiotherapists (18 males; mean age 31 years, range 26–39) participated, including 13 working primarily as clinicians and 13 with combined clinical and research roles. **Results:** Five themes were identified: (1) disruptions of ACL injury in daily life and sport; (2) managing fear of re-injury and uncertainty in surgical vs. conservative care; (3) guiding rehabilitation through challenges of workload, progression, adherence and supportive tools; (4) variability in protocols, assessment tools, and available resources; and (5) returning to sport is more than just passing a test. These themes demonstrate that ACL injuries rehabilitation in Saudi Arabia is shaped by physical and psychological readiness, cultural expectations, and disparities in resources. **Conclusions:** Physiotherapists described ACL rehabilitation as a long-term process that needs an integration of physical, psychological, and contextual factors. This study's findings highlight the need for resource-sensitive, standardized guidelines and the inclusion of psychological readiness assessments within rehabilitation processes. This study provides context-specific evidence that can be used to inform the development of culturally responsive, evidence-based approaches to strengthen ACL rehabilitation in Saudi Arabia.

Keywords: rehabilitation; psychological readiness; return to sport; exercise therapy; fear of re-injury; athletic injury; Saudi Arabia

1. Introduction

Anterior cruciate ligament (ACL) injuries are among the most prevalent and debilitating musculoskeletal conditions in sport [1]. Globally, more than two million ACL injuries occur annually, with incidence rate among athletes exceeding 350 per 100,000 person-years, which is higher compared to the general population [2–5]. Athletes engaged in pivoting and high-intensity sports are particularly vulnerable to ACL injuries, which may result in long-term mechanical/health consequences such as knee instability, early knee osteoarthritis onset, reduced sport performance, and/or psychological distress [6–8]. Rehabilitation plays a critical role in ACL recovery; however, outcomes remain inconsistent, particularly regarding return to sport success rates and long-term knee health [9,10].

In Saudi Arabia, ACL injuries have become a growing sport injury concern, especially among soccer players and young athletes [11]. Prevalence rates of ACL injury in Saudi population have been reported as high as 26.2% [11–14]. Prior research suggest that ACL ruptures account for up to 20% of all sports-related knee injuries, with a steady increase in ACL reconstruction procedures has been observed in major hospitals over the last decade [14–17]. While surgical management for ACL rupture is common (especially for athletes), post-operative rehabilitation outcomes remain variable [18,19]. This variability could be due to several factors such as differences in clinician expertise, lack of access to specialized rehabilitation services, discontinuity of care, and/or disparities between public and private healthcare sectors in terms of the implementation of clinical practice guidelines [18–21]. In addition to the previous variability, the Saudi healthcare context is also influenced by cultural factors (e.g., family and community expectation) as well as systemic factors such as healthcare structure and resource availability [22].

Globally, there is growing recognition that successful ACL rehabilitation must address not only physical restoration but also psychological and contextual factors [9,23]. However, clinical implementation often deviates from evidence-based standards [18,23]. For example, a 2023 qualitative study of 19 physiotherapists in the United Kingdom highlighted significant variability in ACL rehabilitation delivery, describing access to care as a "location lottery" shaped by disparities in training, resources, and multidisciplinary coordination [24]. Similarly, Piussi et al. reported that sports physiotherapists' often feel underprepared to address the psychological burden of ACL injury, despite acknowledging its importance in rehabilitation success [25]. These previous findings highlight the need for more context-specific research in healthcare systems such as Saudi Arabia's where structural and cultural challenges remain underexplored.

Physiotherapists play a critical role in ACL rehabilitation, but little is known about their perceptions and experiences of clinical practice within the Saudi healthcare system. ACL injuries impose substantial societal and economic costs, often exceeding USD 10,000 per case when considering surgery, rehabilitation, and work absenteeism [26,27]. Global and regional disparities in access to specialized rehabilitation and inconsistent adherence to evidence-based practice further complicate recovery, particularly outside main urban centers [28,29]. In Saudi Arabia, limited access to specialized rehabilitation services further compounds these challenges, leading to delayed return to sport or work. Understanding these perspectives is vital given the broader public health, economic, and service implications of ACL injuries such as the costs of delayed return to sport or work, unequal access to specialized rehabilitation, and the psychological consequences of prolonged inactivity.

Therefore, this qualitative study aimed to explore how sport physiotherapists in Saudi Arabia perceive and manage ACL injuries and to identify the contextual and systemic factors influencing rehabilitation practice. We proposed that psychological and structural factors shape physiotherapists' application of return to sport criteria, which may contribute to variability in clinical decision-making.

2. Methods

2.1. Study Design

A descriptive qualitative design was employed to explore the perceptions and experiences of sport physiotherapists involved in the ACL rehabilitation in Saudi Arabia. The study was approved by the Institutional Review Board at Majmaah University (Approval #: MUREC-Dec.25/COM-2024/67). All participants provided informed consent prior to interviews. This study was reported in accordance with the COnsolidation criteria for REporting Qualitative research (COREQ) (Supplementary File) [30].

2.2. Participants and Recruitment

Eligible participants were licensed sport physiotherapists currently practicing in Saudi Arabia with at least 2 years of experience managing individuals with ACL injuries. Inclusion criteria were: (1) age $\geq$ 18 years, (2) qualified as a sport physiotherapist, (3) minimum of two years' post-qualification clinical experience in ACL rehabilitation, and (4) proficiency in English and/or Arabic.

To capture diverse insightful perspectives from participants, recruitment sought variations across sex, years of experience, clinical settings (i.e., public, private, and sport club), and geographical regions [31]. Recruitment took place from January to July of 2025 using purposeful and snowball sampling techniques. Study announcements were distributed through social media platforms (e.g., X and LinkedIn) where a brief description of the study and a short eligibility survey were provided. Eligible respondents who completed the eligibility survey and met the selection criteria were contacted via email or phone call, according to their preferred method indicated in the short survey and invited to participate in semi-structured interviews. Additionally, interviewed physiotherapists were asked to recommend colleagues with ACL injuries expertise.

2.3. Sample

Twenty-six physiotherapists participated in this study. Their characteristics are presented below in Table 1.

Table 1. Participant characteristics (total n = 26).

Characteristic	Number (%)
Sex: Male	18 (69)
Age: Mean (range) years	31 (26–39)
Current employment role	
Clinician	13 (50)
Clinician and researcher	13 (50)
Years of clinical experience	
≤5	14 (54)
6–10	9 (35)
≥11	3 (11)
Sector of current clinical practice	
Governmental/semi-governmental	13 (50)
Private	13 (50)

Table 1. *Cont.*

Characteristic	Number (%)
Highest academic qualification	
Bachelor's degree	16 (62)
Master's degree	7 (27)
Doctor of Philosophy	3 (11)
Number of non-surgical ACL cases seen in last month	
1–5	21 (81)
6–10	4 (15)
>10	1 (4)
Number of post-surgical ACL cases seen in the last month	
1–5	15 (58)
6–10	7 (27)
>10	2 (8)
None	2 (8)

ACL = Anterior cruciate ligament. Unless otherwise stated, data are N (%).

2.4. Data Collection

Semi-structed interviews were conducted via Zoom call (Version 6.5.9, San Jose, CA, USA: Zoom Video Communications Inc.) using an interview guide (Supplementary File). The interview guide, eligibility notice, and invitation script are provided in a Supplementary File. The interview guide was developed collaboratively by the authorship team including senior physiotherapy researchers with experience in ACL injuries management, have Master of Musculoskeletal rehabilitation and PhDs in physiotherapy and have previously published qualitative research [32–35]. The interview guide facilitated open discussion regarding sport physiotherapists' experiences with ACL injury rehabilitation. The guide included broad, exploratory prompts specifically designed to elicit participants' perspectives on patient needs, rehabilitation practices, contextual challenges, and return to sport considerations. The guide was piloted with two expert sport physiotherapists to assess clarity, relevance, and flow, and minor revisions were made accordingly. Demographic data were collected on age, sex, current employment role (e.g., researcher, clinician), years of clinical experience, practice sector (governmental or private), highest qualification, and the number of surgical and non-surgical ACL cases seen in the past month.

At the start of each interview, the interviewers explained study procedures, addressed any participants queries and clarified confidentiality, the voluntary nature of participation, and the right to withdraw at any time. To reduce social desirability and confirmation bias, participants were assured of confidentiality, informed that there were no right or wrong answers, and interviews used neutral, non-judgmental prompts and non-leading open-ended questions. The Interviews were conducted by two final year female Doctor of Physical Therapy students (LA and NA) who had received extensive qualitative research training from senior qualitative researchers (First, second and third authors) and were supervised by the first author (SAA). Prior to this study, the interviewers had no prior relationship with participants, and no field notes were taken during interviews. Interviews were audio-recorded and lasted between 16 and 41 min and only the interviewer and participant attended (except the first 2 interviews which were observed by the first author to ensure clarity and appropriateness of data collection process). At the end of each interview, participants were asked to share any additional thoughts or ideas that have not been covered during the interview. All interviews were conducted once, and no repeated interviews were required.

2.5. Data Analysis

Interviews were conducted in Arabic, audio-recorded, professionally transcribed verbatim and translated into English by two senior and bilingual authors (First and third authors), who have Master of Musculoskeletal Physical Therapy and PhDs in physiotherapy and have previously conducted qualitative research. Transcriptions were independently cross-checked for accuracy and appropriateness, after which the authors met to compare and resolve any discrepancies. The interview data were analyzed using the six-stage model reflexive thematic analysis described by Braun and Clarke [36,37]. This model involved familiarizing, finding, analyzing, categorizing, comparing, and describing codes to generate themes that capture the phenomena under investigation and addressed the research aim [36,38].

Coding was conducted line-by-line to identify potential themes in accordance with the aim of this study. The third author (SSB) independently coded the first five interviews and developed a coding workbook using Microsoft Excel, which was independently reviewed by the first author (SAA) to ensure accuracy and to provide additional modifications. The codes were then checked and verified by the second author (SAA) who has experience in qualitative research, as this step is to ensure clarity and appropriateness of the codes generated. The third author (SSB) then coded the full dataset and produced an Excel spreadsheet of codes and emerging themes. The first author (SAA) independently reviewed and refined codes and themes and discrepancies were resolved through discussion. Data saturation was deemed to have been achieved when additional interview data produced little to no change in the emerging codes from the analysis [36]. Investigator triangulation was employed to enhance the rigor of the analysis and ensure a complete and in-depth interpretation of the data.

All research team reviewed and agreed upon the final list of themes identified. For respondent validation [39], preliminary themes were shared with participants for feedback and verification. Feedback received confirmed that the themes accurately represented participants' perspectives, supporting the credibility and trustworthiness of the findings. All de-identified data were securely stored on a password-protected server with restricted access to the research team only.

2.6. Researcher Reflexivity

The authorship team comprised physiotherapists and academics with expertise in musculoskeletal rehabilitation, qualitative methods, and sports physiotherapy. Their shared professional background provided valuable insight into ACL injury rehabilitation but also carried potential preconceptions about clinical practice in Saudi settings. To address this, reflexive discussions were maintained throughout data collection and analysis to identify and challenge assumptions. Regular peer debriefing enhanced interpretive rigor and transparency. This reflexive stance acknowledges researcher influence as integral to qualitative inquiry and contributes to the study's credibility and trustworthiness [40].

3. Results

3.1. Identified Themes That Describe the Sport Physiotherapists Perception Managing Individuals with ACL Injuries

Five overarching themes were identified from the analysis of interviews with sport physiotherapists managing individuals with ACL injuries: (1) disruptions of ACL injury in daily life and sport; (2) managing fear of re-injury and uncertainty in surgical vs. conservative care; (3) guiding rehabilitation through challenges of workload, progression, adherence and supportive tools; (4) variability in protocols, assessment tools, and available resources;

and (5) returning to sport is more than just passing a test. Each theme is described in detail in the sections below with subthemes (*italicized*) for clarity.

3.1.1. Theme 1: Disruptions of ACL Injury in Daily Life and Sport

Sport physiotherapists consistently described ACL injuries as profoundly disruptive, affecting patients' daily routines, sporting identities, and social participation. Several participants observed that their patients struggled with basic activities such as kneeling, sitting cross-legged, or praying, which often limited engagement in both daily and cultural practices. The disruption was particularly evident among athletes, as one participant noted: *"An ACL injury affects the quality of life... especially for those involved in sports"* (P1).

Many sport physiotherapists highlighted the psychological consequences of ACL injuries, describing patients' fear, frustration, and uncertainty about recovery, often asking questions whether they would return to sport or trust their knee again. For elite athletes, some participants reported that prolonged time away from sport had major negative impacts on identity and livelihood: *"being off the field for 6 to 9 months causes a huge psychological impact on athletes"* (P23).

Social consequences were felt by many sport physiotherapists, who observed that their patients often avoided family or community gatherings to escape questions such as *"Will you stop playing football?"* (P25). Being away from the team environment was perceived as particularly discouraging for athletes. While financial burdens were generally minimal in public hospitals (government-funded care), many participants acknowledged broader economic impacts on patients and the healthcare system. Collectively, these disruptions covered physical, psychological, social, and economic domains (*Physical disruption, psychological effect, social consequences, Economic impact;* Table 2).

Table 2. Subthemes and quotes for Theme 1: "Disruptions of ACL injury in daily life and sport".

Subtheme	Illustrative Quote
Physical disruption	"ACL injury affects patients both physically and psychologically" (P9)
	"Regular activities like sitting cross-legged or prayer can become painful and difficult." (P3)
	"I believe it has a significant impact... it affects their daily tasks, work duties, and responsibilities at home." (P17)
	"ACL injuries impact athletes significantly...It can hinder their performance and return to competitive sports." (P5)
Psychological effect	"The main fear is not being able to return to their sport... some athletes assume they'll have to quit completely..." (P18)
	"ACL injury means being off the field for 6 to 9 months, which causes a huge psychological impact. Some athletes even go through abnormal levels of stress." (P23)
Social consequences	"Some patients feel ashamed to be seen with crutches or feel weak. I remember one patient refused to attend a family gathering because he didn't want to bring his crutch. In athletes, the impact is even greater." (P23)
	"Socially, the injury can prevent the patient from fulfilling home or social responsibilities, leading to reduced interactions and isolation." (P13)
Economic impact	"Economically, it has a burden on both the patient and the healthcare system." (P11)

3.1.2. Theme 2: Managing Fear of Re-Injury and Uncertainty in Surgical vs. Conservative Care

Participants frequently expressed that fear of re-injury often dominated clinical reasoning and strongly influenced patients' treatment decisions. Fear was described as a psychological barrier shaping decision-making—particularly when selecting between surgical and conservative options. Several sport physiotherapists noted that their patients often carried lasting memories of the initial trauma, describing *"hearing a pop in the knee"* (P11) or saying that *"their knee feels disconnected"* (P11). The persistent fear of re-injury often limited patients' engagement in rehabilitation and, in some cases, led them to pursue surgical reconstruction despite available conservative options. One physiotherapist explained that *"the main fear is not being able to return to their sport... some assume they'll have to quit completely"* (P18). Another participant added that *"fear of re-injury is the most common psychological barrier... patients are often afraid of going through the same injury again"* (P10), emphasizing that confidence in the knee extends beyond structural healing and remains central to treatment decision-making.

Uncertainty about long-term outcomes was also reported by several participants. They explained that their patients frequently asked whether they could ever fully recover, whether osteoarthritis would inevitably develop, or whether surgery could guarantee a successful return to sport. Sport physiotherapists noticed that many patients carried unrealistic expectations, particularly regarding surgical outcomes: *"some of the patients want surgery because they believe it will solve everything, but the reality is much more complicated"* (P7).

These anxieties were not limited to elite athletes; recreational and physically active individuals expressed similar concerns about long-term limitations. Several sport physiotherapists described their role as an ongoing negotiation—providing reassurance while correcting misconceptions about both surgical and non-surgical pathways. Ultimately, treatment decisions were often shaped as much by fear, uncertainty, and psychological stress as by medical advice (*fear of re-injury, uncertainty about outcomes, psychological stress;* Table 3).

Table 3. Subthemes and quotes for Theme 2: "Managing fear of re-injury and uncertainty in surgical vs. conservative care".

Subtheme	Illustrative Quote
Fear of re-injury	"Fear of re-injury is the biggest challenge." (P10)
	"Fear of re-injury is the most common thing we hear, even more than pain." (P14)
	"They always ask... 'will I be the same again?' they don't trust the knee like before." (P18)
Psychological stress	"Athletes lose months of their career, and with that comes anxiety, stress, and sometimes depression." (P23)
	"The fear is not only physical... it's emotional, because their career and identity are on the line." (P19)
	"Patients worry a lot about re-injury, become cautious, reduce their movement, and often avoid sports or even daily activities like going up stairs or praying. It has a major psychological impact. (P16)
Uncertainty about outcomes	"Non-surgical cases recover quickly but often carry more fear of re-injury." (P5)
	"Most patients are unsure what surgery or conservative treatment will bring; they're worried about life after treatment." (P22)
	"There's always the question of what will happen after surgery... will they recover fully, or will they develop knee arthritis later?" (P7)
	"Pressure from family or peers to undergo surgery, especially when others had positive outcomes causes emotional conflict if the patient is unsure about the operation. (P5)

3.1.3. Theme 3: Guiding Rehabilitation Through Challenges of Workload, Progression, Adherence, and Supportive Tools

Several sport physiotherapists consistently emphasized that ACL rehabilitation is long, exercise-driven, and requires sustained commitment from patients. Exercise was described as the cornerstone of management: *"from my side, the most important intervention is exercise... especially early on"* (P18). Early rehabilitation typically involved Isometric and endurance strengthening, progressing to concentric, eccentric, and plyometric drills. Adjunctive modalities such as electrotherapy, hydrotherapy, blood-flow restriction, or shockwave were occasionally applied, but always secondary to progressive loading.

Managing progression through phases was described as uneven and clinically challenging. Initial priorities included reducing swelling, restoring quadriceps activation, and regaining range of motion, particularly knee extension. Many participants repeatedly emphasized extension as decisive for outcomes: *"the hardest issue is achieving full extension. Flexion comes back, but extension must be addressed early"* (P9). Failure to restore extension promptly was associated with adhesions, fibrosis, or even the need for secondary surgery.

Weight-bearing strategies varied according to injury characteristics and surgical details. Some participants encouraged early loading when clinically appropriate: *"if the ACL tear is isolated, early weight-bearing is encouraged... gradual progression is essential in all cases"* (P9). In contrast, others delayed weight-bearing following meniscal repair or when graft-related restrictions were present.

Rehabilitation trajectories differed between surgical and non-surgical patients. Some sport physiotherapists observed that non-surgical cases often progressed more quickly and regain muscle strength sooner, while surgical patients followed longer timelines and were often more cautious: *"surgical patients usually need six months; non-surgical may recover in one or two"* (P4). Despite this, surgery was frequently perceived to provide greater long-term stability in the knee joint.

Adherence throughout rehabilitation phases was seen as the most persistent challenge, caused by fear of movement, competing responsibilities, or limited understanding of goals: *"patient adherence to the treatment plan is my top concern... lack of commitment can significantly delay recovery"* (P14). Miscommunication between surgeons and physiotherapists regarding rehabilitation phases and timeline was reported as a limiting factor that can further complicate adherence.

Supportive tools, particularly knee braces, were used selectively. Few participants prescribed them in the early post-surgical phase to provide confidence and protect the joint: *"braces are helpful early on for safety and maintaining extension"* (P6). Others discouraged routine use, cautioning against dependency and stiffness: *"personally, I'm not a fan of knee braces unless there's a strong reason.... they can limit recovery if overused"* (P2).

Post-surgical complications, including swelling, arthrofibrosis, cyclops lesions, and infections, were reported as significant barriers to progress, reinforcing the need for early, structured, and closely monitored rehabilitation.

Overall, sport physiotherapists described ACL rehabilitation as a negotiated, exercise-driven process shaped by progression management, adherence challenges, use of supportive tools, and risks of complications. These findings clustered around the following subthemes: (*common interventions, progression of therapy, weight-bearing strategies, surgical versus non-surgical recovery, post-surgical complications, adherence challenges, and regaining knee extension;* Table 4).

Table 4. Subthemes and quotes for Theme 3: "Guiding rehabilitation through challenges of workload, progression, adherence and supportive tools".

Subtheme	Illustrative Quote
Common interventions (exercise as cornerstone)	"From my side, the most important intervention is exercise... especially early on." (P18)
	"Isometric and endurance strengthening are the foundation before progressing to concentric or eccentric training." (P19)
	"We follow standard protocols but may include modalities like hydrotherapy, electrotherapy, and muscle stimulation... but 95% is exercise." (P20)
	"I mostly rely on exercise; in early stages, I add electrical stimulation or blood flow restriction if needed." (P12)
Progression of therapy	"If extension is not restored in the first two months, the case becomes much harder." (P11)
	"Each phase builds to the next... strength, then balance, then sport drills." (P23)
	"Acute focuses on swelling and ROM; subacute is transition; chronic cases are more functional and goal driven." (P7)

Table 4. *Cont.*

Subtheme	Illustrative Quote
Weight-bearing strategies	"If the ACL tear is isolated, early weight-bearing is encouraged. Gradual progression is essential in all cases." (P9)
	"Unless there's a meniscus repair, early weight-bearing helps patients return to walking sooner." (P11)
	"If meniscus is repaired, we restrict weight-bearing for 4–6 weeks." (P3)
	"If symptoms are under control, I support early weight-bearing, especially for athletes." (P16)
Surgical versus non-surgical recovery	"Surgical patients usually need six months; non-surgical may recover in one or two." (P4)
	"Non-surgical patients often recover faster, with better muscle strength and fewer complications." (P5)
	"Non-surgical cases progress quickly, but surgery provides more long-term stability." (P22)
	"Patients without surgery regain strength faster, but surgical patients are more stable in the long term." (P13)
Post-surgical complications	"The hardest issue is achieving full extension. Flexion comes back, but extension must be addressed early." (P9)
	"Loss of extension even 5 degrees is serious. Delay full extension makes it much harder." (P18)
	"Arthrofibrosis or cyclops lesions sometimes require a second surgery." (P9)
	"Complications such as infections, I encountered a case of necrosis after surgery." (P10)
Adherence challenges	"Non-compliance with rehab plans, fear of movement, and poor understanding of goals are common barriers." (P25)
	"Some stop coming once pain reduces, which interrupts progression." (P12)
	"The biggest barrier is adherence and lack of motivation... these delay recovery." (P21)
Supportive tools	"Braces are helpful early on for safety and maintaining extension... they give patients confidence." (P6)
	"Post-surgery, braces may help short-term but should not be used long-term." (P21)
	"I support using them early on for confidence, but only for short-term." (P24)

3.1.4. Theme 4: Variation in Protocols, Assessment Tools and Resources

Many sport physiotherapists consistently reported wide variation in how ACL rehabilitation protocol was delivered, both within and across clinical settings *"protocols vary between hospitals and private clinics. Generally, implementation in private clinics is better, especially in terms of time and flexibility."* (P19). While some reported that they adhere to internationally recognized guidelines, others relied mainly on personal experience, leading to inconsistent management practices. One participant reflected, *"protocols vary from therapist to therapist. I personally follow the Melbourne Protocol...which I see as reliable for gradual rehabilitation"* (P9). This lack of a unified approach was seen as a major barrier to ensuring consistent quality of care.

It is reported that there was discrepancy in ACL assessment practices. Although a number of clinicians employed objective measures such as hop tests, strength assessment, or kinesiophobia scales many acknowledged that decisions were often based on clinical observation rather than standardized testing. Limited time and restricted access to specialized equipment, particularly in high-volume government hospitals, were reported as key challenges.

Many sport physiotherapists reported that the resource disparities have influenced rehabilitation practices. Several participants in private centers reported access to advanced equipment and technologies, whereas those in public hospitals frequently encountered shortages of even basic tools. These differences not only affected rehabilitation trajectories but also shaped clinicians' perception of their ability to provide optimal care. These accounts highlight an ongoing challenge of inconsistency in ACL injury rehabilitation and underscore the need for standardized clinical guidelines. Overall, accounts revealed marked inconsistency in protocols, outcome measures, resource limitations, highlighting the need for standardized, context-sensitive clinical guidelines that account for variations across healthcare settings (*Protocol variability in practice, outcome measures, resource limitations;* Table 5).

Table 5. Subthemes and quotes for Theme 4: "Variation in protocols, assessment tools and resources".

Subtheme	Illustrative Quote
Protocol variability in practice	"No unified protocol... I adapt between Aspetar and Melbourne." (P2)
	"Government hospitals stick to rigid monthly progressions; private settings allow flexibility." (P19)
	"Protocols differ from therapist to therapist, and that leads to inconsistency." (P2)
	"Some places follow strict guidelines; others go by experience... it's very mixed." (P16)
	"Some protocols are outdated, and patients get confused when advice changes between settings." (P24)
Outcome measures	"We use hop tests, balance measures, goniometers, depending on stage of rehabilitation." (P7)
	"For psychology, I use the Tampa Scale for Kinesiophobia... it matters as much as strength." (P21)
	"We use hop tests, isokinetic measures, and sometimes VALD systems, but there's no unified approach." (20)
Resource limitations	"Some clinics don't even have the basic tools... protocols stay on paper." (P25)

3.1.5. Theme 5: Returning to Sport Is More than Just Passing a Test

Return to sport was consistently viewed as a process that extends beyond passing a physical test, with fear of re-injury emerging as a key determinant of psychological readiness and confidence rather than a treatment barrier. While measures such as hop tests and strength assessments were regarded as essential benchmarks, many physiotherapists reported that psychological readiness often lagged behind physical recovery. As one participant explained, *"they may pass all the tests, but still tell you they don't feel ready"* (P14). This mismatch between physical clearance and perceived readiness created ongoing challenges in clinical decision-making.

External pressures further complicated the process. Athletes were often urged to return prematurely by coaches, clubs, or families, even when they were not psychologically prepared. One participant noted, *"some athletes rush because they don't want to lose their spot on the team"* (P15). These competing demands often placed sport physiotherapists in the difficult position of balancing immediate performance with long-term safety.

Many of our participants stressed that successful return to sport required more than biomechanical recovery. Confidence in the knee, trust in performance, and gradual reintegration into competition were seen as equally critical. As one therapist summarized, *"returning to sport is not just about the knee...it's about the whole athlete being ready again"* (P15). Collectively, these accounts underscore that return to sport cannot be reduced to test results alone but must incorporate physical readiness, psychological preparedness, and the broader social and cultural context (*Physical readiness, psychological preparedness, external pressures, social and cultural context;* Table 6).

Table 6. Subthemes and quotes for Theme 5: "Returning to sport is more than just passing a test".

Subtheme	Illustrative Quote
Physical readiness	"Even after good physical recovery, athletes hesitate to return to pivoting sports." (P15)
	"ACL injuries significantly impact athletes' ability to return at the same level they once played." (P19)
Psychological preparedness	"Fear of the knee failing is the top concern, even when physical tests look good." (P9)
	Psychological readiness is a major factor (P25)
	"Many athletes are cleared physically, but mentally they're not ready to trust their knee again." (P23)
	"It's our job as physiotherapists to reintroduce sport-specific activities like ball catching, sudden change direction, and jumping... to rebuild that trust." (P11)

Table 6. *Cont.*

Subtheme	Illustrative Quote
External pressures	"Coaches often push for quicker return to play… we have to advocate for safety." (P12)
Social and cultural context	"Sometimes family pressure or social expectations influence the decision more than clinical tests." (P13)
	"In some cases, cultural habits play a role… like avoiding certain movements even after clearance." (P21)

4. Discussion

This is the first qualitative study that explored the perspectives of sports physiotherapists on the management of ACL injuries working in Saudi Arabia. This study findings revealed that sport physiotherapists view ACL rehabilitation as a complex, multidimensional process that extends beyond physical recovery and incorporates psychological, social and contextual considerations. Participants emphasized that the disruption ACL injuries caused in daily and sporting activities, the impact of fear of re-injury and uncertainty in treatment decisions, the difficulties of sustaining progression and adherence within long rehabilitation pathways, and the variability in protocols, assessment tools, and resources across settings. Sport physiotherapists also stressed that returning to sport requires more than passing physical tests, as psychological preparedness and cultural context are equally decisive. The five main themes highlighted the clinical and contextual realities of ACL rehabilitation in Saudi Arabia and extended recent qualitative research from Europe and Australia [24,25,41,42]. These themes offer insights into the complex realities of clinical practice and point out key areas for improvement in care delivery and policy development.

4.1. Theme 1: Disruptions of ACL Injury in Daily Life and Sport

Based on participants' responses, ACL injuries were described as extending beyond the clinic environment, disrupting daily life and requiring ongoing adaptation. Sport physiotherapists observed that their patients with ACL injuries often struggled with restrictions in basic activities, altered social roles, and psychological adjustment and in some cases financial stability. This is similar to the recent work describing ACL reconstruction as a "life-shaping event" rather than a single surgical episode [41,42]. Such disruption is not only peripheral but central, shaping how athletes engage in rehabilitation from the outset. The psychological burden of ACL injury was particularly notable among athletes, where long rehabilitation timelines challenged identity and career prospects [43,44]. These disruptions highlight the importance of adopting a biopsychosocial approach in ACL rehabilitation. Recognizing that recovery is not only biomechanical but also highly individualized and contextual [45–47].

4.2. Theme 2: Managing Fear of Re-Injury and Uncertainty in Surgical vs. Conservative Care

A major finding of this study was that the fear of re-injury emerged as a central factor influencing decision-making, often persisted despite favorable physical progress, consistent with previous studies [48,49]. Our participants noted that readiness to return to sport was not always aligned with test results and was frequently shaped by uncertainty and external pressures from coaches or families. These observations mirror evidence that psychological readiness is strongly associated with return to sport status, with those who return typically reporting higher ACL-return to sport scores than non-returners, and that paths of readiness may stagnate for long periods without targeted input [50,51]. Importantly, prior qualitative research has indicated how fear is constructed and maintained, underscoring why it can dominate decisions even when physical criteria are met [50]. A 2025 study suggested that the timing of measuring psychological readiness is important: administering the ACL–return-to-sport questionnaire after completing physical performance tests, may provide more realistic appraisal of self-confidence than pre-test questionnaires [52]. Therefore, sport physiotherapists play a dual role, not just as providers of physical rehabilitation, but also as emotional supporters and educators. They are responsible for addressing misunderstandings, providing reassurance, and guiding patients to make informed, evidence-based decisions rather than fear [53,54].

4.3. Theme 3: Guiding Rehabilitation Through Challenges of Workload, Progression, Adherence, and Supportive Tools

Study participants reflected on the tension between criterion-based rehabilitation and the practical realities of adherence. Fluctuating motivation, socioeconomic barriers, and competing responsibilities often disrupted structured progression, despite physiotherapist follow contemporary guidelines that emphasize criteria-based loading, progressive strength training, and staged decision points across the continuum [23]. This clinical picture is consistent with broader evidence on the adherence barriers in ACL rehabilitation, including logistical constraints, low self-efficacy, and environmental pressures [55,56]. Highlighting the need to embed behavior-change strategies and supportive tools into routine care [55,57].

4.4. Theme 4: Variation in Protocols, Assessment Tools and Resources

A key systemic challenge identified in this study was the variation in assessment practices and resource availability, which added further complexity in ACL rehabilitation. Sport physiotherapists described inconsistent use of hop tests, strength measures, and movement-quality ratings, reflecting a broader lack of alignment on benchmarks and clearance criteria. This inconsistency has also been noted internationally. This aligns with international evidence showing substantial heterogeneity in return-to-sport testing and decision-making, even among expert clinicians [24,58]. A recent Delphi consensus study further highlights the need for standardized, multimodal assessment protocols to guide safe progression [58]. In addition, mounting evidence cautions that hop-test limb-symmetry indices can overestimate functional recovery relative to strength testing and that adding movement-quality ratings improves decision signal beyond distance-based metrics [59,60]. Taken together, these findings support the move toward multimodal, serial testing rather than one-off pass/fail decisions [61].

4.5. Theme 5: Returning to Sport Is More than Just Passing a Test

Participants consistently reported that returning to sport is a complex, staged process that goes beyond simply passing physical performance tests, with psychological readiness often lags behind physical recovery. Sport physiotherapists emphasized how contextual factors including athlete identity, competitive demands, and coach or family influence, shape return to sport decision as much as physical criteria. These observations align with a very recent review and a qualitative study similarly suggesting that objective test batteries are necessary but insufficient, and that readiness must be interpreted alongside psychological, social and contextual information across staged decision-making [41,61]. Within the Saudi context, where competitive sport participation is rapidly expanding and social expectations can exert strong influence, these contextual factors may be particularly salient in shaping return to sport trajectories.

4.6. Strengths and Limitations Pertain to the Current Study

This qualitative study followed the COREQ reporting guidelines [30], applied investigator triangulation and respondent validation, thereby increasing the trustworthiness of the study findings. The inclusion of sport physiotherapists from diverse clinical practice settings across both public and private healthcare settings in Saudi Arabia, provided insightful information about how ACL rehabilitation is adapted, strengthening the transferability of results.

However, several limitations should be considered. The purposive and snowball sampling approach may have introduced selection bias, participants with particular interest overrepresented, potentially limiting the diversity of perspectives. Each participant was interviewed only once, which may have limited the depth of inquiry. Field notes were not collected during interviews, potentially reducing contextual richness and may limit reflexivity regarding non-verbal cues. Although interviews were conducted by final-year DPT students who received training and regular supervision from senior qualitative researchers, their limited level of experience may have influenced the depth of probing during interviews. Additionally, as interviews were conducted primarily in Arabic, subtle nuances may have been lost during translation despite bilingual verification. Further, this study is based on data from Saudi sport physiotherapist only and does not include the views of athletes or coaches. Nonetheless, findings of this study provide important insights into sport physiotherapists' experiences and perceptions that can support and guide the development of culturally tailored, patient-centered strategies for ACL injury management in Saudi Arabia. Future research should incorporate perspectives of athletes with ACL injuries and coaches and evaluate implementation strategies across healthcare sectors.

4.7. Implication for Practice

Sport physiotherapists experience and perceptions voiced in this study highlight several clinical implications that could strengthen ACL rehabilitation and return-to-sport outcomes. Incorporating a standardized measure of psychological readiness, such as the Anterior Cruciate Ligament–Return to Sport after Injury (ACL-RSI) scale, at planned stages of recovery may help identify athletes at risk of premature return [62]. Adopting criteria-based progression checklists that include strength, hop performance, and sport-specific tasks, rather than relying solely on time-based milestones, may support safer and more individualized rehabilitation. Clinicians who use criteria-based checklists tend to have better outcomes and lower re-injury rates than those relying mainly on arbitrary time milestones [21,62,63]. Ongoing professional development and interprofessional training are also needed to promote consistent, evidence-based practice across different healthcare settings (public and private) [62]. These steps would facilitate the alignment of clinical care with national priorities to improve rehabilitation standards and optimize outcomes for athletes in Saudi Arabia.

5. Conclusions

This study showed that sports physiotherapists in Saudi Arabia view ACL rehabilitation as a complex process shaped by lived disruption of sport and daily activities, fear of re-injury, adherence challenges, variability in practice, and the complexity of return to sport decisions. Sport physiotherapists emphasized that successful rehabilitation required more than applying standardized protocols, instead advocating for integration of physical, psychological, and contextual factors. The study findings highlight current practice challenges and emphasize the need for evidence-based guidance that can be adapted effectively within the Saudi healthcare system.

Supplementary Materials: The following supporting information can be downloaded at: https://www.mdpi.com/article/10.3390/jcm14207301/s1, The interview guide (English and Arabic).

Author Contributions: Study conception and design, S.A.A. (Sultan A. Alanazi), S.A.A. (Samia A. Alamrani), S.S.B., L.A., N.A., N.Z.A., M.A., A.D.A., A.M.A. (Ahmed M. Almansour), A.A. and A.M.A. (Aqeel M. Alenazi); data collection, S.A.A. (Sultan A. Alanazi), L.A., and N.A.; analysis and interpretation of results, S.A.A. (Sultan A. Alanazi), S.A.A. (Samia A. Alamrani), S.S.B., L.A. and N.A.; manuscript drafting and reviewing, S.A.A. (Sultan A. Alanazi), S.A.A. (Samia A. Alamrani), S.S.B., L.A., N.A., N.Z.A., M.A., A.D.A., A.M.A. (Ahmed M. Almansour), A.A. and A.M.A. (Aqeel M. Alenazi). All authors have read and agreed to the published version of the manuscript.

Funding: This research was supported by Majmaah University (Project number: R-2025-2070). The funders had no role in data collection, analysis and interpretation, decision to publish, or preparation of the manuscript.

Institutional Review Board Statement: The study was approved by the Institutional Review Board at Majmaah University (Approval #: MUREC-Dec.25/COM-2024/67). Date of ethical approval is 25 December 2024.

Informed Consent Statement: All participants provided informed consent prior to participation.

Data Availability Statement: The datasets analyzed in the current study are available from the corresponding author on reasonable request.

Acknowledgments: The authors would like to thank the physiotherapists who participated in this study. The author extends the appreciation to the Deanship of Postgraduate Studies and Scientific Research at Majmaah University for funding this research work through project number (R-2025-2070). The author extends the appreciation to Princess Nourah bint Abdulrahman University Researchers Supporting Project number (PNURSP2025R539), Princess Nourah bint Abdulrahman University, Riyadh, Saudi Arabia for funding this research.

Conflicts of Interest: There are no conflicts of interest to disclose.

References

1. Ardern, C.L.; Taylor, N.F.; Feller, J.A.; Webster, K.E. Fifty-five per cent return to competitive sport following anterior cruciate ligament reconstruction surgery: An updated systematic review and meta-analysis including aspects of physical functioning and contextual factors. *Br. J. Sports Med.* **2014**, *48*, 1543. [CrossRef] [PubMed]
2. Gans, I.; Retzky, J.S.; Jones, L.C.; Tanaka, M.J. Epidemiology of Recurrent Anterior Cruciate Ligament Injuries in National Collegiate Athletic Association Sports: The Injury Surveillance Program, 2004–2014. *Orthop. J. Sports Med.* **2018**, *6*, 2325967118777823. [CrossRef]
3. Nordenvall, R.; Bahmanyar, S.; Adami, J.; Stenros, C.; Wredmark, T.; Felländer-Tsai, L. A population-based nationwide study of cruciate ligament injury in Sweden, 2001–2009: Incidence, treatment, and sex differences. *Am. J. Sports Med.* **2012**, *40*, 1808–1813. [CrossRef]
4. Granan, L.P.; Forssblad, M.; Lind, M.; Engebretsen, L. The Scandinavian ACL registries 2004–2007: Baseline epidemiology. *Acta Orthop.* **2009**, *80*, 563–567. [CrossRef]
5. Sanders, T.L.; Maradit Kremers, H.; Bryan, A.J.; Larson, D.R.; Dahm, D.L.; Levy, B.A.; Stuart, M.J.; Krych, A.J. Incidence of Anterior Cruciate Ligament Tears and Reconstruction: A 21-Year Population-Based Study. *Am. J. Sports Med.* **2016**, *44*, 1502–1507. [CrossRef] [PubMed]
6. Filbay, S.R.; Culvenor, A.G.; Ackerman, I.N.; Russell, T.G.; Crossley, K.M. Quality of life in anterior cruciate ligament-deficient individuals: A systematic review and meta-analysis. *Br. J. Sports Med.* **2015**, *49*, 1033–1041. [CrossRef]
7. Øiestad, B.E.; Engebretsen, L.; Storheim, K.; Risberg, M.A. Knee osteoarthritis after anterior cruciate ligament injury: A systematic review. *Am. J. Sports Med.* **2009**, *37*, 1434–1443. [CrossRef]
8. Ardern, C.L.; Taylor, N.F.; Feller, J.A.; Webster, K.E. A systematic review of the psychological factors associated with returning to sport following injury. *Br. J. Sports Med.* **2013**, *47*, 1120–1126. [CrossRef] [PubMed]
9. van Melick, N.; van Cingel, R.E.H.; Brooijmans, F.; Neeter, C.; van Tienen, T.; Hullegie, W.; Nijhuis-van der Sanden, M.W.G. Evidence-based clinical practice update: Practice guidelines for anterior cruciate ligament rehabilitation based on a systematic review and multidisciplinary consensus. *Br. J. Sports Med.* **2016**, *50*, 1506. [CrossRef]
10. Bernhardsson, S.; Larsson, M.E.H.; Johansson, K.; Öberg, B. "In the physio we trust": A qualitative study on patients' preferences for physiotherapy. *Physiother. Theory Pract.* **2017**, *33*, 535–549. [CrossRef]
11. Alqarni, F.S.; Alshehri, K.O.; Alotaibi, T.M.; Alsulami, A.N.; Alshehri, A.O.; Aseri, K.S. The prevalence and determinants of anterior cruciate ligament rupture among athletes practicing football in Jeddah Avenues 2020. *J. Family Med. Prim. Care* **2022**, *11*, 4528–4535. [CrossRef]

12. Almaawi, A.; Awwad, W.; Bamugaddam, A.; Alasheikh, M.; Muaddi, M.; Almutair, O.; Alomar, A.Z. Prevalence of knee injuries among male college students in Riyadh, Kingdom of Saudi Arabia. *J. Orthop. Surg. Res.* **2020**, *15*, 126. [CrossRef]
13. Dafalla, S.; Bokhari, Y.; Yazbik, R.; Ali, A.; Sheikh, K.; Alnaggar, A. Prevalence of anterior cruciate ligament injury and other ligament injuries among the Saudi community in Jeddah city, Saudi Arabia. *Int. J. Radiol. Imaging Technol.* **2020**, *6*, 62. [CrossRef]
14. Albaker, A.B.; Bahkali, A.B.; Bassi, M.M.; Alhassun, J.A.; Alyami, B.H.; Alanazi, B.S.; Alnakhli, Z.A.; Alzahrani, K. The prevalence rate of anterior cruciate ligaments reconstruction among population in Saudi Arabia. *Med. Sci.* **2023**, *27*, 1–9. [CrossRef]
15. Khired, Z.A.; Alshahrani, H.S.; Altayyib, N.M.; Alsuayri, A.H.; Alamri, A.D.; Alahmari, A.S.; Alqarni, M.A.; Alsaadi, S.K. Prevalence and risk factors of anterior cruciate ligament injuries among football team players in Bisha City, Saudi Arabia. *Int. J. Med. Dev. Ctries.* **2023**, *7*, 1325–1332. [CrossRef]
16. Alyami, A.H.; Darraj, H.; Hamdi, S.; Saber, A.; Bakri, N.; Maghrabi, R.; Hakami, K.M.; Darraj, A. Awareness of Anterior Cruciate Ligament Injury-Preventive Training Programs among Saudi Athletes. *Clin. Pract.* **2023**, *13*, 656–665. [CrossRef]
17. Grassi, A.; Carulli, C.; Innocenti, M.; Mosca, M.; Zaffagnini, S.; Bait, C. New Trends in Anterior Cruciate Ligament Reconstruction: A Systematic Review of National Surveys of the Last 5 Years. *Joints* **2018**, *6*, 177–187. [CrossRef]
18. Greenberg, E.M.; Greenberg, E.T.; Albaugh, J.; Storey, E.; Ganley, T.J. Rehabilitation Practice Patterns Following Anterior Cruciate Ligament Reconstruction: A Survey of Physical Therapists. *J. Orthop. Sports Phys. Ther.* **2018**, *48*, 801–811. [CrossRef]
19. Devana, S.K.; Solorzano, C.; Nwachukwu, B.; Jones, K.J. Disparities in ACL Reconstruction: The Influence of Gender and Race on Incidence, Treatment, and Outcomes. *Curr. Rev. Musculoskelet. Med.* **2022**, *15*, 1–9. [CrossRef]
20. Alshehri, Y.S. Current views on preoperative rehabilitation practice after anterior cruciate ligament injury among licensed physical therapists in Saudi Arabia: An online-based cross-sectional survey. *Medicine* **2024**, *103*, e37861. [CrossRef]
21. Myer, G.D.; Paterno, M.V.; Ford, K.R.; Quatman, C.E.; Hewett, T.E. Rehabilitation after anterior cruciate ligament reconstruction: Criteria-based progression through the return-to-sport phase. *J. Orthop. Sports Phys. Ther.* **2006**, *36*, 385–402.
22. Alshehri, Y.S.; Aljohani, M.M.; Alzahrani, H.; Alzhrani, M.; Alkhathami, K.M.; Alshahrani, A.; Khaled, O.A. Current rehabilitation practices and return to sports criteria after anterior cruciate ligament reconstruction: A survey of physical therapists in Saudi Arabia. *J. Sport Rehabil.* **2023**, *33*, 114–120.
23. Kotsifaki, R.; Korakakis, V.; King, E.; Barbosa, O.; Maree, D.; Pantouveris, M.; Bjerregaard, A.; Luomajoki, J.; Wilhelmsen, J.; Whiteley, R. Aspetar clinical practice guideline on rehabilitation after anterior cruciate ligament reconstruction. *Br. J. Sports Med.* **2023**, *57*, 500. [CrossRef]
24. Dunphy, E.; Button, K.; Murray, E.; Hamilton, F.L. Beyond guidelines: A qualitative clinical stakeholder study of optimal management of anterior cruciate ligament rehabilitation. *Musculoskelet. Care* **2023**, *21*, 117–129.
25. Piussi, R.; Krupic, F.; Senorski, C.; Svantesson, E.; Sundemo, D.; Johnson, U.; Hamrin Senorski, E. Psychological impairments after ACL injury–Do we know what we are addressing? Experiences from sports physical therapists. *Scand. J. Med. Sci. Sports* **2021**, *31*, 1508–1517. [CrossRef]
26. Filbay, S.R.; Skou, S.T.; Bullock, G.S.; Le, C.Y.; Räisänen, A.M.; Toomey, C.; Ezzat, A.M.; Hayden, A.; Culvenor, A.G.; Whittaker, J.L.; et al. Long-term quality of life, work limitation, physical activity, economic cost and disease burden following ACL and meniscal injury: A systematic review and meta-analysis for the OPTIKNEE consensus. *Br. J. Sports Med.* **2022**, *56*, 1465–1474. [CrossRef]
27. Filbay, S.R.; Grindem, H. Evidence-based recommendations for the management of anterior cruciate ligament (ACL) rupture. *Best Pract. Res. Clin. Rheumatol.* **2019**, *33*, 33–47.
28. Crawford, T.; Parsons, J.; Webber, S.; Fricke, M.; Thille, P. Strategies to Increase Access to Outpatient Physiotherapy Services: A Scoping Review. *Physiother Can.* **2022**, *74*, 197–207. [CrossRef]
29. Alfaqeeh, G.; Cook, E.J.; Randhawa, G.; Ali, N. Access and utilisation of primary health care services comparing urban and rural areas of Riyadh Providence, Kingdom of Saudi Arabia. *BMC Health Serv. Res.* **2017**, *17*, 106. [CrossRef]
30. Tong, A.; Sainsbury, P.; Craig, J. Consolidated criteria for reporting qualitative research (COREQ): A 32-item checklist for interviews and focus groups. *Int. J. Qual. Health Care* **2007**, *19*, 349–357. [CrossRef]
31. Moser, A.; Korstjens, I. Series: Practical guidance to qualitative research. Part 3: Sampling, data collection and analysis. *Eur. J. Gen. Pract.* **2018**, *24*, 9–18. [CrossRef]
32. Alanazi, S.A.; Vicenzino, B.; Maclachlan, L.R.; Smith, M.D. "It's like a nail being driven in the ankle": A qualitative study of individuals' lived experiences to inform a core domain set for ankle osteoarthritis. *Musculoskelet. Sci. Pract.* **2023**, *66*, 102813. [CrossRef]
33. Alanazi, S.A.; Vicenzino, B.; Smith, M.D. Concerns beyond ankle symptoms predominate healthcare professionals' views of patients with ankle osteoarthritis: A qualitative study. *Musculoskelet. Sci. Pract.* **2024**, *72*, 102946. [CrossRef]
34. Alamrani, S.; Gardner, A.; Falla, D.; Russell, E.; Rushton, A.B.; Heneghan, N.R. Outcome measures for young people with adolescent idiopathic scoliosis: A qualitative exploration of healthcare professionals' perceptions and practices. *PLoS ONE* **2024**, *19*, e0297339. [CrossRef]

35. Alamrani, S.; Gardner, A.; Falla, D.; Russell, E.; Rushton, A.B.; Heneghan, N.R. Content validity of the Scoliosis Research Society questionnaire (SRS-22r): A qualitative concept elicitation study. *PLoS ONE* **2023**, *18*, e0285538. [CrossRef]
36. Braun, V.; Clarke, V. Using thematic analysis in psychology. *Qual. Res. Psychol.* **2006**, *3*, 77–101. [CrossRef]
37. Braun, V.; Clarke, V. Reflecting on reflexive thematic analysis. *Qual. Res. Sport Exerc. Health* **2019**, *11*, 589–597. [CrossRef]
38. Braun, V.; Clarke, V. *Thematic Analysis*; American Psychological Association: Washington, DC, USA, 2012.
39. Mays, N.; Pope, C. Qualitative research in health care. Assessing quality in qualitative research. *BMJ* **2000**, *320*, 50–52. [CrossRef]
40. Pezalla, A.E.; Pettigrew, J.; Miller-Day, M. Researching the researcher-as-instrument: An exercise in interviewer self-reflexivity. *Qual. Res.* **2012**, *12*, 165–185. [CrossRef]
41. Fältström, A.; Gustafsson, T.; Wärnsberg, N.; Sonesson, S.; Hermansen, A. Athletes' perspectives on return to sport after anterior cruciate ligament reconstruction and their strategies to reduce reinjury risk: A qualitative interview study. *BMC Sports Sci. Med. Rehabil.* **2024**, *16*, 131. [CrossRef]
42. Piussi, R.; Brandt, E.; Johansson, A.; Snaebjörnsson, T.; Thomeé, R.; Samuelsson, K.; Hamrin Senorski, E. The Patient-Physiotherapist Tango: A Personalized Approach to ACL Recovery–A Qualitative Interview Study. *Int. J. Sports Phys. Ther.* **2024**, *19*, 1589–1599.
43. Clement, D.; Arvinen-Barrow, M.; Fetty, T. Psychosocial responses during different phases of sport-injury rehabilitation: A qualitative study. *J. Athl. Train.* **2015**, *50*, 95–104. [CrossRef]
44. Liew, B.X.W.; Feller, J.A.; Webster, K.E. Understanding the psychological mechanisms of return to sports readiness after anterior cruciate ligament reconstruction. *PLoS ONE* **2022**, *17*, e0266029.
45. Slater, D.; Kvist, J.; Ardern, C.L. Biopsychosocial Factors Associated with Return to Preinjury Sport After ACL Injury Treated Without Reconstruction: NACOX Cohort Study 12-Month Follow-up. *Sports Health* **2023**, *15*, 176–184.
46. Kaye, J.A.; Spence, D.; Alexanders, J. Using a Biopsychosocial Approach Within ACL Rehabilitation: An Exploration of Student Physiotherapists' Perceptions and Experiences. *Physiother Theory Pract.* **2022**, *38*, 1718–1730.
47. Truong, L.K.; Mosewich, A.D.; Holt, C.J.; Le, C.Y.; Miciak, M.; Whittaker, J.L. Psychological, social and contextual factors across recovery stages following a sport-related knee injury: A scoping review. *Br. J. Sports Med.* **2020**, *54*, 1149–1156. [CrossRef]
48. Hsu, C.J.; Meierbachtol, A.; George, S.Z.; Chmielewski, T.L. Fear of Reinjury in Athletes. *Sports Health* **2017**, *9*, 162–167.
49. Bullock, G.S.; Sell, T.C.; Zarega, R.; Reiter, C.; King, V.; Wrona, H.; Mills, N.; Ganderton, C.; Duhig, S.; Räisäsen, A.; et al. Kinesiophobia, Knee Self-Efficacy, and Fear Avoidance Beliefs in People with ACL Injury: A Systematic Review and Meta-Analysis. *Sports Med.* **2022**, *52*, 3001–3019. [CrossRef]
50. Xiao, M.; van Niekerk, M.; Trivedi, N.N.; Hwang, C.E.; Sherman, S.L.; Safran, M.R.; Abrams, G.D. Patients Who Return to Sport After Primary Anterior Cruciate Ligament Reconstruction Have Significantly Higher Psychological Readiness: A Systematic Review and Meta-analysis of 3744 Patients. *Am. J. Sports Med.* **2023**, *51*, 2774–2783.
51. Sell, T.C.; Zerega, R.; King, V.; Reiter, C.R.; Wrona, H.; Bullock, G.S.; Mills, N.; Räisänen, A.; Ledbetter, L.; Collins, G.S.; et al. Anterior Cruciate Ligament Return to Sport after Injury Scale (ACL-RSI) Scores over Time After Anterior Cruciate Ligament Reconstruction: A Systematic Review with Meta-analysis. *Sports Med. Open* **2024**, *10*, 49.
52. Larson, D.; Rohrberg, J.; Lorenz, D.; Clark, N. Administering the ACL-RSI Before or After ACL Functional Testing: Does It Matter? *Int. J. Sports Phys. Ther.* **2025**, *20*, 770–778. [CrossRef] [PubMed]
53. Little, C.; Lavender, A.P.; Starcevich, C.; Mesagno, C.; Mitchell, T.; Whiteley, R.; Bakhshayesh, H.; Beales, D. Understanding Fear after an Anterior Cruciate Ligament Injury: A Qualitative Thematic Analysis Using the Common-Sense Model. *Int. J. Environ. Res. Public Health* **2023**, *20*, 2920. [CrossRef]
54. Zadro, J.R.; Pappas, E. Time for a Different Approach to Anterior Cruciate Ligament Injuries: Educate and Create Realistic Expectations. *Sports Med.* **2019**, *49*, 357–363. [CrossRef]
55. Walker, A.; Hing, W.; Lorimer, A. The Influence, Barriers to and Facilitators of Anterior Cruciate Ligament Rehabilitation Adherence and Participation: A Scoping Review. *Sports Med. Open* **2020**, *6*, 32. [CrossRef]
56. Fang, C.J.; Miller, J.A.; Yergensen, C.J.; Hall, M., Jr.; Kanhere, A.P.; Vera, A.M.; Bratton, A. Racial/Ethnic Disparities Exist Among Patients Who Undergo Anterior Cruciate Ligament Reconstruction in Socioeconomic Status, Perception of Health Status and Literacy. *Arthrosc. Sports Med. Rehabil.* **2025**, *7*, 101000. [CrossRef]
57. Walker, A.; Hing, W.; Gough, S.; Lorimer, A. 'Such a massive part of rehab is between the ears'; barriers to and facilitators of anterior cruciate ligament reconstruction rehabilitation: A qualitative focus group analysis. *BMC Sports Sci. Med. Rehabil.* **2022**, *14*, 106. [CrossRef]
58. van Melick, N.; Dietvorst, M.; van Oort, M.; Claessens, R.L.A.; Janssen, R.P.A.; Bogie, R.; Claussen, W.; Greenberg, E.M.; Grindem, H.; Kearney, S.; et al. Anterior Cruciate Ligament Rehabilitation for the 10- to 18-Year-Old Adolescent Athlete: Practice Guidelines Based on International Delphi Consensus. *Orthop. J. Sports Med.* **2023**, *11*, 23259671231172454. [CrossRef]
59. Simonsson, R.; Sundberg, A.; Piussi, R.; Högberg, J.; Senorski, C.; Thomeé, R.; Samuelsson, K.; Della Villa, F.; Hamrin Senorski, E. Questioning the rules of engagement: A critical analysis of the use of limb symmetry index for safe return to sport after anterior cruciate ligament reconstruction. *Br. J. Sports Med.* **2025**, *59*, 376–384. [CrossRef]

60. Weber, M.; Müller, M.; Mathieu-Kälin, M.; Caminada, S.; Häberli, M.; Baur, H. Evaluation of hop test movement quality to enhance return to sport testing. A cross-sectional study. *Front. Sports Act. Living* **2024**, *6*, 1305817. [CrossRef] [PubMed]
61. Welling, W. Return to sports after an ACL reconstruction in 2024–A glass half full? A narrative review. *Phys. Ther. Sport* **2024**, *67*, 141–148. [CrossRef] [PubMed]
62. Cavanaugh, J.T.; Powers, M. ACL Rehabilitation Progression: Where Are We Now? *Curr. Rev. Musculoskelet. Med.* **2017**, *10*, 289–296. [CrossRef] [PubMed]
63. Joreitz, R.; Lynch, A.; Popchak, A.; Irrgang, J. Criterion-Based Rehabilitation Program with Return to Sport Testing Following Acl Reconstruction: A Case Series. *Int. J. Sports Phys. Ther.* **2020**, *15*, 1151–1173. [CrossRef] [PubMed]

Journal of
Clinical Medicine

MDPI

Article

Can PRP Enhance Hamstring Recovery Post-ACL Reconstruction? Retrospective Insights from Non-Professional Athletes

Roxana Mihaela Munteanu [1,2,3], Andrei Marian Feier [4,5,*], Bogdan Voicu [2], Arpad Solyom [3,6], Pia Simona Făgăraş [2] and Tudor Sorin Pop [4,5]

1 Doctoral School, George Emil Palade University of Medicine, Pharmacy, Science, and Technology of Targu Mures, 540142 Targu Mures, Romania; roxana-mihaela.munteanu@umfst.ro
2 Department M2 Functional and Complementary Sciences, Epidemiology, Ethics and Socio-Human Sciences, George Emil Palade University of Medicine, Pharmacy, Science, and Technology of Targu Mures, 540139 Targu Mures, Romania; drbogdanv@gmail.com (B.V.)
3 OKF Medical Center, 540139 Targu Mures, Romania; arpad.solyom@umfst.ro
4 Department M4 Clinical Sciences, Orthopedics and Traumatology I, George Emil Palade University of Medicine, Pharmacy, Science, and Technology of Targu Mures, 540139 Targu Mures, Romania; tudor.pop@umfst.ro
5 Department of Orthopaedics and Traumatology, Clinical County Hospital of Mureș, 540139 Targu Mures, Romania
6 Department M3 Clinical Sciences, Orthopedics and Traumatology II, George Emil Palade University of Medicine, Pharmacy, Science, and Technology of Targu Mures, 540139 Targu Mures, Romania
* Correspondence: andrei.feier@umfst.ro

Abstract

Background and Objectives: Hamstring strength deficits are common after ACL reconstruction and may impair stability and increase reinjury risk. Despite structured rehabilitation, early postoperative asymmetries frequently persist. Platelet-rich plasma (PRP) has emerged as a potential biologic adjunct that may enhance tissue healing and facilitate muscle strength recovery. This study aimed to evaluate the efficacy of intra-articular PRP injections on hamstring strength restoration in non-professional athletes undergoing ACLR. **Materials and Methods**: This retrospective cohort study analyzed 68 non-professional athletes who underwent primary ACLR between 2020 and 2024. Participants followed a standardized, phase-appropriate rehabilitation program and were allocated to either a PRP group (n = 34; five intra-articular PRP injections every 4 weeks starting at week 4 postoperatively) or a control group (n = 34; rehabilitation alone). Data were analyzed with linear mixed-effects models to examine group, time, and group-by-time interactions. **Results**: Both groups improved over time, but PRP influenced faster hamstring strength recovery and greater symmetry. At 20 weeks, the PRP group achieved higher concentric strength (15.6 ± 4.3 vs. 13.6 ± 3.5; $p = 0.040$) and markedly reduced asymmetry (isometric: –1.1 vs. 0.6; $p < 0.001$; concentric: –0.6 vs. 1.9; $p < 0.001$). **Conclusions**: The addition of serial PRP injections to a structured rehabilitation protocol after ACLR influenced faster hamstring strength recovery and improved interlimb symmetry compared to rehabilitation alone. These findings suggest that PRP may serve as a potential biologic adjunct to optimize postoperative outcomes and facilitate a safer return to sport in non-professional athletes.

Keywords: anterior cruciate ligament reconstruction; hamstring recovery; platelet-rich plasma; muscle strength; rehabilitation

1. Introduction

Anterior cruciate ligament reconstruction (ACLR) is widely performed in active individuals, yet postoperative deficits in hamstring strength remain a persistent challenge, particularly when hamstring autografts are used [1–3]. Hamstring function plays an important role in lower-limb stability, gait control, and athletic performance, and incomplete recovery affects biomechanics, reduced dynamic stability, and an increased risk of reinjury during return-to-sport activities [4,5]. Despite structured rehabilitation protocols, many patients experience prolonged or incomplete restoration of knee flexor strength, emphasizing the need for strategies that may optimize postoperative muscle recovery [6].

Restoration of hamstring strength is clinically relevant not only for performance but also for joint protection [4]. The hamstrings act as dynamic synergists of the ACL by limiting anterior tibial translation, and strength deficits—especially at deeper flexion angles—may persist long after surgery [7]. Current rehabilitation approaches target multiple strength qualities, including maximal, eccentric, and multiplanar capacity [4], yet asymmetries frequently remain during the early return-to-sport phase [8]. These deficits can affect the quadriceps-to-hamstring (Q/H) strength ratio, an important marker of neuromuscular readiness and reinjury risk [9].

Given these challenges, biologic augmentation has been explored as a potential adjunct to enhance postoperative recovery [10]. Platelet-rich plasma (PRP) is an autologous concentrate rich in growth factors such as PDGF, TGF-β, VEGF, and IGF-I, ref. [11] which may modulate inflammation, support tissue remodeling, and influence the intra-articular environment after ACLR [12].

Although PRP has demonstrated potential benefits in conditions such as tendinopathy [13], rotator cuff repair [14], and osteoarthritis [15], its role in ACL reconstruction remains unclear. Evidence across studies is heterogeneous: some report improvements in pain or graft maturation [16], whereas others—including recent randomized clinical trials—find no significant clinical benefit in postoperative function or knee symptoms [17].

Importantly, few studies have examined whether intra-articular PRP may influence postoperative hamstring muscle recovery specifically [17,18].

While PRP has been proposed to modulate neuromuscular inhibition and periarticular tissue healing, its effect on objective strength outcomes after ACLR is not well established, and data regarding interlimb strength symmetry remain limited [16]. Thus, the clinical relevance of PRP in supporting hamstring strength restoration during rehabilitation has not been adequately investigated [19].

To address this gap, the present retrospective cohort study evaluated whether serial intra-articular PRP injections, administered in conjunction with a standardized postoperative rehabilitation program, were associated with improved hamstring strength recovery and interlimb symmetry in non-professional athletes following ACLR.

2. Materials and Methods

2.1. Study Design

This retrospective cohort study included 68 subjects who underwent ACLR between 2020 and 2024. Participants were divided into two groups: a treatment group that followed a standardized rehabilitation protocol and received PRP infiltrations, and a control group that followed the same protocol without PRP administration. Because this was a retrospective study, group allocation was not randomized. Patients were assigned to the PRP or control group based on the treatment they had already received as part of routine clinical practice. All eligible patients were enrolled consecutively according to the order of presentation, ensuring naturalistic sampling without investigator influence. Controls were drawn from the same clinical population and met the same inclusion criteria as the PRP group. The inclusion criteria were patients who underwent primary ACL reconstruction between 2020 and 2024, non-professional (amateur) athletes engaged in regular physical activity, no concomitant ligament injuries (isolated ACL tear). Exclusion criteria included the presence of cardiovascular or musculoskeletal disorders, use of corticosteroid therapy, or occurrence of postoperative injuries during the rehabilitation period. The exclusion criteria were the missing data on muscle strength. Although strict matching was not performed, the two groups were comparable in terms of age, sex, graft type, and baseline hamstring strength. Collected data included patient age, sex, body mass index (BMI), graft type, general health status, and current medication.

A total of 82 patients who underwent primary ACL reconstruction were screened for eligibility. Fourteen patients were excluded due to incomplete rehabilitation data (n = 8), concomitant meniscal repair requiring restricted loading (n = 4), or missing follow-up strength measurements (n = 2). The remaining 68 patients were included in the analysis: 34 who received PRP injections in addition to rehabilitation and 34 who underwent standard rehabilitation only.

A detailed flow diagram illustrating patient inclusion, exclusion, and follow-up is provided in Figure 1.

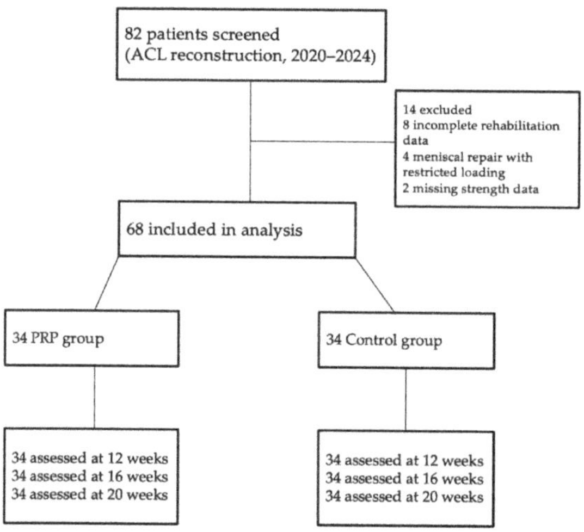

Figure 1. STROBE flow diagram of patient selection and follow-up. Flow of participants from initial screening through inclusion, allocation to PRP or control groups, and assessment at each follow-up point, including reasons for exclusion and missing data.

This retrospective cohort study included consecutively enrolled non-professional athletes who underwent ACL reconstruction at OKF Medical Center Târgu Mures. All eligible patients meeting the inclusion and exclusion criteria were analyzed.

This retrospective study was approved by the Ethics Committee for Scientific Research of the George Emil Palade University of Medicine, Pharmacy, Science and Technology of Târgu Mureș (approval nr. 3562/20 January 2025).

2.2. Rehabilitation Protocol

All participants completed the same standardized rehabilitation program consisting of 3–4 supervised sessions per week. The intervention included progressive phases targeting restoration of knee mobility, neuromuscular activation, progressive strengthening, proprioceptive and balance training, plyometric exercises, activity-specific and sport-specific drills.

Progression was based on predefined clinical criteria (pain < 3/10, full extension, adequate quadriceps control).

Rehabilitation sessions were delivered by licensed physiotherapists. Therapists were not blinded to PRP allocation. Rehabilitation adherence was 100%, with all subjects completing the prescribed sessions.

2.3. PRP Intervention

The experimental group received five intra-articular injections of autologous leukocyte-poor platelet-rich plasma (PRP). Injections were administered at weeks 4, 8, 12, 16, and 20 postoperatively by the orthopedic surgeon. Each injection consisted of 5 mL of P-PRP. The schedule of PRP injections and functional testing sessions is illustrated in Figure 2.

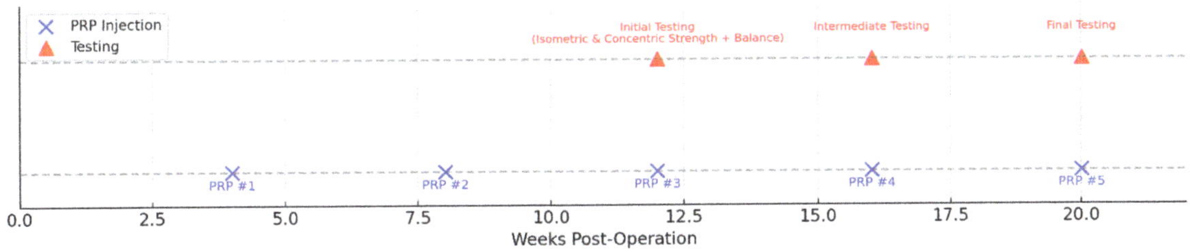

Figure 2. Timeline of PRP injections and outcome assessments following ACLR. Five intra-articular PRP injections were administered at approximately 4, 8, 12, 16, and 20 weeks postoperatively (blue "×"). Functional testing sessions (red triangles) were scheduled at three key phases: Initial Testing (around week 10; isometric and concentric quadriceps and hamstrings strength combined with static balance assessment), Intermediate Testing (around week 15; progressive strength and functional control evaluation), and Final Testing (around week 20; comprehensive return-to-sport assessment). This timeline illustrates the structured integration of biologic augmentation and objective performance monitoring during postoperative rehabilitation.

PRP was prepared using the double-spin protocol described by Dhurat et al. [11]. Centrifugation was performed using a specialized centrifuge (XC SPINPLUS, Shanghai, China) in a two-step (double-spin) process.

A total of 30 mL venous blood was drawn into citrate-dextrose tubes, centrifuged at 1200 rpm for 10 min, followed by a second spin at 3000 rpm for 10 min. This yielded 3–5 mL of leukocyte-poor PRP, injected intra-articularly without exogenous activation.

The use of multiple PRP doses was supported by literature indicating that repeated administrations enhance cumulative biological effects. Tao et al. [20] demonstrated superior outcomes with three sequential injections, while Corsini et al. [21] highlighted the importance of achieving sufficient cumulative platelet dosing for optimal anti-inflammatory and reparative activity.

2.4. Outcome Measures

Primary outcomes included: Maximal isometric hamstring strength, Maximal concentric hamstring strength, Limb strength asymmetry, calculated as:

$$\text{Asymmetry (\%)} = [(\text{Injured limb} - \text{Healthy limb})/\text{Healthy limb}] \times 100.$$

Positive values indicate greater strength in the injured limb, whereas negative values indicate a deficit compared to the healthy limb. These parameters represent surrogate indicators of early functional recovery.

Evaluations were performed at 12, 16, and 20 weeks postoperatively, corresponding to key rehabilitation phases: 12 weeks: early strengthening following graft integration, 16 weeks: advanced neuromuscular training phase, 20 weeks: late-phase functional progression. This timing is supported by prior evidence by San Jose et al., showing persistent hamstring deficits during the first 3–6 postoperative months [22].

2.5. Strength Testing Procedures

Strength assessments were performed using the Kineto Intelligent Load rehabilitation robot. Participants completed a standardized warm-up consisting of 10 min cycling at moderate intensity, open- and closed-chain activation exercises, hamstring-specific drills: leg curls, Romanian deadlifts, hip bridges.

For the Isometric Max Strength Balance Test, the subject was placed in a standing position in front of the device, with ankle cuffs connecting them to the machine. The subject was instructed to perform a knee flexion up to 90 degrees and to hold the position for 5 s, ensuring they exerted maximal force to maintain the flexion. The test was performed once on both the affected and unaffected limb.

For the Concentric Max Strength Balance Test, the subject was also in a standing position, with ankle cuffs, in front of the device, and was asked to perform 5 knee flexions, focusing on the lifting phase, thus emphasizing concentric contraction, using both the affected and unaffected limb.

All evaluations were supervised by the same physiotherapist to ensure consistent technique and avoid compensatory movements.

2.6. Statistical Analysis

Descriptive statistics were calculated for all demographic, clinical, and outcome variables. Continuous variables are reported as mean $\pm$ standard deviation, and categorical variables as counts and percentages. Due to missing data for BMI this parameter was excluded from statistical analysis. Complete case analysis was performed using linear mixed-effects models fitted by Restricted Maximum Likelihood (REML) estimation to account for the longitudinal study design and repeated measures within participants. Patient-specific random intercepts and slopes for time were included to model individual variability in baseline strength and recovery trajectories. Fixed effects included treatment group, time, age, sex, and graft type (hamstring vs. patellar tendon). Primary outcomes were isometric and concentric hamstring strength of the affected limb, while secondary outcomes examined strength asymmetry between healthy and affected limbs. Group-by-time interaction terms were included to test differential recovery rates between treatment arms. Model assumptions were verified through residual diagnostics, and all models achieved successful convergence. Statistical significance was set at $\alpha = 0.05$, and analyses were conducted using Python's statsmodels package (version 0.14.0). Between-group comparisons at each time point were performed using independent *t*-tests with pooled standard deviations; *p*-values were annotated as ns ($p \geq 0.05$), * ($p < 0.05$), ** ($p < 0.01$), or *** ($p < 0.001$). Since this is a retrospective study, no a priori sample size calculation was conducted, but a post hoc power analysis was performed with G*Power software (University of Düsseldorf, Düsseldorf, Germany, version 3.1.9.7.). The post hoc calculated power ($1 - \beta$) was 0.95 for the REML analysis comparing hamstring force (primary outcome) recovery with an effect size d = 0.41 ($\alpha = 0.05$, two-tailed), measured across 3 timepoints in two groups (n = 34 each). This showed a strong statistical power for detecting group differences caused by PRP intervention. Effect sizes (Cohen's d) were calculated for final assessments to quantify between-group differences as negligible ($|d| < 0.2$), small (0.2–0.5), medium (0.5–0.8), or large (>0.8).

3. Results

The study population comprised 68 participants (50 males, 18 females; age range 18–54 years) with predominantly hamstring autografts (n = 61, 89.7%). The demographic and baseline characteristics of the participants were analyzed (Table 1), and no statistically significant differences were found between the PRP-treated and control groups regarding age, sex distribution, body mass index, or graft source. Both groups were therefore considered homogeneous and comparable for subsequent analyses.

Table 1. Baseline characteristics of the PRP and control groups.

Parameter	Group	Mean	SD	Count/Ratio	Mean Difference	p-Value
Age (years)	Control	31.3	8.6	—	1.2	0.564
	PRP	30.1	8.6	—		
Sex (m/f)	Control	—	—	25/9	0	1.000
	PRP	—	—	25/9		
BMI (kg/m^2)	Control	23.8	0.7	—	−1	0.382
	PRP	24.8	0.6	—		
Graft type (hamstring/patellar)	Control	—	—	30/4	−1/1	0.689
	PRP	—	—	31/3		

All patients were monitored clinically after each PRP injection and during routine rehabilitation visits. No cases of infection, synovitis, or significant joint effusion were observed following any of the five intra-articular PRP injections. Four patients (11.8%) reported mild, transient post-injection pain or swelling lasting less than 48 h, which resolved without medical intervention. No procedure-related complications were recorded.

Linear mixed-effects analysis revealed significant time effects across all models ($p < 0.001$), indicating overall recovery in both treatment groups. Crucially, significant group-by-time interactions were observed for both isometric and concentric strength measures ($p < 0.001$), demonstrating superior recovery rates in the experimental group. The experimental group showed 1.34 units (95% CI: 0.90–1.78) faster isometric strength recovery and 1.61 units (95% CI: 1.15–2.07) faster concentric strength recovery per time point compared to controls. Analysis of strength asymmetry revealed significant group differences, with the experimental group achieving better limb symmetry (isometric asymmetry: $\beta = -0.54$, $p = 0.027$; concentric asymmetry: $\beta = -0.65$, $p = 0.053$). Male participants consistently demonstrated higher absolute strength values across all measures (effect size: 2.0–5.0 units, $p < 0.001$), while age and graft type did not affect the outcomes (all $p > 0.05$). The affected limb strength improved by 2.3–3.0 units per time point, while strength asymmetry decreased by 1.9–2.4 units per time point, indicating successful rehabilitation progress. All mixed-effects models converged successfully with log-likelihood values ranging from −350.4 to −392.9, and residual diagnostics confirmed appropriate model assumptions.

Statistical analysis revealed that concentric strength showed a statistically significant between-group difference at the final assessment, with the experimental group achieving 15.62 ± 4.30 units versus 13.62 ± 3.54 units in the control group ($p = 0.040$). Isometric strength exhibited a strong trend toward significance at the final time point, with means of 16.29 ± 4.32 versus 14.50 ± 4.42 ($p = 0.097$) (Figure 3). Effect sizes for these primary outcomes ranged from small to medium (Cohen's d = 0.41–0.51).

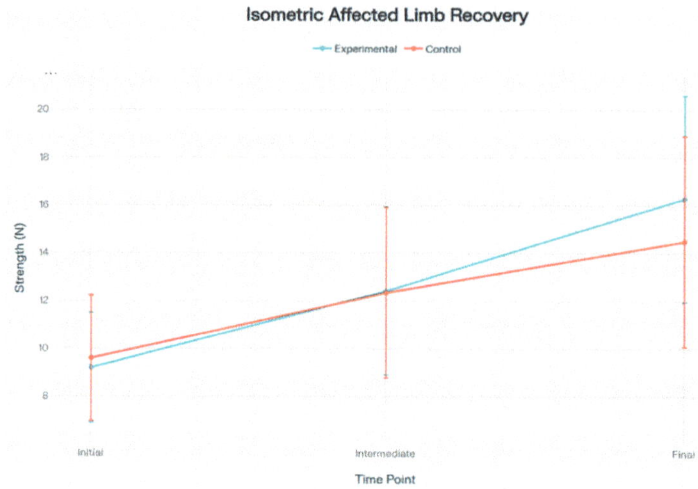

(A)

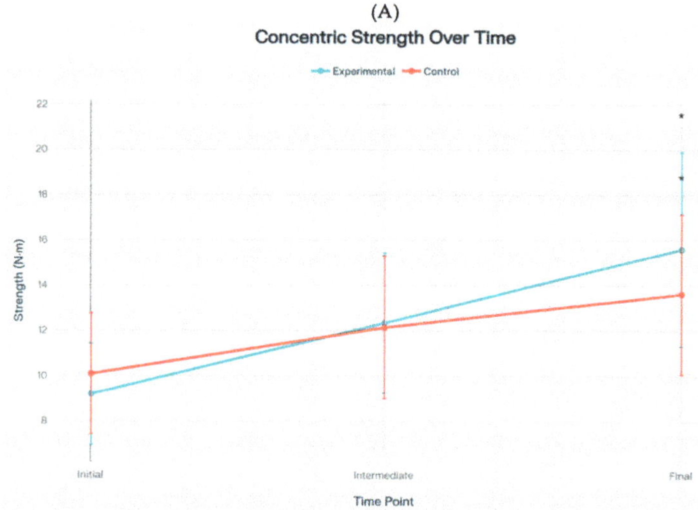

(B)

Figure 3. Recovery of hamstring strength in the affected limb over time. (**A**) Isometric strength measurements at initial, intermediate, and final assessments (**B**) Concentric strength measurements at initial, intermediate, and final assessments. Data presented as mean ± standard deviation (n = 34 per group). Statistical comparisons between groups at each time point: ns = non-significant, * $p < 0.05$.

However, both isometric and concentric asymmetry measures demonstrated statistically significant group differences at the final assessment ($p < 0.001$). The PRP group showed near-zero or slightly negative asymmetry values—indicating that the operated limb approached or marginally exceeded the contralateral limb—with isometric asymmetry of −1.13 ± 0.96 versus 0.64 ± 0.76, and concentric asymmetry of −0.57 ± 1.08 versus 1.93 ± 1.75 (Figure 3). These asymmetry outcomes were associated with large effect sizes (Cohen's d = −1.72 to −2.04) (Figure 4). The effect size analysis demonstrated small to medium differences in affected limb strength, while asymmetry outcomes showed large effect sizes in the experimental group (Figure 5).

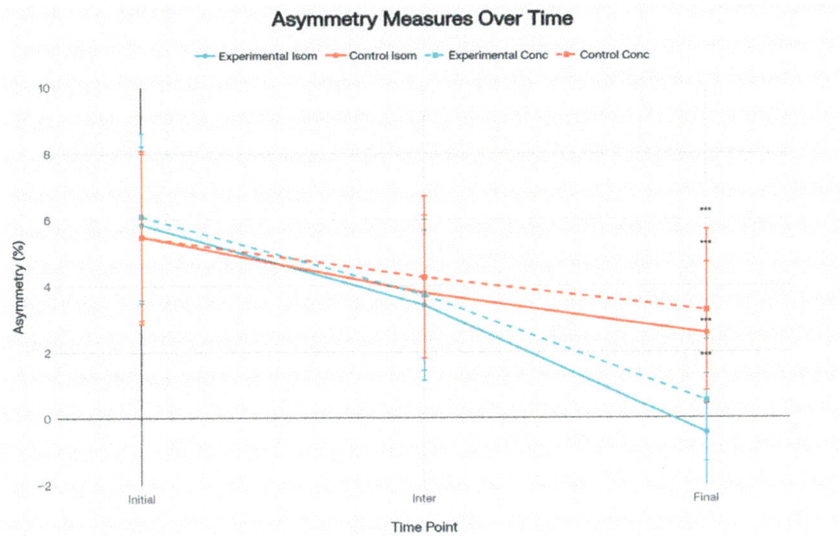

Figure 4. Recovery of strength symmetry between limbs over time. Isometric asymmetry is represented by solid lines, and concentric asymmetry by dashed lines. The control group is shown in red, and the PRP group in blue. Lower values indicate better interlimb symmetry. Data are presented as mean ± SD. The PRP group demonstrated statistically significant but moderate improvements in symmetry at the final assessment for both isometric ($p < 0.001$) and concentric ($p < 0.001$) measures. Negative values in the PRP group indicate that the operated limb achieved strength levels slightly exceeding those of the contralateral limb. *** indicates a statistically significant difference between groups ($p < 0.0002$).

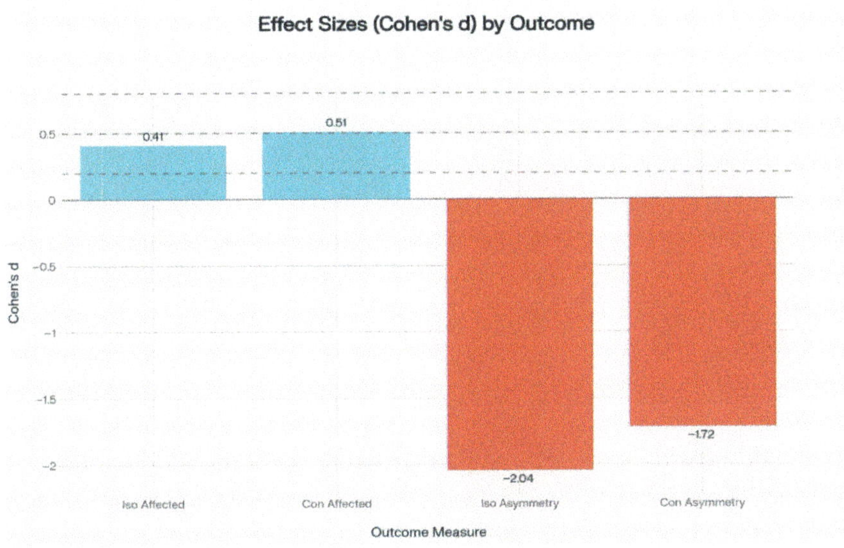

Figure 5. Effect sizes (Cohen's d) comparing experimental vs. control groups at final assessment. Primary outcomes (affected limb strength) showed small to medium effect sizes, while secondary outcomes (asymmetry measures) demonstrated large effect sizes favoring the experimental intervention. Reference lines indicate effect size thresholds: small (0.2), medium (0.5), and large (0.8).

4. Discussion

4.1. Main Findings

The main finding of this study was that the addition of PRP to a standardized postoperative rehabilitation program influenced statistically significant but modest improvements in hamstring strength recovery and interlimb symmetry in non-professional athletes after ACLR. Participants receiving PRP showed faster strength gains and a more complete restoration of symmetry compared with those undergoing rehabilitation alone, independent of age, sex, or graft type.

While our findings suggest that PRP influences hamstring strength recovery, the effect size was modest, and the results should be interpreted as exploratory. Further prospective, randomized studies are needed to confirm these observations.

Given the retrospective nature of this study, causality cannot be established, and the observed effects should be interpreted with caution.

4.2. Comparison with Existing Literature

Persistent hamstring strength deficits after ACLR are well documented. A previous review, by Thomas et al. [2] have reported that residual hamstring strength deficits ACLR can persist in 9–27% of patients even three years postoperatively. In contrast, our PRP-treated cohort achieved near-complete restoration of hamstring strength and interlimb symmetry within 20 weeks, suggesting that adjunctive biologic stimulation may accelerate muscle recovery and potentially reduce the long-term persistence of strength deficits described in the literature.

Recent longitudinal work by Datta et al. [23] demonstrated that hamstring strength and functional parameters improve progressively up to 18 months after ACLR with semitendinosus–gracilis autografts, reflecting the natural, gradual course of recovery. In our cohort, the addition of platelet-rich plasma to a standardized rehabilitation program appeared to accelerate this trajectory, allowing patients to achieve near-complete hamstring strength restoration and interlimb symmetry within 20 weeks. These findings suggest that biologic augmentation may shorten the otherwise prolonged recovery window described in conventional rehabilitation pathways.

Desouza et al. [24] conducted a randomized controlled trial on grade 2 hamstring injuries and demonstrated that PRP can accelerate return-to-sport time and promote faster tissue healing in acute muscle damage. Even though our investigation focused on post-ACLR hamstring recovery rather than acute injuries, the accelerated restoration of strength and improved limb symmetry observed in our PRP-treated group parallels the enhanced healing reported in traumatic hamstring tears, supporting the notion that PRP may facilitate muscle regeneration and functional recovery across different clinical contexts.

While some studies have suggested potential benefits of intra-articular PRP administration on tissue healing or early strength recovery after ACL reconstruction, several systematic reviews and retrospective analyses have failed to demonstrate consistent or clinically meaningful effects. For instance, a comprehensive meta-analysis on the clinical use of PRP in knee disorders concluded that, among the available evidence, ACL reconstruction represents the only area showing no significant differences between PRP-treated and control groups, indicating that PRP has not yet been proven beneficial in this context [18]. These contrasting results highlight the substantial heterogeneity in PRP preparation methods, platelet and leukocyte concentrations, and injection protocols, which may account for the variability in clinical outcomes across studies.

Although a recent randomized controlled trial investigating intra-articular PRP after ACLR reported no significant improvements in patient-reported knee symptoms or overall joint function at 12 months [17], our study specifically targeted objective hamstring strength recovery and demonstrated meaningful benefits in both strength restoration and limb symmetry. This suggests that PRP's impact may be more readily detectable in direct muscle performance metrics than in broader subjective functional scores.

4.3. Potential Mechanism

Recent evidence suggests that intra-articular PRP may influence not only graft healing and joint homeostasis but also neuromuscular recovery through its biological effects on the intra-articular environment. Gill et al. report that PRP contains high concentrations of growth factors such as PDGF, TGF-β, VEGF, and IGF-1, which exert potent anti inflammatory and angiogenic effects that enhance tissue repair and modulate neural pathways involved in arthrogenic muscle inhibition (AMI). By reducing synovial inflammation and improving the biochemical milieu around the reconstructed ACL, PRP may help restore normal afferent input from joint receptors, thereby facilitating better muscle activation patterns and faster strength recovery [25].

Although PRP was administered intra-articularly, its potential influence on periarticular muscle recovery may be mediated by indirect mechanisms. Andia et al. showed that intra-articular PRP can reduce local inflammation and modulate cytokine activity within the joint, which can decrease arthrogenic muscle inhibition—an important factor limiting postoperative muscle activation. Moreover, growth factors released from the synovial environment may exert paracrine effects on periarticular tissues, facilitating neuromuscular recovery [13].

Experimental evidence also supports a neurotrophic mechanism: combined PRP and brain-derived neurotrophic factor (BDNF) treatments have been shown to enhance neural regeneration and improve locomotor performance in animal models [26]. In line with these findings, PRP has been proposed as a modulator of joint neurobiology, contributing to reduced pain and improved proprioception.

These biological mechanisms may partly explain our findings, where participants receiving serial intra-articular PRP injections achieved faster restoration of hamstring strength and improved inter-limb symmetry at 20 weeks.

4.4. Limitations

This study has several limitations. First, its retrospective design and relatively small sample size (n = 68) limit causal inference, and the absence of randomization or blinding introduces a risk of selection and performance bias, although groups were comparable at baseline and followed the same rehabilitation protocol. The 20-week follow-up captures only short-term recovery, without information on long-term strength, functional outcomes, or reinjury risk. Additionally, potential confounders such as individual variations in muscle mass, baseline performance, or subtle differences in rehabilitation execution could not be fully controlled.

A further limitation concerns graft type distribution: only a small number of participants received patellar tendon autografts, preventing a reliable analysis of potential PRP-by-graft-type interactions and reducing statistical power for subgroup comparisons. Muscle strength assessments were performed using the Kineo Intelligent Load system rather than a validated isokinetic dynamometer; because reliability metrics (ICC, SEM, MDC) for our specific test protocol are not yet established, the findings should be interpreted as device-specific and may not be directly generalizable to other measurement systems.

Limb dominance was not recorded, which may influence interlimb comparisons, particularly in cases where the injured limb exceeded the contralateral limb in strength. Finally, no imaging or biomarker assessments were available to objectively verify intra-articular or musculotendinous effects of PRP, meaning the proposed biological mechanisms remain hypothetical.

Because this was a retrospective study, an immortal time bias may be present. Although all patients in the PRP group received the injection at the same standardized postoperative time point, there is an inherent period between surgery and the PRP administration during which patients had to remain event-free to be eligible for treatment. This time-related bias should be considered when interpreting the results.

Future research should include randomized controlled trials with larger samples, standardized PRP preparation protocols, validated strength testing procedures, and extended follow-up to determine the long-term clinical relevance of biologic augmentation after ACL reconstruction.

5. Conclusions

The experimental rehabilitation protocol incorporating PRP was associated with modest but statistically significant improvements in both primary and secondary outcomes, including enhanced interlimb symmetry (the most clinically relevant parameter), and a trend toward greater strength restoration in the operated limb compared with the contralateral side. Improvements were observed consistently across both isometric and concentric muscle actions, suggesting a potential supportive role of PRP during early postoperative rehabilitation. These superior outcomes were observed exclusively in the group that received PRP, whereas the control group following rehabilitation alone did not demonstrate comparable improvements.

Author Contributions: Conceptualization, R.M.M. and T.S.P.; methodology, R.M.M. and A.M.F.; software, P.S.F.; validation, B.V., T.S.P. and A.S.; formal analysis, R.M.M. and P.S.F.; investigation, R.M.M. and A.M.F.; resources, B.V. and A.S.; data curation, R.M.M. and P.S.F.; writing—original draft preparation, R.M.M. and A.M.F.; writing—review and editing, T.S.P.; visualization, T.S.P., B.V. and A.S.; supervision, T.S.P. and A.M.F.; project administration, R.M.M. and T.S.P. All authors have read and agreed to the published version of the manuscript.

Funding: This research received no external funding.

Institutional Review Board Statement: The study was conducted in accordance with the Declaration of Helsinki and approved by the Institutional Review Board (or Ethics Committee) of George Emil Palade University of Medicine, Pharmacy, Science and Technology of Târgu Mures, (nr. 3562, date 20 January 2025) for studies involving humans.

Informed Consent Statement: Informed consent was obtained from all subjects involved in the study. Written informed consent has been obtained from the patient(s) to publish this paper.

Data Availability Statement: The data presented in this study are available on request from the corresponding author.

Acknowledgments: We are grateful for the support offered by the OKF Medical Center in Târgu Mures team.

Conflicts of Interest: The authors declare no conflicts of interest.

References

1. Cimino, F.; Volk, B.S.; Setter, D. Anterior cruciate ligament injury: Diagnosis, management, and prevention. *Am. Fam. Physician* **2010**, *82*, 917–922. [PubMed]
2. Thomas, A.C.; Villwock, M.; Wojtys, E.M.; Palmieri-Smith, R.M. Lower extremity muscle strength after anterior cruciate ligament injury and reconstruction. *J. Athl. Train.* **2013**, *48*, 610–620. [CrossRef]

3. Lee, O.S.; Lee, Y.S. Changes in hamstring strength after anterior cruciate ligament reconstruction with hamstring autograft and posterior cruciate ligament reconstruction with tibialis allograft. *Knee Surg. Relat. Res.* **2020**, *32*, 27. [CrossRef]
4. Buckthorpe, M.; Danelon, F.; La Rosa, G.; Nanni, G.; Stride, M.; Della Villa, F. Recommendations for Hamstring Function Recovery After ACL Reconstruction. *Sports Med.* **2021**, *51*, 607–624. [CrossRef] [PubMed]
5. Georgoulis, A.D.; Ristanis, S.; Moraiti, C.O.; Paschos, N.; Zampeli, F.; Xergia, S.; Georgiou, S.; Patras, K.; Vasiliadis, H.S.; Mitsionis, G. ACL injury and reconstruction: Clinical related in vivo biomechanics. *Orthop. Traumatol. Surg. Res.* **2010**, *96*, S119–S128. [CrossRef]
6. Suydam, S.M.; Cortes, D.H.; Axe, M.J.; Snyder-Mackler, L.; Buchanan, T.S. Semitendinosus Tendon for ACL Reconstruction: Regrowth and Mechanical Property Recovery. *Orthop. J. Sports Med.* **2017**, *5*, 2325967117712944. [CrossRef]
7. Bouzekraoui Alaoui, I.; Moiroux-Sahraoui, A.; Mazeas, J.; Kakavas, G.; Biały, M.; Douryang, M.; Forelli, F. Impact of Hamstring Graft on Hamstring Peak Torque and Maximum Effective Angle After Anterior Cruciate Ligament Reconstruction: An Exploratory and Preliminary Study. *Bioengineering* **2025**, *12*, 465. [CrossRef]
8. Grindem, H.; Snyder-Mackler, L.; Moksnes, H.; Engebretsen, L.; Risberg, M.A. Simple decision rules can reduce reinjury risk by 84% after ACL reconstruction: The Delaware-Oslo ACL cohort study. *Br. J. Sports Med.* **2016**, *50*, 804–808. [CrossRef] [PubMed]
9. van Dyk, N.; Bahr, R.; Whiteley, R.; Tol, J.L.; Kumar, B.D.; Hamilton, B.; Farooq, A.; Witvrouw, E. Hamstring and Quadriceps Isokinetic Strength Deficits Are Weak Risk Factors for Hamstring Strain Injuries: A 4-Year Cohort Study. *Am. J. Sports Med.* **2016**, *44*, 1789–1795. [CrossRef]
10. Dallo, I.; Chahla, J.; Mitchell, J.J.; Pascual-Garrido, C.; Feagin, J.A.; LaPrade, R.F. Biologic Approaches for the Treatment of Partial Tears of the Anterior Cruciate Ligament: A Current Concepts Review. *Orthop. J. Sports Med.* **2017**, *5*, 2325967116681724. [CrossRef] [PubMed]
11. Dhurat, R.; Sukesh, M. Principles and Methods of Preparation of Platelet-Rich Plasma: A Review and Author's Perspective. *J. Cutan. Aesthetic Surg.* **2014**, *7*, 189–197. [CrossRef]
12. Kon, E.; Di Matteo, B.; Altomare, D.; Iacono, F.; Kurpyakov, A.; Lychagin, A.; Timashev, P.; Kalinsky, E.; Lipina, M. Biologic agents to optimize outcomes following ACL repair and reconstruction: A systematic review of clinical evidence. *J. Orthop. Res.* **2022**, *40*, 10–28. [CrossRef]
13. Andia, I.; Maffulli, N. Platelet-rich plasma for muscle injury and tendinopathy. *Sports Med. Arthrosc. Rev.* **2013**, *21*, 191–198. [CrossRef]
14. Castricini, R.; Longo, U.G.; De Benedetto, M.; Panfoli, N.; Pirani, P.; Zini, R.; Maffulli, N.; Denaro, V. Platelet-rich plasma augmentation for arthroscopic rotator cuff repair: A randomized controlled trial. *Am. J. Sports Med.* **2011**, *39*, 258–265. [CrossRef]
15. Meheux, C.J.; McCulloch, P.C.; Lintner, D.M.; Varner, K.E.; Harris, J.D. Efficacy of Intra-articular Platelet-Rich Plasma Injections in Knee Osteoarthritis: A Systematic Review. *Arthroscopy* **2016**, *32*, 495–505. [CrossRef]
16. Eslami, S.; Fattah, S.; Taher, S.A.; Rezasoltani, Z. Platelet-rich plasma therapy or arthroscopic surgery on repair of anterior cruciate ligament rupture. *Eur. J. Transl. Myol.* **2022**, *32*, 10538. [CrossRef] [PubMed]
17. Ye, Z.; Chen, H.; Qiao, Y.; Wu, C.; Cho, E.; Wu, X.; Li, Z.; Wu, J.; Lu, S.; Xie, G.; et al. Intra-Articular Platelet-Rich Plasma Injection After Anterior Cruciate Ligament Reconstruction: A Randomized Clinical Trial. *JAMA Netw. Open* **2024**, *7*, e2410134. [CrossRef] [PubMed]
18. Trams, E.; Kulinski, K.; Kozar-Kaminska, K.; Pomianowski, S.; Kaminski, R. The Clinical Use of Platelet-Rich Plasma in Knee Disorders and Surgery-A Systematic Review and Meta-Analysis. *Life* **2020**, *10*, 94. [CrossRef] [PubMed]
19. Seijas, R.; Ares, O.; Catala, J.; Alvarez-Diaz, P.; Cusco, X.; Cugat, R. Magnetic resonance imaging evaluation of patellar tendon graft remodelling after anterior cruciate ligament reconstruction with or without platelet-rich plasma. *J. Orthop. Surg.* **2013**, *21*, 10–14. [CrossRef]
20. Tao, X.; Aw, A.A.L.; Leeu, J.J.; Bin Abd Razak, H.R. Three Doses of Platelet-Rich Plasma Therapy Are More Effective Than One Dose of Platelet-Rich Plasma in the Treatment of Knee Osteoarthritis: A Systematic Review and Meta-analysis. *Arthroscopy* **2023**, *39*, 2568–2576. [CrossRef]
21. Corsini, A.; Perticarini, L.; Palermi, S.; Bettinsoli, P.; Marchini, A. Re-Evaluating Platelet-Rich Plasma Dosing Strategies in Sports Medicine: The Role of the "10 Billion Platelet Dose" in Optimizing Therapeutic Outcomes-A Narrative Review. *J. Clin. Med.* **2025**, *14*, 2714. [CrossRef] [PubMed]
22. San Jose, A.T.; Maniar, N.; Timmins, R.G.; Beerworth, K.; Hampel, C.; Tyson, N.; Williams, M.D.; Opar, D.A. Explosive hamstrings strength asymmetry persists despite maximal hamstring strength recovery following anterior cruciate ligament reconstruction using hamstring tendon autografts. *Knee Surg. Sports Traumatol. Arthrosc.* **2023**, *31*, 299–307. [CrossRef] [PubMed]
23. Tanmay, D.; Pritam, R. Change in hamstring parameters by isokinetic analysis after arthroscopic ACL reconstruction using hamstring graft—A prospective study. *J. Orthop. Rep.* **2025**, *5*, 100709. [CrossRef]

24. Desouza, C.; Shetty, V. Efficacy of platelet-rich plasma in grade 2 hamstring muscle injuries: Results from a randomized controlled trial. *Eur. J. Orthop. Surg. Traumatol.* **2025**, *35*, 259. [CrossRef]
25. Gill, S.S.; Cenci, G.; Falcinelli, S.; Marzano, F.; Carriero, B.; Filippi, N.; Pace, V. Platelet rich plasma and anterior cruciate ligament repair. *World J. Orthop.* **2025**, *16*, 693–704. [CrossRef]
26. Zhao, T.; Yan, W.; Xu, K.; Qi, Y.; Dai, X.; Shi, Z. Combined treatment with platelet-rich plasma and brain-derived neurotrophic factor-overexpressing bone marrow stromal cells supports axonal remyelination in a rat spinal cord hemi-section model. *Cytotherapy* **2013**, *15*, 792–804. [CrossRef]

Journal of
Clinical Medicine

MDPI

Article

Short-Term Outcome of Combined Anterior Cruciate Ligament Reconstruction and Anterolateral Ligament Reconstruction with Suture Tape Augmentation

Chieh-An Chuang [1,2,3], You-Hung Cheng [2,3,4], Cheng-Pang Yang [2,3,4], Chen-Heng Hsu [2,3,4], Chung-Yu Chen [2,3,4], Yi-Hsuan Lin [2,3,4] and Huan Sheu [2,3,4,*]

1 Department of Orthopaedic Surgery, Keelung Chang Gung Memorial Hospital, Keelung 204, Taiwan; b9702055@cgmh.org.tw
2 Department of Orthopaedic Surgery, Bone and Joint Research Center, Linkou Chang Gung Memorial Hospital, Taoyuan 333423, Taiwan
3 Comprehensive Sports Medicine Center, Linkou Chang Gung Memorial Hospital, Taoyuan 333423, Taiwan
4 Department of Orthopaedic Surgery, Linkou Chang Gung Memorial Hospital, Taoyuan 333423, Taiwan
* Correspondence: mp1333@cgmh.org.tw; Tel.: +886-3-3281200 (ext. 2163)

Abstract

Background: Persistent rotational instability and graft failure remain major challenges following anterior cruciate ligament reconstruction (ACLR). The addition of anterolateral ligament reconstruction (ALLR) and suture tape augmentation may enhance graft protection and early stability. This study aimed to assess the short-term clinical outcomes of combined ACLR and ALLR with suture tape augmentation, hypothesizing that this technique would yield favorable results in patients with ACL injury. **Methods**: Twenty-four patients (16 males, 8 females; mean age 30.8 years) with high grade pivot shift who underwent combined ACLR and ALLR with suture tape augmentation between 2022 and 2024 were retrospectively reviewed. Objective assessments included pivot-shift grading and anterior tibial translation (ATT) using a GNRB arthrometer. Patient-reported outcome measures (PROMs) comprised the International Knee Documentation Committee (IKDC), Marx activity score, and Single Assessment Numeric Evaluation (SANE) scores. Subgroup analysis compared graft diameters < 8 mm versus ≥8 mm. **Results**: The mean follow-up period was 23.4 months. Significant improvements were observed postoperatively in IKDC (45.9→83.7), Marx (4.4→9.9), SANE (49.2→85.2), and ATT (4.7→1.1 mm) (all $p < 0.001$). Full range of motion was regained at a mean of 3.2 months. Twenty-one patients presented no pivot shift and three with grade one postoperatively. No significant differences were found between the small (<8 mm) and large (≥8 mm) graft groups. MRI at one year showed intact grafts without adverse reactions. **Conclusions**: Combined ACL and anterolateral ligament reconstruction with suture tape augmentation demonstrated promising short-term stability and functional recovery without significant complications. This technique may enhance biomechanical reinforcement of both ACL and ALL grafts and represents a viable option for patients with smaller graft diameters.

Keywords: anterior cruciate ligament reconstruction; anterolateral ligament; sutures; treatment outcome; patient reported outcome measures; internal brace

1. Introduction

Anterior cruciate ligament (ACL) injury is among the most common sports-related knee injuries, particularly in athletes engaged in pivoting activities [1]. Although ACL

 https://doi.org/10.3390/jcm14238283

reconstruction (ACLR) remains the gold standard for restoring knee stability and function, persistent rotational laxity and graft failure continue to pose challenges [2]. Reported failure rates of 10–15% in young athletes underscore the need for ongoing refinement of surgical techniques to optimize long-term outcomes [3].

The anterolateral ligament (ALL) has been reported to be an important secondary stabilizer against anterolateral rotational instability [4,5]. Studies have shown that combined ACLR and ALL reconstruction (ALLR) improves rotational control [6,7]. Furthermore, combined ACLR and ALLR has been reported to decrease graft failure rate and revision rates of ACLR compared with isolated ACLR [8,9]. These findings have fueled increasing interest in incorporating ALLR into ACLR procedures, particularly for high-risk patients [10].

On the other hand, suture tape augmentation (STA) has emerged as a promising innovation aimed at improving knee laxity and protecting the graft during its early healing phase [11,12]. Acting as an "internal brace", STA provides additional reinforcement to reduce micromotion and elongation under load with added graft stiffness [13–15]. Studies have reported encouraging outcomes for ACLR with STA, including improved stability and potentially reduced early graft failure [16].

More recently, STA has also been applied to ALL repair or reconstruction techniques in ACL-injured patients [17,18]. Different ALL reconstruction techniques have been described in the literature, including the traditional two-limb construct and the single-limb construct [19,20]. When performing combined ACLR and ALLR, the graft—often the gracilis tendon used for the ALL—may be relatively small in diameter or insufficient in length for a two-limb construct. The addition of suture tape augmentation can provide supplementary support for the single-limb gracilis graft, particularly in cases with smaller graft diameters.

As a result, while combined ACLR and ALLR have demonstrated improved control of rotational instability, the addition of suture tape augmentation in both ACL and ALL may provide further biomechanical reinforcement that protects the graft complex, particularly during the healing phase. Accordingly, the integration of ACLR, ALLR, and STA in a single procedure represents a biomechanically complementary strategy designed to enhance early stability, promote graft protection, and potentially improve short-term clinical outcomes. The aim of the study was to evaluate the short-term clinical outcomes of combined ACLR and ALLR with STA in patients presenting with ACL deficiency and pivot instability. We hypothesized that this combined strategy could provide promising early stability and favorable functional outcomes without complications.

2. Materials and Methods

2.1. Study Design and Patient Selection

This retrospective study reviewed patients who underwent combined anterior cruciate ligament reconstruction (ACLR) and anterolateral ligament reconstruction (ALLR) between 2022 and 2024. Patients were included if they presented with a high-grade pivot shift preoperatively; underwent combined ACLR and ALLR with suture tape augmentation; had at least one year of postoperative follow-up; and had complete medical records with patient-reported outcome measures (PROMs). Exclusion criteria included absence of a high-grade pivot shift, follow-up of less than one year, or incomplete clinical or PROMs data.

2.2. Clinical and Demographic Data Collection

Demographic and clinical information was collected, including age, sex, body mass index (BMI), time since surgery, graft diameter, tibial slope, meniscal injury, and cartilage status. Objective evaluations comprised the pivot-shift test grading, GNRB® system (GNRB) for anterior tibial translation (ATT) [21], and assessment of knee range of motion (ROM). PROMs included Marx activity score, the International Knee Documentation Committee

(IKDC) score, and Single Assessment Numeric Evaluation (SANE). The assessment and grading of the pivot-shift test followed previously published criteria, with grades classified as 0 (normal), 1 (glide), 2 (clunk), and 3 (locked subluxation) [22]. A high-grade pivot shift was defined as a pivot-shift test graded as 2 or 3. Return to preinjury activity level was evaluated based on both the Marx Activity Rating Scale and patient self-report. It was defined as the resumption of the same level of sports participation as before injury, with a postoperative Marx score equal to or higher than the preinjury value. For subgroup analysis, a post hoc grouping was performed. Patients were divided according to graft diameter into those with grafts smaller than 8 mm and those with grafts measuring 8 mm or greater.

2.3. Surgical Technique

All reconstructions were performed using hamstring autografts. The graft was prepared by tripling the semitendinosus tendon and combining it with a single strand of gracilis tendon. Both tendons were sutured together to create a continuous construct, forming a four-strand ACL graft (three strands of semitendinosus and one of gracilis) and a single-strand gracilis extension for the ALL. A suture tape (FiberTape, Arthrex, Naples, FL, USA) was taken from Biocomposite Swivelock C anchor (Swivelock C; Arthrex) and was incorporated along the ACL and ALL grafts as an internal brace, as shown in Figure 1.

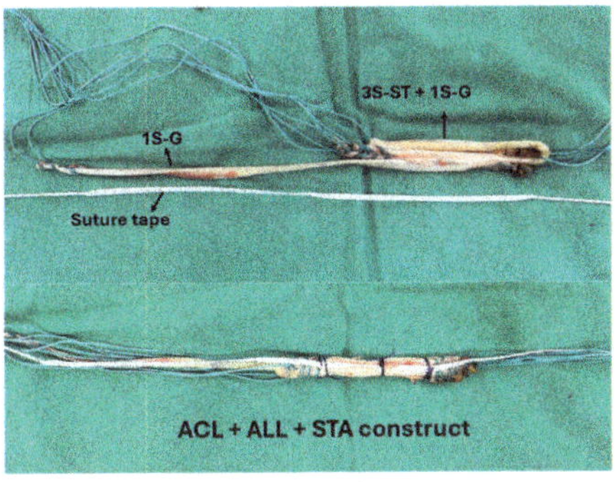

Figure 1. Continuous graft of combined ACL, ALL and suture tape augmentation, before and after suture integration. 3S-ST: 3-stranded semitendinosus tendon; 1S-G: 1-stranded gracilis tendon; G: Gracilis tendon; ACL: Anterior cruciate ligament; ALL: Anterolateral ligament; STA: Suture tape augmentation.

Both femoral and tibial tunnels were prepared using an outside-in technique. The femoral tunnel entry point was positioned proximal and posterior to the lateral epicondyle, with the exit directed toward the posterolateral aspect of the lateral femoral condyle at the anatomic anteromedial (AM) bundle footprint. The tibial tunnel for the ALL was located midway between Gerdy's tubercle and the fibular head, approximately 1 cm below the joint line. After tunnel preparation, the graft was passed from tibia to femur, and the ALL portion was routed distally beneath the iliotibial band to the tibial tunnel, as illustrated in Figure 2a–c. The ALL graft was then passed into the tibial tunnel. Graft fixation was performed using bioabsorbable interference screws. The ACL graft was tensioned and fixed at 30° of knee flexion under the reverse Lachman test, with manual assistance to ensure appropriate tension. The ALL graft was fixed at full knee extension with the tibia in a neutral rotational position [23]. The suture tape was fixed alongside the grafts and finally tied together at the tibial incision site to reinforce the construct. The final intra-articular configuration is demonstrated in Figure 3.

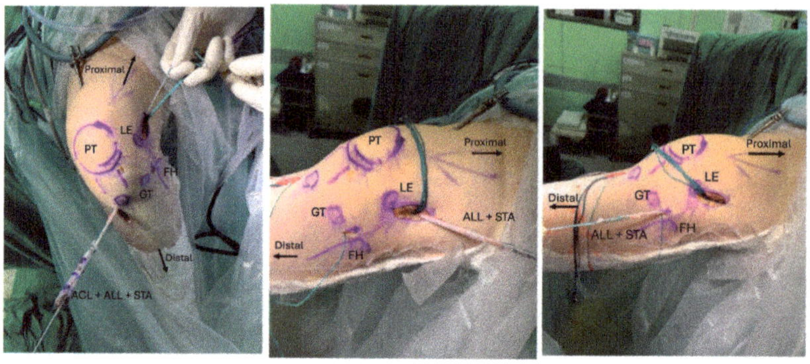

(a) (b) (c)

Figure 2. Demonstration of combined ACL and ALL and suture tape passage (**a**) Graft passage trantibial into the knee (**b**) ALL and suture tape passed out of the femur tunnel over proximal and posterior to the femoral lateral epicondyle. (**c**) ALL and suture tape passed underneath the IT band to tibial ALL point between Gerdy's tubercle and fibula head. PT: patella; LE: lateral epicondyle; GT: Gerdy's tubercle; FH: fibula head; ACL: Anterior cruciate ligament; ALL: Anterolateral ligament; STA: Suture tape augmentation.

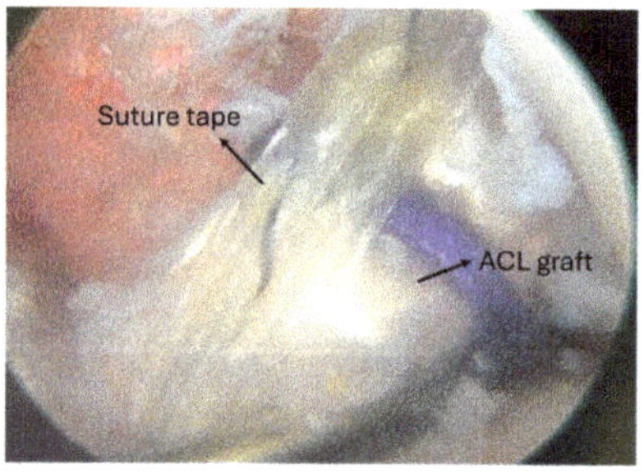

Figure 3. Demonstration of ACL graft and suture tape augmentation intra-articularly.

2.4. Postoperative Rehabilitation Protocol

Postoperative rehabilitation was standardized and adjusted according to the presence of concomitant meniscal repair. Continuous passive motion was initiated immediately after surgery to promote early joint mobility. Patients without meniscal repair ambulated with crutches for the first two weeks, progressed to full weightbearing thereafter, and did not require a brace. Jogging was permitted at three months postoperatively, sprinting and competitive exercises at six months, and unrestricted return to sports at approximately nine months. For patients who underwent meniscal repair, a range-of-motion brace was applied for six weeks. Knee flexion was limited to 0–60° during the first four weeks and advanced to full range of motion thereafter. Partial weightbearing with crutches was maintained for four weeks, followed by gradual progression as tolerated.

2.5. MRI Evaluation

Postoperative MRI follow-up was performed approximately one year after surgery, depending on patient willingness. The graft was evaluated using proton density sequences.

2.6. Statistical Analysis

All statistical analyses were performed using SPSS software (version 23.0; IBM Corp., Armonk, NY, USA) and Microsoft Excel 2016 (Microsoft Corp., Redmond, WA, USA). Categorical variables were analyzed using Fisher's exact test, and continuous variables were compared using the Mann–Whitney U test or unpaired t-test as appropriate. Wilcoxon signed-rank test was used for non-parametric data. Statistical significance was set at a p-value less than 0.05.

3. Results

A total of 29 patients who underwent combined ACLR and ALLR with suture tape augmentation were identified during the study period. Three patients were excluded due to follow-up of less than one year, and two patients did not complete the PROMs questionnaire. Consequently, 24 patients met the inclusion criteria and were included in the final analysis. The cohort comprised 16 males and 8 females, with a mean age of 30.8 ± 12.8 years (range, 14–50 years). The mean follow-up period was 23.4 ± 6.4 months (range, 12–34 months). Patient demographic and clinical characteristics are summarized in Table 1. All patients presented with a positive pivot-shift test before surgery, including 10 patients with grade 2 and 14 patients with grade 3 instability, indicating significant rotational laxity. Seven patients had ACL graft diameters smaller than 8 mm. Concomitant meniscal injuries were found in 11 patients—eight involving lateral meniscus tears, three with medial meniscus tears and two with concomitant tears. All meniscal tears were treated with arthroscopic repair at the time of reconstruction.

Table 1. Patient characteristics.

Age (years)	30.8 ± 12.8
Gender (M/F)	16/8
BMI (kg/m^2)	20.3 ± 2.0
Side (R/L)	11/13
Graft size (mm)	8.4 ± 0.8
Time from injury (months)	3.9 (2–14) ± 2.3
Follow-up (months)	23.4 (12–34) ± 6.4
Pre-op Pivot grade II/III	10/14
STSD-ATT by GNRB (mm)	4.7 ± 0.7
Medial cartilage injury (n, %)	4 (16.7%)
Lateral cartilage injury (n, %)	3 (12.5%)
Medial meniscus tear (n, %)	3 (12.5%)
Lateral meniscus tear (n, %)	8 (33.3%)

BMI: body mass index; STSD: side-to-side difference; ATT: anterior tibia translation.

The preoperative and postoperative clinical assessments and patient-reported outcome measures (PROMs) are presented in Table 2. At the final follow-up, patients achieved favorable functional recovery, with mean postoperative IKDC, Marx score and SANE of 83.7 ± 4.8, 9.9 ± 1.6, and 85.2 ± 4.8, respectively. Full range of motion was regained in all patients at an average of 3.2 months postoperatively. Averaged ATT measured by GNRB improved significantly from 4.7 ± 0.7 mm to 1.1 ± 0.4 mm. There were 3 patients who presented with grade 1 pivot shift and 21 with no pivot shift noted post-operatively. Fourteen patients (58.3%) successfully returned to their preinjury activity level within one year after surgery. When patients were stratified by graft diameter (<8 mm vs. ≥8 mm), the baseline demographic characteristics are detailed in Table 3, and the postoperative outcomes and PROMs are summarized in Table 4. Patients in the smaller graft diameter group presented with significantly lower BMI. There were no statistically significant differences between the two groups in postoperative GNRB measurements, pivot-shift grading, or PROMs (all $p > 0.05$).

Table 2. Pre-operative and post-operative PROMs, pivot grade, and ATT.

	Pre-Op (Mean ± SD)	Post-Op (Mean ± SD)	*p*-Value
IKDC	45.9 ± 7.9	83.7 ± 4.8	<0.001
Marx	4.4 ± 1.0	9.9 ± 1.6	<0.001
SANE	49.2 ± 9.7	85.2 ± 4.8	<0.001
Pivot grade (0:1:2:3)	0:0:10:14	21:3:0:0	<0.001
STSD-ATT (mm)	4.7 ± 0.7	1.1 ± 0.4	<0.001

IKDC: International Knee Documentation Committee; SANE: Single Assessment Numeric Evaluation; STSD: side-to-side difference; ATT: anterior tibia translation.

Table 3. Pre-operative patient comparison between graft size <8 mm and ≥8 mm.

	<8 mm (n = 7)	≥8 mm (n = 17)	*p*-Value
Age (years)	25.6 ± 14.5	34.4 ± 11.5	0.182
Gender (F/M)	4/3	5/12	0.417
BMI (kg/m^2)	18.7 ± 1.8	20.9 ± 1.8	0.019
Side (L/R)	3/4	10/7	0.793
Graft size (mm)	7.4 ± 0.2	8.9 ± 0.6	<0.001
Pivot grade (0:1:2:3)	0:0:3:4	0:0:7:10	0.373
STSD-ATT (mm)	4.7 ± 0.8	4.8 ± 0.7	0.782
IKDC	45.4 ± 7.6	46.1 ± 8.2	0.860
Marx	4.9 ± 1.1	4.2 ± 0.9	0.169
SANE	50.7 ± 8.9	48.5 ± 10.3	0.610

BMI: body mass index; STSD: side-to-side difference; ATT: anterior tibia translation; IKDC: International Knee Documentation Committee; SANE: Single Assessment Numeric Evaluation.

Table 4. Post-operative PROMs, Pivot test grade, and STSD-ATT by GNRB compared by graft size.

	<8 mm (n = 7)	≥8 mm (n = 17)	*p*-Value
IKDC	82.3 ± 4.2	84.3 ± 5.1	0.334
Marx	9.6 ± 2.2	10.1 ± 1.4	0.605
Sane	86.4 ± 5.6	84.7 ± 4.5	0.485
Pivot grade (0:1:2:3)	6:1:0:0	15:2:0:0	0.881
STSD-ATT (mm)	1.0 ± 0.5	1.1 ± 0.4	0.502

STSD: side-to-side difference; ATT: anterior tibia translation; IKDC: International Knee Documentation Committee; SANE: Single Assessment Numeric Evaluation.

A single postoperative complication occurred in an 18-year-old patient who developed a knee infection 10 days after reconstruction. The patient presented with knee swelling and erythema and was successfully treated with arthroscopic debridement followed by a two-week course of antibiotics, without recurrence of infection.

Among the 24 patients, 7 patients underwent postoperative magnetic resonance imaging (MRI) one year after surgery. All MRIs demonstrated intact ACL and ALL grafts with normal signal intensity and no significant tunnel widening (>2 mm) was observed in the measured tunnels. Two patients exhibited small cyst-like lesions at the tibial tunnel of ACL, but both were asymptomatic and did not require further intervention. No graft failure or loss of knee stability was observed during the follow-up period.

4. Discussion

The results of this study support the hypothesis that combined anterior cruciate ligament reconstruction and anterolateral ligament reconstruction with suture tape augmentation yields promising short-term functional outcomes in patients with ACL injury and pivot-shift instability. The mean postoperative IKDC, Marx activity score, and SANE were 83.7 ± 4.8, 9.9 ± 1.6, and 85.2 ± 4.8, respectively. Full range of motion was restored at an average of 3.2 months postoperatively. There were no significant differences in outcomes between patients with graft diameters < 8 mm and those with grafts ≥ 8 mm. No complications regarding suture tape augmentation, such as foreign body reaction, were observed. Despite the promising outcomes, studies with larger case series, inclusion of control groups, and longer follow-up periods are needed in the future to assess graft protection and durability and validate the reliability of this treatment approach.

Persistent rotational instability after ACL injury has been associated with an increased risk of progressive gonarthrosis, underscoring the essential role of the ACL and rotational knee stability in maintaining joint health and preventing degenerative changes [24]. Combined ACL and ALL reconstruction has gained increasing popularity, particularly in patients at higher risk of residual rotational instability or revision surgeries [25,26]. Recent meta-analyses and randomized controlled trials have reported that combined ACL and ALL reconstruction offers superior control of knee laxity, lower graft failure rates, and higher return-to-sport and graft survival rates [27,28]. The addition of an ALL reconstruction or a lateral extra-articular tenodesis is especially beneficial in high-risk patients, such as young athletes, patients exhibiting high-grade pivot shift, or those with anatomic risks for ACL failure [29–31]. All patients in our series presented with significant pivot shift, making them appropriate candidates for combined ACL and ALL reconstruction. After the operation, pivot shift changed from 14 patients with grade III and 10 with grade II preoperatively to 3 with grade I and 21 with grade 0 postoperatively. These findings are in line with previous studies that combined ACLR and ALLR to restore the rotation instability effectively. On the other hand, side to side difference in ATT measured from GNRB reported significant improvement from 4.7 ± 0.7 preoperatively to 1.1 ± 0.4 mm postoperatively. The results were similar to a previous study by Cheng et al., who conducted a study reporting outcome measures of GNRB for ACLR and ALLR [32]. These findings suggested that the augmentation of suture tape in both ACL and ALL constructs may enhance initial stability during the early healing phase. In the present series, no cases of graft failure were observed within the mean follow-up period of two years, consistent with previously reported short-term outcomes.

Suture tape augmentation in ACL reconstruction has been shown in both biomechanical and clinical studies to enhance graft strength, reduce elongation, and provide a "load-sharing" or "safety-belt" effect during early rehabilitation [33–37]. Clinical series have reported low complication rates and satisfactory patient-reported outcomes, with evidence of improved short-term function and decreased re-rupture risk [35,38,39]. Gao et al. reported that ACLR with STA is associated with a reduced graft failure rate and increased RTS rate compared with standard ACLR without additional reoperations or complications [40]. Potential concerns include over-constraint, stress shielding, and delayed graft maturation. Nevertheless, neither animal nor human studies have shown significant differences in ligamentization, histological appearance, or intra-articular complications between augmented and non-augmented grafts [33,41]. Our results were in line with previous studies, with no MRI evidence of tunnel stress shielding or intra-articular abnormal signal change around the ACL graft observed. Regarding the cyst-like lesions observed in two patients on postoperative MRI, these small lesions were located around the tibial tunnel and adjacent to the bioabsorbable screw. They were asymptomatic and were most likely related to the degradation process of the bioabsorbable material rather than the suture tape's reaction within the bone tunnel. Similar findings have been described in the literature, where bioabsorbable fixation devices were associated with tibial cyst formation after ACL reconstruction [42]. Although these lesions are generally benign and self-limiting, recognizing this imaging appearance is important for accurate interpretation of postoperative MRI findings. Finally, no over-constraint-related range of motion deficits were noted, and all patients regained full range of motion by an average of 3.2 months postoperatively. This might be due to combined STA in ACLR and ALLR allowing early stability and therefore early rehabilitation.

In terms of postoperative rehabilitation, this study adopted the protocol described by Chiu et al., emphasizing early range-of-motion recovery, progressive weight-bearing, and functional training [18]. With recent advances in mechatronic rehabilitation systems integrating robotic assistance and sensor-based feedback, combining such feedback-guided technologies with current rehabilitation strategies could further enhance motion accuracy and neuromuscular re-education [43]. This integration may enable ACL-reconstructed patients to regain natural gait and athletic performance more precisely and efficiently.

Graft diameter is another critical determinant of ACL reconstruction outcomes. Previous studies have demonstrated that hamstring autografts smaller than 8 mm are associated with higher failure and revision rates compared with larger grafts [44,45]. Meta-analyses have shown that each 0.5 mm increase in graft diameter significantly reduces failure risk, and grafts $\geq$ 8 mm are generally preferred [45,46]. Mariscalco et al. further reported that smaller hamstring autograft size predicted poorer KOOS Sport and Recreation scores at two years postoperatively [47]. On the other hand, a biomechanical study conducted by Bachmaier et al. suggested that STA could reduce the possibility of graft tears, especially for grafts with small diameters [48]. Interestingly, in the present study, no significant difference was found between patients with grafts <8 mm and $\geq$8 mm in terms of short-term functional outcomes. Both groups demonstrated reliable postoperative stability, with anterior tibial translation (ATT) measuring 1.0 mm and 1.4 mm, respectively. In this study, suture tape augmentation was integrated with both the ACL and ALL grafts, indicating that the reconstructed ACL was reinforced not only by the internal brace within the joint but also by the "ALL–suture tape" construct outside the notch. Therefore, despite smaller graft diameters, satisfactory outcomes could be achieved, as the combined effect of ALL reconstruction and suture tape augmentation likely provided sufficient biomechanical reinforcement to compensate for reduced graft size.

This study has several limitations. First, it was a retrospective study with a relatively small sample size. Second, the mean follow-up period was approximately two years, with a minimum of one year; thus, the results should be considered preliminary. Longer-term follow-up is necessary to evaluate durability, graft maturation, and late complications. Third, there was no control group of isolated ACL reconstruction or ACL plus ALL reconstruction without suture tape augmentation for comparison. Finally, postoperative MRI follow-up was available in only around 30% of patients (7/24), which may have limited the detection of subclinical intra-articular reactions or bone tunnel changes related to the suture tape.

5. Conclusions

Combined ACL and ALL reconstruction with suture tape augmentation showed promising short-term results in patients with high-grade pivot shift. The technique was safe, with no range of motion limitation or graft-related complications, and may be a viable option for patients with smaller graft diameters. However, larger prospective comparative studies with extended follow-up are warranted to validate these findings and to further determine the potential advantages of this technique over standard reconstruction methods.

Author Contributions: Conceptualization, C.-A.C., C.-P.Y. and Y.-H.L.; methodology, C.-H.H., C.-P.Y. and Y.-H.L.; validation, C.-A.C.; formal analysis, C.-A.C., C.-Y.C. and Y.-H.C.; investigation, C.-A.C. and Y.-H.C.; resources, C.-A.C., C.-Y.C., C.-H.H., Y.-H.C. and Y.-H.L.; data curation, C.-Y.C. and Y.-H.L.; writing—original draft preparation, C.-A.C.; writing—review and editing, C.-A.C., H.S.,

C.-P.Y., Y.-H.C.,Y.-H.L. and C.-Y.C.; visualization, C.-A.C.; supervision, H.S. and C.-P.Y. All authors have read and agreed to the published version of the manuscript.

Funding: This research received no external funding.

Institutional Review Board Statement: The study was conducted in accordance with the Declaration of Helsinki, and approved by the Institutional Review Board of Chang Gung Medial Foundation (No. 202300134B0, dated 6 February 2023).

Informed Consent Statement: Patient consent was waived due to the retrospective nature of the study.

Data Availability Statement: The datasets generated during or analyzed during the current study are available from the corresponding author on reasonable request.

Conflicts of Interest: The authors declare no conflicts of interest.

Abbreviations

The following abbreviations are used in this manuscript:

ACL	Anterior cruciate ligament
ACLR	Anterior cruciate ligament reconstruction
ALLR	Anterolateral ligament reconstruction
STA	Suture tape augmentation
ATT	Anterior tibial translation
PROMs	Patient-reported outcome measures
IKDC	International Knee Documentation Committee
SANE	Single Assessment Numeric Evaluation
MRI	Magnetic resonance imaging
ROM	Range of motion
BMI	Body mass index

References

1. Mall, N.A.; Chalmers, P.N.; Moric, M.; Tanaka, M.J.; Cole, B.J.; Bach, B.R., Jr.; Paletta, G.A., Jr. Incidence and trends of anterior cruciate ligament reconstruction in the United States. *Am. J. Sports Med.* **2014**, *42*, 2363–2370. [CrossRef]
2. Grassi, A.; Zicaro, J.P.; Costa-Paz, M.; Samuelsson, K.; Wilson, A.; Zaffagnini, S.; Condello, V.; Committee, E.A. Good mid-term outcomes and low rates of residual rotatory laxity, complications and failures after revision anterior cruciate ligament reconstruction (ACL) and lateral extra-articular tenodesis (LET). *Knee Surg. Sports Traumatol. Arthrosc.* **2020**, *28*, 418–431. [CrossRef] [PubMed]
3. Samitier, G.; Marcano, A.I.; Alentorn-Geli, E.; Cugat, R.; Farmer, K.W.; Moser, M.W. Failure of Anterior Cruciate Ligament Reconstruction. *Arch. Bone Jt. Surg.* **2015**, *3*, 220–240. [PubMed]
4. Ahn, J.H.; Patel, N.A.; Lin, C.C.; Lee, T.Q. The anterolateral ligament of the knee joint: A review of the anatomy, biomechanics, and anterolateral ligament surgery. *Knee Surg. Relat. Res.* **2019**, *31*, 12. [CrossRef]
5. Kang, K.T.; Koh, Y.G.; Park, K.M.; Choi, C.H.; Jung, M.; Shin, J.; Kim, S.H. The anterolateral ligament is a secondary stabilizer in the knee joint: A validated computational model of the biomechanical effects of a deficient anterior cruciate ligament and anterolateral ligament on knee joint kinematics. *Bone Jt. Res.* **2019**, *8*, 509–517. [CrossRef]
6. Mogos, S.; D'Ambrosi, R.; Antonescu, D.; Stoica, I.C. Combined Anterior Cruciate Ligament and Anterolateral Ligament Reconstruction Results in Superior Rotational Stability Compared with Isolated Anterior Cruciate Ligament Reconstruction in High Grade Pivoting Sport Patients: A Prospective Randomized Clinical Trial. *J. Knee Surg.* **2023**, *36*, 54–61.
7. Mathew, M.; Dhollander, A.; Getgood, A. Anterolateral Ligament Reconstruction or Extra-Articular Tenodesis: Why and When? *Clin. Sports Med.* **2018**, *37*, 75–86. [CrossRef]
8. Han, J.H.; Kim, S.H.; Jung, M.; Moon, H.S.; Chung, K. Combined Anterior Cruciate Ligament and Anterolateral Ligament Reconstruction Shows Reduced Graft Failure Rates and Superior Residual Rotational Stability Regardless of Anterolateral Ligament Reconstruction Graft: A Systematic Review. *J. Clin. Med.* **2025**, *14*, 2237. [CrossRef]
9. Na, B.R.; Kwak, W.K.; Seo, H.Y.; Seon, J.K. Clinical Outcomes of Anterolateral Ligament Reconstruction or Lateral Extra-articular Tenodesis Combined with Primary ACL Reconstruction: A Systematic Review with Meta-analysis. *Orthop. J. Sports Med.* **2021**, *9*, 23259671211023099. [CrossRef]

10. Yang, C.P.; Chen, M.Z.; Wang, C.L.; Chao-Yu Chen, A.; Hsu, K.Y.; Chan, Y.S.; Chiu, J.C. Double-bundle ACL combined with ALL reconstruction for patients at high risk of ACL failure: Clinical and radiological results. *BMC Musculoskelet. Disord.* **2024**, *25*, 594. [CrossRef]
11. Wilson, W.T.; Hopper, G.P.; Byrne, P.A.; MacKay, G.M. Anterior Cruciate Ligament Repair with Internal Brace Ligament Augmentation. *Surg. Technol. Int.* **2016**, *29*, 273–278. [PubMed]
12. He, J.; Kanto, R.; Fayed, A.M.; Price, T.M.; DiNenna, M.A.; Linde, M.A.; Smolinski, P.; van Eck, C.F. Augmenting ACL Repair with Suture Tape Improves Knee Laxity: A Biomechanical Study. *Orthop. J. Sports Med.* **2023**, *11*, 23259671221146013. [CrossRef] [PubMed]
13. Lu, W.; Deng, Z.; Essien, A.E.; Arthur Vithran, D.T.; Opoku, M.; Li, Y.; Xiao, W. Clinical Research Progress of Internal Brace Ligament Augmentation Technique in Knee Ligament Injury Repair and Reconstruction: A Narrative Review. *J. Clin. Med.* **2023**, *12*, 1999. [CrossRef] [PubMed]
14. Jackson, G.R.; Opara, O.; Tuthill, T.; Khan, Z.A.; Hevesi, M.; Mameri, E.; Jawanda, H.; Batra, A.K.; Schundler, S.; McCormick, J.; et al. Suture Augmentation in Orthopaedic Surgery Offers Improved Time-Zero Biomechanics and Promising Short-Term Clinical Outcomes. *Arthroscopy* **2023**, *39*, 1357–1365. [CrossRef]
15. Wicks, E.D.; Stack, J.; Rezaie, N.; Zeini, I.M.; Osbahr, D.C. Biomechanical Evaluation of Suture Tape Internal Brace Reinforcement of Soft Tissue Allografts for ACL Reconstruction Using a Porcine Model. *Orthop. J. Sports Med.* **2022**, *10*, 23259671221091252. [CrossRef]
16. Daniel, A.V.; Smith, P.A. Less Subsequent Revision Anterior Cruciate Ligament Reconstruction Following Primary Bone-Patellar Tendon-Bone Anterior Cruciate Ligament Reconstruction with Suture Tape Augmentation-A Retrospective Comparative Therapeutic Trial with 5-Year Follow-Up. *Arthroscopy* **2024**, *40*, 2455–2464. [CrossRef]
17. Heusdens, C.H.W.; Hopper, G.P.; Dossche, L.; Mackay, G.M. Anterolateral Ligament Repair with Suture Tape Augmentation. *Arthrosc. Tech.* **2018**, *7*, e1311–e1314. [CrossRef]
18. Chiu, C.H.; Chi, J.E.; Huang, P.H.; Chang, S.S.; Hsu, K.Y.; Chao-Yu Chen, A.; Chan, Y.S. Anatomic Double-Bundle ACL Reconstruction with Extra-articular Anterolateral Ligament Reconstruction and Internal Brace. *Arthrosc. Tech.* **2021**, *10*, e789–e796. [CrossRef]
19. Sonnery-Cottet, B.; Daggett, M.; Helito, C.P.; Fayard, J.M.; Thaunat, M. Combined Anterior Cruciate Ligament and Anterolateral Ligament Reconstruction. *Arthrosc. Tech.* **2016**, *5*, e1253–e1259. [CrossRef]
20. Thiebat, G.; Maggioni, L.M.; De Pamphilis, R.; Manzini, C.; Panzeri, A.; Pungitore, M. Gracilis Anatomic Anterolateral Ligament Reconstruction: Technical Note. *Arthrosc. Tech.* **2025**, *14*, 103475. [CrossRef]
21. Robert, H.; Nouveau, S.; Gageot, S.; Gagniere, B. A new knee arthrometer, the GNRB: Experience in ACL complete and partial tears. *Orthop. Traumatol. Surg. Res.* **2009**, *95*, 171–176. [CrossRef] [PubMed]
22. Vaudreuil, N.J.; Rothrauff, B.B.; de Sa, D.; Musahl, V. The Pivot Shift: Current Experimental Methodology and Clinical Utility for Anterior Cruciate Ligament Rupture and Associated Injury. *Curr. Rev. Musculoskelet. Med.* **2019**, *12*, 41–49. [CrossRef] [PubMed]
23. Saithna, A.; Thaunat, M.; Delaloye, J.R.; Ouanezar, H.; Fayard, J.M.; Sonnery-Cottet, B. Combined ACL and Anterolateral Ligament Reconstruction. *JBJS Essent. Surg. Tech.* **2018**, *8*, e2. [CrossRef]
24. Passaretti, A.; Colò, G.; Bulgheroni, A.; Vulcano, E.; Surace, M.F. Gonarthrosis and ACL lesion: An intraoperative analysis and correlations in patients who underwent total knee arthroplasty. *Minerva Orthop.* **2024**, *75*, 331–336. [CrossRef]
25. Boksh, K.; Sheikh, N.; Chong, H.H.; Ghosh, A.; Aujla, R. The Role of Anterolateral Ligament Reconstruction or Lateral Extra-articular Tenodesis for Revision Anterior Cruciate Ligament Reconstruction: A Systematic Review and Meta-analysis of Comparative Clinical Studies. *Am. J. Sports Med.* **2024**, *52*, 269–285. [CrossRef]
26. Jung, S.H.; Park, J.S.; Jung, M.; Chung, K.; Ha, T.H.; Choi, C.H.; Kim, S.H. Combined Anterolateral Ligament Reconstruction Results in Better Knee Stability and More Satisfactory Subjective Outcomes in Non-Athlete Patients Undergoing Revision Anterior Cruciate Ligament Reconstruction. *J. Clin. Med.* **2024**, *13*, 4087. [CrossRef]
27. Mercurio, M.; Cofano, E.; Gasparini, G.; Galasso, O.; Familiari, F.; Sanzo, V.; Ciolli, G.; Corona, K.; Cerciello, S. Isolated ACL Reconstruction Versus Combined ACL and Anterolateral Ligament Reconstruction: Functional Outcomes, Return to Sport, and Survivorship: An Updated Meta-analysis of Comparative Studies. *Am. J. Sports Med.* **2025**, *53*, 971–980. [CrossRef]
28. Ariel de Lima, D.; de Lima, L.L.; de Souza, N.G.R.; de Moraes Perez, R.A.; Sobrado, M.F.; Guimaraes, T.M.; Helito, C.P. Clinical outcomes of combined anterior cruciate ligament and anterolateral ligament reconstruction: A systematic review and meta-analysis. *Knee Surg. Relat. Res.* **2021**, *33*, 33. [CrossRef]
29. Kawanishi, Y.; Kobayashi, M.; Yasuma, S.; Fukushima, H.; Kato, J.; Murase, A.; Takenaga, T.; Yoshida, M.; Kuroyanagi, G.; Kawaguchi, Y.; et al. Anterolateral ligament reconstruction in addition to primary double-bundle anterior cruciate ligament reconstruction for grade 3 pivot shift improves residual knee instability during surgery. *J. Exp. Orthop.* **2021**, *8*, 51. [CrossRef]
30. Madhan, A.S.; Ganley, T.J.; McKay, S.D.; Pandya, N.K.; Patel, N.M. Trends in Anterolateral Ligament Reconstruction and Lateral Extra-articular Tenodesis with ACL Reconstruction in Children and Adolescents. *Orthop. J. Sports Med.* **2022**, *10*, 23259671221088049. [CrossRef]

31. Peng, W.L.; Chen, Y.J.; Hung, Y.C.; Ho, C.S.; Chiu, C.H.; Chen, A.C.; Chan, Y.S.; Hsu, K.Y.; Yang, C.P. Single-bundle ACL combined with ALL reconstruction yields comparable outcomes in patients with varied anatomical risk factors for ACL graft failure. *BMC Musculoskelet. Disord.* **2024**, *25*, 625. [CrossRef] [PubMed]
32. Cheng, Y.H.; Chiu, C.H.; Chen, A.C.; Chan, Y.S.; Hsu, K.Y. Outcomes of Combined Anterior Cruciate Ligament and Anterolateral Ligament Reconstruction According to GNRB Arthrometer Measurement. *Medicina* **2023**, *59*, 366. [CrossRef] [PubMed]
33. Mackenzie, C.E.A.; Huntington, L.S.; Tulloch, S. Suture Tape Augmentation of Anterior Cruciate Ligament Reconstruction Increases Biomechanical Stability: A Scoping Review of Biomechanical, Animal, and Clinical Studies. *Arthroscopy* **2022**, *38*, 2073–2089. [CrossRef] [PubMed]
34. Maginnis, C.; Root, C.; Schiavo, J.H.; Ierulli, V.K.; Vopat, B.; Mulcahey, M.K. Analysis of Graft Types Augmented with an Internal Brace for ACL Reconstruction: A Systematic Review. *Am. J. Sports Med.* **2024**, *52*, 2415–2423. [CrossRef]
35. Wilson, W.T.; Kennedy, M.J.; MacLeod, D.; Hopper, G.P.; MacKay, G.M. Outcomes of Anterior Cruciate Ligament Reconstruction with Independently Tensioned Suture Tape Augmentation at 5-Year Follow-up. *Am. J. Sports Med.* **2023**, *51*, 3658–3664. [CrossRef]
36. Zheng, T.; Cao, Y.; Song, G.; Li, Y.; Zhang, Z.; Feng, Z.; Zhang, H. Suture tape augmentation, a novel application of synthetic materials in anterior cruciate ligament reconstruction: A systematic review. *Front. Bioeng. Biotechnol.* **2022**, *10*, 1065314.
37. Gutiérrez, M.A.; Ortiz, A.V.; Arellano, C.H.; Arza, I.M.; Solís-Mencía, C.A.; D'Orazio, G.T. Seatbelt Anterior Cruciate Ligament Reconstruction: A Variant of Internal Brace in Anterior Cruciate Ligament Reconstruction with an Adjustable Loop. *Arthrosc. Tech.* **2024**, *13*, 102892. [CrossRef]
38. Tavakoli Darestani, R.; Afzal, S.; Pourmojarab, A.; Baroutkoub, M.; Sayyadi, S.; Barati, H. A comparative analysis of suture-augmented and standard hamstring autograft single-bundle ACL reconstruction outcomes: Short-term functional benefits without long-term impact. *BMC Musculoskelet. Disord.* **2023**, *24*, 971. [CrossRef]
39. Novaretti, J.V.; Dias Junior, C.P.P.; Lima, L.S.; Amaro, J.T.; Gomes, D.E.; Cohen, M. Anterior Cruciate Ligament Reconstruction with Internal Brace Augmentation Results in Fewer Reruptures Compared to Reconstruction without Augmentation. *Rev. Bras Ortop.* **2024**, *59*, e868–e875.
40. Gao, Y.; Shi, W.; Zhang, Z.; Bai, W.; Yang, Y.; Ma, Y.; Wang, C.; Wang, J.; Gong, X.; Wang, J. Association of suture augmentation with graft failure and clinical outcomes following anterior cruciate ligament reconstruction: A systematic review and meta-analysis of comparative studies with a minimum 2-year follow-up. *Knee Surg. Sports Traumatol. Arthrosc.* **2025**, *33*, 2799–2814. [CrossRef]
41. Tensho, K.; Iwaasa, T.; Koyama, S.; Shimodaira, H.; Takahashi, T.; Takahashi, J. No Difference in Graft Signal Intensity on Magnetic Resonance Imaging or Clinical Outcome Between Anterior Cruciate Ligament Reconstruction With and Without Suture Augmentation. *Arthroscopy* **2025**, *41*, 1931–1941.e1934. [CrossRef] [PubMed]
42. Barbosa, N.C.; Campos, J.P.; Capelao, V.; Kandhari, V.; Vieira, T.D.; Sonnery-Cottet, B. A comprehensive scoping review of tibial cysts after anterior cruciate ligament reconstruction. *J. Exp. Orthop.* **2021**, *8*, 40. [CrossRef] [PubMed]
43. Ciobanu, I.; Stanculescu (Badea), D.I.; Iliescu, A.; Popescu, A.M.; Seiciu, P.L.; Mikolajczyk, T.; Moldovan, F.; Berteanu, M. The usability pilot study of a mechatronic system for gait rehabilitation. *Procedia Manuf.* **2018**, *22*, 864–871. [CrossRef]
44. Alomar, A.Z.; Nasser, A.S.B.; Kumar, A.; Kumar, M.; Das, S.; Mittal, S. Hamstring graft diameter above 7 mm has a lower risk of failure following anterior cruciate ligament reconstruction. *Knee Surg. Sports Traumatol. Arthrosc.* **2022**, *30*, 288–297. [CrossRef] [PubMed]
45. Snaebjornsson, T.; Hamrin-Senorski, E.; Svantesson, E.; Karlsson, L.; Engebretsen, L.; Karlsson, J.; Samuelsson, K. Graft Diameter and Graft Type as Predictors of Anterior Cruciate Ligament Revision: A Cohort Study Including 18,425 Patients from the Swedish and Norwegian National Knee Ligament Registries. *J. Bone Jt. Surg. Am.* **2019**, *101*, 1812–1820. [CrossRef]
46. Itoh, M.; Itou, J.; Okazaki, K.; Iwasaki, K. Estimation Failure Risk by 0.5-mm Differences in Autologous Hamstring Graft Diameter in Anterior Cruciate Ligament Reconstruction: A Meta-analysis. *Am. J. Sports Med.* **2024**, *52*, 535–543. [CrossRef]
47. Mariscalco, M.W.; Flanigan, D.C.; Mitchell, J.; Pedroza, A.D.; Jones, M.H.; Andrish, J.T.; Parker, R.D.; Kaeding, C.C.; Magnussen, R.A. The influence of hamstring autograft size on patient-reported outcomes and risk of revision after anterior cruciate ligament reconstruction: A Multicenter Orthopaedic Outcomes Network (MOON) Cohort Study. *Arthroscopy* **2013**, *29*, 1948–1953. [CrossRef]
48. Bachmaier, S.; Smith, P.A.; Bley, J.; Wijdicks, C.A. Independent Suture Tape Reinforcement of Small and Standard Diameter Grafts for Anterior Cruciate Ligament Reconstruction: A Biomechanical Full Construct Model. *Arthroscopy* **2018**, *34*, 490–499. [CrossRef]

Journal of
Clinical Medicine

MDPI

Systematic Review

Does Adding LEAP to ACL Reconstruction Reduce Graft Failure? A Systematic Review and Meta-Analysis of Comparative Studies with Minimum Two-Year Follow-Up

Simone Giusti [1], Angelo Matteucci [1], Simone Pavone [2,3,*], Ciro Mignano [1] and Ezio Adriani [1]

[1] UOC Traumatologia Dello Sport e Chirurgia Articolare, Università Cattolica del Sacro Cuore, Largo Francesco Vito 1, 00168 Rome, Italy; simonegiustiwork@gmail.com (S.G.); ciromignanotri@gmail.com (C.M.)

[2] IRCCS Humanitas Research Hospital, Via Manzoni 56, Rozzano, 20089 Milan, Italy

[3] Department of Biomedical Sciences, Humanitas University, Via Rita Levi Montalcini 4, Pieve Emanuele, 20072 Milan, Italy

* Correspondence: simone.pavone@outlook.com

Abstract

Background: Anterior cruciate ligament (ACL) reconstruction (ACLR) is the gold-standard treatment for ACL rupture; however, graft failure remains a significant concern, particularly in young, active, or high-risk patients. The addition of a Lateral Extra-Articular Procedure (LEAP) has been proposed to enhance rotational stability and reduce the risk of graft rupture. This systematic review and meta-analysis aimed to determine whether adding LEAP to primary ACLR reduces graft failure rates compared to isolated ACLR, with a minimum follow-up of two years. **Methods:** A comprehensive literature search was conducted across PubMed, Scopus, Embase and Cochrane Library databases in accordance with PRISMA guidelines. Eighteen comparative studies with a minimum 24-month follow-up were included, encompassing 7336 patients (3857 undergoing isolated ACLR and 3479 undergoing ACLR with LEAP). The primary outcome was graft failure rate. Data were analyzed using the Mantel–Haenszel method with a fixed-effects model to calculate pooled risk ratios (RR) and 95% confidence intervals (CI). **Results:** Pooled analysis demonstrated a significant increase in graft rupture risk in the ACLR-alone group compared to ACLR + LEAP (RR 2.72; 95% CI: 2.23–3.32; $p < 0.00001$), with negligible heterogeneity ($I^2 = 0\%$). LEAP was particularly beneficial in high-risk populations such as young athletes and individuals with high-grade pivot shift or ligamentous laxity. Secondary outcomes showed improved rotational stability and comparable patient-reported outcomes and complication rates between groups. **Conclusions:** ACLR alone presents a higher risk of graft failure in comparison with the ALCR + LEAP technique. Furthermore, the addition of LEAP to ACLR improves rotational stability without increasing complications. LEAP should be selectively considered in patients with high-risk profiles or persistent intraoperative instability. These findings support the incorporation of LEAP as a valuable adjunct in modern ACL reconstruction strategies.

Keywords: ACL reconstruction; sports medicine; lateral extra-articular procedure; LEAP; graft failure; knee stability; meta-analysis

1. Introduction

Anterior cruciate ligament (ACL) tears are among the most common knee injuries, affecting more than 150,000 people each year, most of whom are athletes. Anterior cruciate ligament (ACL) reconstruction has become the gold standard for the treatment of ACL injuries. Over the years, various reconstruction techniques have been proposed and gradually improved. Among the various surgical techniques proposed, lateral extra-articular procedures (LEAP) are often used to address residual femoral rotation and the potential knee instability that may persist following anterior cruciate ligament (ACL) reconstruction [1]

Several recent studies have investigated the benefits of combining LEAP with ACLR, suggesting potential advantages in selected patient populations [2]. Currently, LEAP is typically indicated in the majority of cases involving high-grade rotational instability, anterolateral ligament injury, high-risk patients such as young athletes that practice pivoting sports (soccer, basketball, rugby) or those with ligamentous laxity, revision ACL reconstructions, and persistent rotational instability despite adequate intra-articular repair, although it is not routinely performed by all surgeons [1].

The aim of our systematic review and meta-analysis is to assess whether adding LEAP to primary ACL reconstruction significantly reduces graft failure rates compared to isolated ACLR, at a minimum follow-up of two years. Our analysis focuses on providing evidence-based guidance on the necessity and appropriateness of LEAP, considering that its routine application may not confer additional protective benefits and could represent an unnecessary surgical intervention in many cases.

2. Methods and Materials

This systematic review and meta-analysis adhered to the guidelines outlined in the Preferred Reporting Items for Systematic Reviews and Meta-analyses (PRISMA) The PRISMA checklist is provided in Supplementary Materials. The protocol for this systematic review and meta-analysis was prospectively registered in PROSPERO (ID: CRD420251158621).

2.1. Eligibility Criteria

(1) Cohort studies, Randomized clinical trials, Systematic reviews, Randomized comparative studies, Meta-analyses, Randomized controlled trials, Retrospective comparative studies, Retrospective propensity-matched cohort study, Retrospective cohort studies, Prospective randomized controlled trials, Retrospective cohort; propensity-matched case–control studies;
(2) Studies written in the English language;
(3) Studies on patients who underwent ACL reconstruction, with or without Lateral Extra-articular Procedures (LEAP);
(4) Only studies with patients who underwent ACL reconstruction with a minimum 24 months follow-up were considered;
(5) Only studies presenting graft rupture rate, in percentage (%) or in absolute value;

2.2. Exclusion Criteria

(1) Case reports, reviews, letters to the editor, cadaveric studies, commentaries, and editorials;
(2) All studies with Level of Evidence = 4 or 5;
(3) Mean age < 14 years;
(4) Studies older than 8 years (1 May 2018–1 May 2025);
(5) Revision reconstruction;

Data on type of graft used (Hamstring Tendons (HT), Bone-Patellar-Tendon Bone (BTB), Quadriceps Tendon (QT)), type of femoral tunnel practised (trans-tibial, modified trans-tibial or antero-medial tunnel) and type of bundle (single or double bundle) were not considered as exclusion criteria.

2.3. Information Sources and Search Strategy

A comprehensive search of PubMed, Scopus, Embase and the Cochrane Library was performed. Two reviewers (M.A. and P.S.) independently gathered studies, and then the results were cross-checked and merged for analysis.

All search results were independently screened by title/abstract and then by full text against predefined criteria (clinical studies reporting graft rupture rate after ACL reconstruction, in percentage or in absolute values).

A total of 214 records were identified through database searching. After removal of 7 duplicates and screening of titles and abstracts, 177 studies were excluded. 37 full-text articles were assessed for eligibility, of which 19 were excluded for reasons such as non-comparative design, follow-up shorter than 2 years, or pediatric cohorts. 18 studies met the inclusion criteria and were included in the final qualitative and quantitative synthesis.

2.4. Data Items

Extracted data consisted of the following:

(1) Study information: author, publication year, title, study type, level of evidence, purpose, and main conclusions;
(2) Population details: sample size, sex distribution (when possible), mean age, and therapeutic protocol (ACL reconstruction, with or without LEAP);
(3) Methodology specifics: type of graft (when possible), graft rupture rate (directly in percentage % or indirectly, as event occurred/number of participants);

2.5. Risk of Bias

P.S. and M.C. performed the risk-of-bias assessment independently and in duplicate, using tools appropriate to study design: RoBANS for non-randomized studies and RoB 2 for randomized trials. Any disagreements were resolved by discussion; if consensus was not reached, a third reviewer (M.A.) adjudicated. RoBANS comprises six domains—(a) patient selection, (b) confounding variables, (c) measurement of exposure, (d) blinding of outcome assessment, (e) incomplete outcome data, and (f) selective outcome reporting—each rated Low, High, or Unclear risk. RoB 2 includes five domains—(1) randomization process, (2) deviations from intended interventions (effect of assignment), (3) missing outcome data, (4) measurement of the outcome, and (5) selection of the reported result—with signaling questions supporting domain judgments (Low risk, Some concerns, High risk).

Overall judgment rules followed standard criteria: Low risk if all domains were Low; Some concerns if no domain was High but $\geq$1 domain raised concerns; High risk if $\geq$1 domain was High or multiple concerns substantially lowered confidence.

Risk of bias was assessed for the 18 included studies: five RCTs (assessed with RoB 2) and thirteen non-randomized studies (assessed with RoBANS). Among the RCTs, Heard et al. [3], Getgood et al. [4], and Porter et al. [5] were judged Low risk across all RoB 2 domains, while El-Azab et al. and Lucidi et al. raised some concerns in certain domains, resulting in an overall judgment of some concerns.

RoBANS assessments indicated heterogeneous risk-of-bias patterns among non-randomized studies. Patient selection, exposure ascertainment, completeness of outcome data, and selective reporting were generally judged at low risk. However, confounding and outcome assessment frequently raised concerns, primarily due to unmeasured confounders and the absence of blinding procedures, which could influence outcome evaluation. Notably, Monaco et al. [6], Viglietta et al. [7], Serna et al. [8], Mahmoud et al. [9], and Rowan et al. [10], were low across all RoBANS domains (overall low risk). Risk of bias due to missing results was assessed visually using funnel plot: suggested slight asymmetry, indicating a possible risk of publication bias.

Visual summaries are provided in Figures 1 and 2.

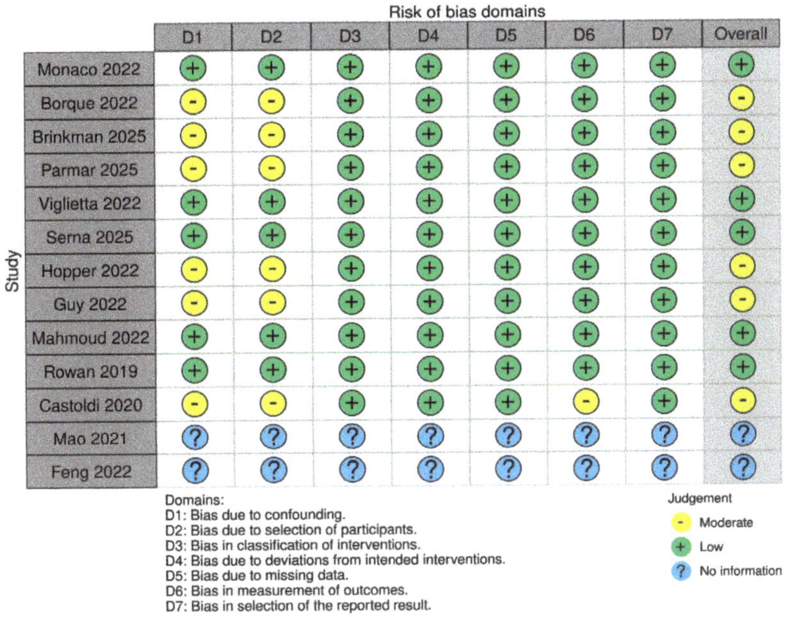

Figure 1. Risk of Bias—Non-Randomized Studies (RoBANS) by robvis [6–18].

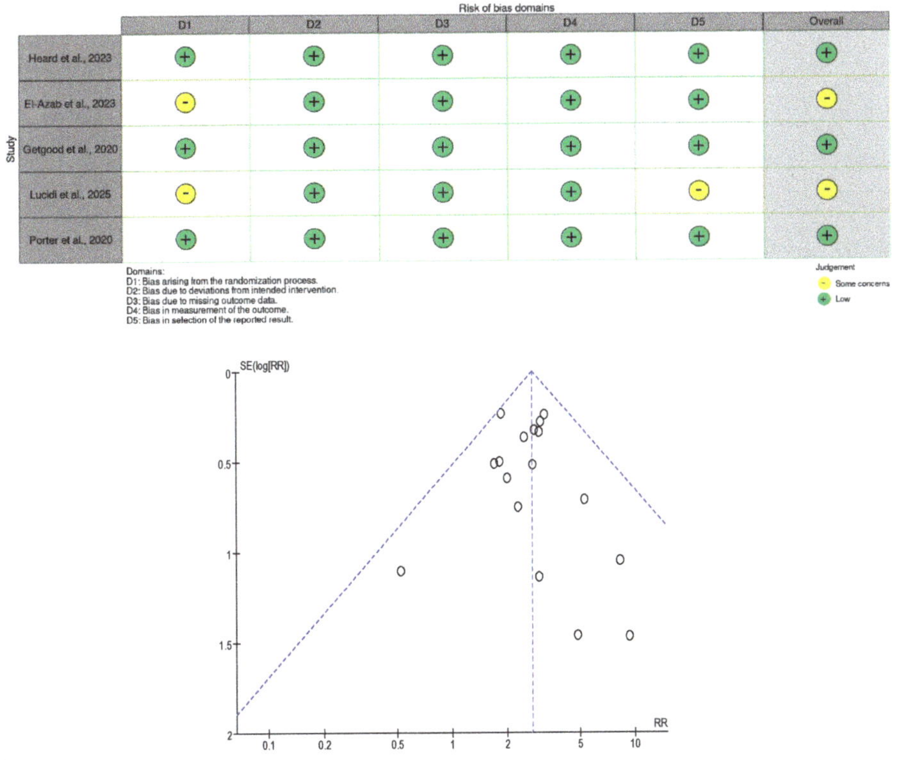

Figure 2. Risk of Bias—Randomized Controlled Trials (RoB 2) by robvis [3–5,19,20]. Risk of Publication Bias—Funnel plot.

2.6. Data Analysis

Patients from the included studies were categorized into two groups based on the type of technique practiced (LEAP or non-LEAP).

Successively, each single event was extracted from the rupture's percentage. When they occurred, results were rounded to excess or defect. If a study presented more graft-harvesting techniques, they were summed, and considered as a single result.

Our aim was to calculate the risk ratio of each group, and then a comparison was made between the two sets of data.

All events were inserted in Review Manager software (RevMan, version 5.4.1, Cochrane, London, UK), using dichotomous data with Mantel-Haenzsel statistical method, risk ratio on fixed effect ($I^2 = 0\%$), IC 95%.

The degree of heterogeneity in graft rupture rate was assessed with the I^2 index, which was interpreted as follows: 0.0–24.9% to indicate no heterogeneity, 25.0–49.9% to indicate low heterogeneity, 50.0–74.9% to indicate moderate heterogeneity, 75.0–100.0% to indicate high heterogeneity. A higher I^2 score implies a larger proportion of variability in the results that could be attributed to heterogeneity [16].

Sensitivity analyses using a random-effects model produced similar pooled estimates (Risk Ratio 2.62, 95% CI 2.14–3.19; $Tau^2 = 0.00$; $Chi^2 = 12.57$, df = 17 ($p = 0.76$); $I^2 = 0\%$, $p < 0.00001$), confirming the robustness of the fixed-effects results.

In addition, the pooled risk difference (random-effects model) was 0.07 (95% CI 0.05–0.09), with moderate heterogeneity ($I^2 = 63\%$). This variability likely reflects differences in baseline event rates across studies rather than inconsistent treatment effects, as the relative effect (RR) was homogeneous ($I^2 = 0\%$).

To address differences in sample size across studies, weighted mean values were used instead of arithmetic mean values. The use of weighted mean values allowed studies with larger sample sizes to contribute more to the computed average compared to studies with small sample sizes.

Certainty of the evidence was not formally assessed using the GRADE approach; however, potential limitations, risk of bias, and inconsistency among included studies were qualitatively discussed to provide an overall appraisal of the confidence in the findings

2.7. Study Selection and PRISMA Flow

The systematic review was conducted in accordance with the Preferred Reporting Items for Systematic Reviews and Meta-Analyses (PRISMA) 2020 guidelines. Study screening and selection were performed independently by two reviewers (S.P. and A.M.). Any disagreements regarding inclusion or exclusion were resolved through discussion. In cases where consensus could not be reached, a third reviewer (C.M.) was consulted, and their decision was considered final. The search strategy identified 214 records, of which 7 duplicates were removed. After screening titles and abstracts, 177 records were excluded. A total of 37 full-text articles were assessed for eligibility, and 19 were excluded for not meeting the predefined inclusion criteria (e.g., not comparative studies, follow-up <2 years, pediatric cohorts). Eighteen studies met all criteria and were included in the final analysis. The study selection process is detailed in the PRISMA flow diagram. (Figure 3).

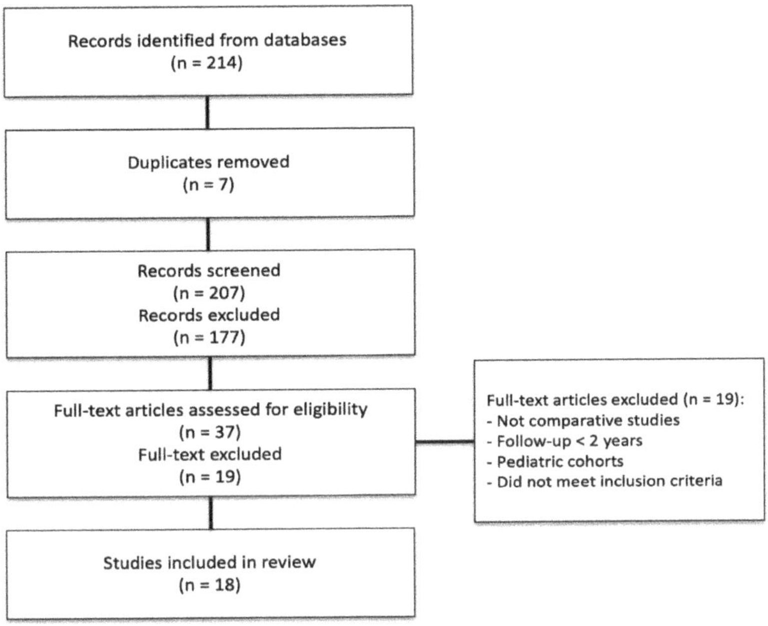

Figure 3. PRISMA 2020 flow diagram summarizing the study selection process. A total of 214 records were identified through database searching. After removal of 7 duplicates and screening of titles and abstracts, 177 studies were excluded. Thirty-seven full-text articles were assessed for eligibility, of which 19 were excluded for reasons such as non-comparative design, follow-up shorter than 2 years, or pediatric cohorts. Eighteen studies met the inclusion criteria and were included in the final qualitative and quantitative analyses.

3. Results

Eighteen comparative studies meeting inclusion criteria were analyzed, encompassing a total of 7336 patients (3857 undergoing isolated ACL reconstruction [ACLR] and 3479 undergoing ACLR with additional lateral extra-articular procedures [ACLR + LEAP]). All included studies reported graft rupture rates at a minimum of 2-year follow-up, with patient populations generally composed of high-risk individuals (e.g., young athletes, those with high-grade pivot shift or generalized ligamentous laxity).

Across individual studies, the incidence of graft failure varied markedly between groups. In 17 of the 18 studies, the addition of LEAP was associated with numerically lower re-rupture rates compared to ACLR alone. For instance, Monaco et al. [6] reported 0% graft failure in the ACLR + LEAP group versus 15% in the ACLR-only group, while Hopper et al. [14] observed a significant difference between 6.0% and 15.5%, respectively ($p = 0.0105$). In contrast, Parmar et al. [13], was the only study reporting a slightly higher failure rate in the LEAP group (4.7% vs. 3%), though the difference was not statistically significant. Several high-quality RCTs (e.g., Getgood et al. [4], Heard et al. [3], El-Azab et al. [19]) consistently demonstrated a relative risk reduction in graft failure with LEAP augmentation (Table 1).

Pooled analysis using a fixed-effect Mantel-Haenszel model showed a significant increase in the risk of graft rupture in the ACLR alone group compared to ACLR + LEAP, with a risk ratio (RR) of 2.72 (95% CI: 2.23 to 3.32; $p < 0.00001$). This suggests that patients undergoing isolated ACLR are nearly three times more likely to experience graft failure compared to those receiving an additional LEAP procedure. The heterogeneity among studies was negligible ($I^2 = 0\%$, $Chi^2 = 12.57$, df = 17; $p = 0.76$), supporting the consistency of this finding across diverse populations and study designs (Figure 4).

Table 1. Graft Rupture.

Study	ACLR	ACLR + LEAP
Monaco et al., 2022 [6]	15%	0%
Borque et al., 2022 [11]	9.5%	3.4%
Heard et al., 2023 [3]	11%	4%
Mao et al., 2021 [17]	12%	3.93%
El-Azab et al., 2023 [19]	6.3%	2.1%
Feng et al., 2022 [18]	11.5%	3.6%
Castoldi et al., 2020 [16]	29%	13%
Getgood et al., 2020 [4]	11.3%	3.7%
Brinkman et al., 2025 [12]	HA 17.9%, QA 1.8%	4.3%
Parmar et al., 2025 [13]	3%	4.7%
Lucidi et al., 2025 [20]	37%	19%
Viglietta et al., 2022 [7]	10.4%	1.2%
Serna et al., 2025 [8]	4.9%	2.6%
Hopper et al., 2022 [14]	15.5%	6%
Guy et al., 2022 [15]	34.0%	6.5%
Mahmoud et al., 2022 [9]	11%	5%
Porter et al., 2020 [5]	14.8%	0%
Rowan et al., 2019 [10]	5%	0%

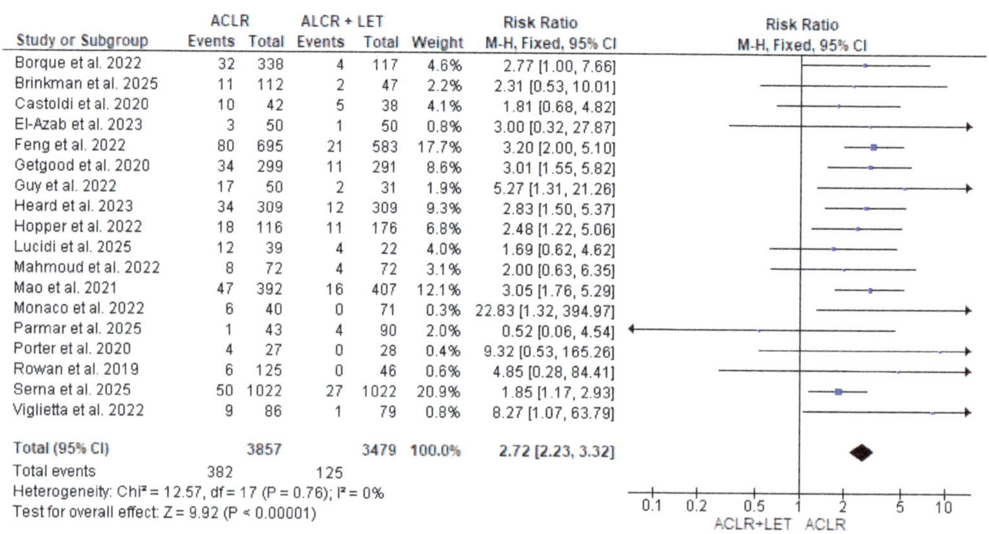

Figure 4. Pooled analysis using a fixed-effect Mantel-Haenszel model showed a significant increase in the risk of graft rupture in the ACLR alone group compared to ACLR + LEAP, with a risk ratio (RR) of 2.72 (95% CI: 2.23 to 3.32; $p < 0.00001$) [3–20].

Overall, the results of this meta-analysis confirm that the addition of LEAP to ACLR significantly reduces the risk of graft failure, particularly in high-risk populations. This benefit appears robust across study design, graft type, and surgical technique, and is achieved without a meaningful increase in adverse events. A summary of the results is included in Table 2.

4. Additional Findings

In addition to graft failure rates, secondary outcomes were consistently reported across the included studies and revealed converging trends favoring the addition of LEAP.

In terms of **rotational stability**, Monaco et al. [6] reported a pivot-shift grade 3 in 11.4% of the ACLR group versus 0% in the ACLR + LEAP group ($p = 0.021$), and a side-to-side anteroposterior laxity >5 mm in 17.1% versus 0% ($p = 0.003$). Similarly, Brinkman et al. [12], found reduced postoperative pivot-shift grades in both the HT + LEAP and QT groups compared to isolated HT (retear rate: 17.9% HT vs. 4.3% HT + LEAP). Viglietta et al. [7] also showed a markedly lower instability rate in the combined ACLR + LEAP group (graft failure: 1.2% vs. 10.4%).

Regarding **patient-reported outcomes**, Getgood et al. [4] and El-Azab et al. [19] observed no statistically significant differences in IKDC or KOOS scores between groups at final follow-up, while Porter et al. [5] documented superior Lysholm scores (96.8 vs. 92.5; $p = 0.004$) and Tegner activity scale (median 8 vs. 7; $p = 0.03$) in the LEAP group. Rowan et al. [10] found that patients receiving LEAP achieved a significantly higher median Lysholm score (98 vs. 90; $p = 0.005$) and returned to sport sooner (6 vs. 8 months; $p < 0.001$).

Return to sport rates were comparable or improved with LEAP augmentation. For instance, Heard et al. [3] and Hopper et al. [14], showed equivalent or better return-to-play metrics in the ACLR + LEAP group. In Rowan et al. [10], 100% of LEAP patients resumed pivoting sports versus 76% in the ACLR group.

Adverse event rates were similar between groups. Heard et al. [3] reported no significant increase in minor surgical or medical complications with LEAP. Mahmoud et al. [9] observed comparable complication profiles (e.g., 3 vs. 4 re-arthroscopies; 0 vs. 1 DVT), and no study reported increased incidence of postoperative stiffness or infection attributable to LEAP.

Finally, while one study (Castoldi et al. [16]) suggested a trend toward increased lateral compartment osteoarthritis after LEAP, no consistent association was found across the remaining long-term follow-up studies. On the contrary, Viglietta et al. [7] reported lower Kellgren–Lawrence OA grades in the LEAP group.

Subgroup Analyses: Risk Populations and Graft Types

Subgroup analyses revealed notable patterns based on patient risk profiles and graft type.

High-risk populations, such as adolescents, elite athletes, and individuals with generalized ligamentous laxity or high-grade pivot shift, consistently benefitted from the addition of LEAP. For instance, in the STABILITY trial (Getgood et al. [4]), which enrolled patients $\leq$25 years old with $\geq$2 high-risk criteria, the 2-year graft rupture rate was significantly reduced in the LEAP group (3.7% vs. 11.3%; $p < 0.01$). Hopper et al. [14] demonstrated a hazard ratio (HR) of 2.678 (95% CI 1.173–4.837; $p = 0.0164$) for graft failure in isolated ACLR, with even stronger effects observed in athletes under 21 years (HR = 2.381; $p = 0.0068$). Rowan et al. [10], focusing on elite athletes, reported 0% re-ruptures in the LEAP group versus 5% in ACLR alone, and Guy et al. [15] showed a failure rate of 6.5% with LEAP versus 34% without in elite skiers ($p = 0.0412$).

In contrast, studies in lower-risk populations or those not explicitly stratified by risk (e.g., Parmar et al. [13], Mahmoud et al. [9]) did not show as pronounced a benefit, and in Parmar's cohort of female soccer players, failure rates were slightly higher in the LEAP group (4.7% vs. 3%), though not significantly.

With regard to **graft type**, several studies stratified outcomes by the source of the autograft. Castoldi et al. [16] used BTB grafts and found a 29% failure rate in ACLR versus 13% in ACLR + LEAP. In contrast, Lucidi et al. [20] compared three techniques: BTB (37% re-rupture), hamstring tendon (25%), and over-the-top HT + LEAP (19%), indicating a potential protective effect of LEAP independent of graft type. Brinkman et al. [12] compared hamstring autografts (HT) and quadriceps tendon autografts (QT), observing a notably higher failure rate in HT (17.9%) compared to QT (1.8%) and showing that combining HA with LEAP (4.3%) substantially reduced this risk. Getgood et al. [4] and Heard et al. [3], both using hamstring autografts, reported improved stability and reduced re-rupture when augmented with LEAP, suggesting a particular benefit in this graft category.

Table 2. Summary of the results.

Publication	Study Design and Level of Evidence	Therapeutic Protocol	Outcomes	Patients' Characteristics	Graft Rupture Rates	Additional Findings	Contra-Lateral YES/NO (Y/N)
Monaco et al., 2022 [6]	Cohort study; Level of evidence, 3	Early adolescent patients who underwent ACLR using a hamstring tendon autograft with (71) or without (40) the Arnold-Coker modification of the MacIntosh procedure; patients with ≥1 additional risk factors for a graft rupture were offered LEAP in addition to ACLR	Graft rupture rates, patient-reported outcome measure scores (KOOS and subjective IKDC), knee stability, return-to-sports rates, reoperation rates, and complications were assessed.	Patients (n): 111 (71 + 40) Age (Y): 16.3 (mean) Follow up: 24–89 months	ACLR: 15% ACLR + LEAP: 0% OR: 15.91 [95% CI, 1.81–139.44]; $p = 0.012$)	Significantly better knee stability with ACLR + LEAP (pivot-shift grade 3: 0.0% vs. 11.4%, respectively; $p = 0.021$) (side-to-side anteroposterior laxity difference >5 mm: 0.0% vs. 17.1%, respectively; $p = 0.003$) and Tegner activity scores (7 vs. 6, respectively; $p = 0.010$).	N/D (not determined)
Borque et al., 2022 [11]	Cohort study; Level of evidence, 3	A consecutive cohort of elite athletes with an isolated ACL tear undergoing autograft patellar or hamstring tendon reconstruction with (117) or without (338) Lemaire LEAP	Graft rupture rate	Patients (n): 455 (117 + 338) Age (Y): 22.5 (mean) Follow up: 24 months	ACLR: 9.5% ACLR + LEAP: 3.4%	The addition of LEAP reduced the risk of undergoing revision by 2.8 times in elite athletes undergoing primary ACLR. This risk reduction did not differ significantly between the patellar tendon and hamstring tendon autografts. With these results, status as an elite athlete should be included in the indications for a LEAP, as they are at increased risk for ACL graft failure.	N/D
Heard et al., 2023 [3]	Randomized clinical trial; Level of evidence, 1	Stability is a randomized clinical trial comparing hamstring tendon ACLR with and without LEAP. Patients aged 14–25 years with an ACL-deficient knee were included. Patients were followed and adverse events documented (type, actions taken, resolution) with visits at 3, 6, 12, and 24 months postoperatively.	Adverse events were categorized as none, minor medical, minor surgical, contralateral ACL rupture, or graft rupture. Patient-reported outcome measures (PROMs) collected at each visit included the Knee Injury and Osteoarthritis Outcome Score (KOOS), International Knee Documentation Committee Score (IKDC), and ACL Quality of Life Questionnaire (ACL-QOL).	Patients (n): 618 (309 + 309) Age (Y): 18.9 (mean) Follow up: 24 months	ACLR: 11% ACLR + LEAP: 4%	The addition of LEAP to hamstring tendon autograft ACLR in young patients at high risk of re-injury resulted in a statistically significant reduction in graft rupture. While the addition of LEAP may increase rates of hardware irritation, there was no significant increase in overall rates of minor medical adverse events, minor surgical events, or overall re-operation rates.	N/D
Mao et al., 2021 [17]	Systematic review; Level of evidence, 2	PubMed, Embase, and the Cochrane Central Register of Controlled Trials databases were searched between inception and 1 July 2020. Level 1 or 2 randomized controlled trials that compared isolated single-bundle ACLR with (407) or without (392) LEAP with ACLR were included.	Data were meta-analyzed for the primary outcome measure of knee stability and the secondary outcome measures of patient-reported outcome scores, return to sports, and graft failure. Dichotomous variables were presented as relative risks (RRs), and continuous variables were presented as mean differences (MDs) and standardized MDs (SMDs).	Patients (n): 799 (392 + 407) Age (Y): 18.8–31.3 (mean) Follow up: 24 months min	ACLR: 12% ACLR + LEAP: 3.93%	The addition of LEAP to single-bundle ACLR appeared to be associated with a statistically significant, clinically relevant reduction in postoperative ALRI in the long term (>2 years) relative to ACLR alone. The adoption of LEAP may also lead to higher postoperative activity levels and a lower incidence of graft failure. For these reasons, the LEAP procedure should be considered in combination with isolated single-bundle ACLR, particularly in patients involved in strenuous sports.	N/D

Table 2. *Cont.*

Publication	Study Design and Level of Evidence	Therapeutic Protocol	Outcomes	Patients' Characteristics	Graft Rupture Rates	Additional Findings	Contra-Lateral YES/NO (Y/N)
El-Azab et al., 2023 [19]	Randomized Comparative Study; Level of evidence, 1	A Prospective Blinded Randomized Controlled study included 100 consecutive patients who underwent ACL-R with hamstring tendon grafts in our Hospital. The patients were allocated into two groups (Group A and B) with randomization; group A received ACL-R with a large-size ACL-graft diameter of 6 strands, and group B received ACL-R of 4 strands combined with lateral extraarticular tenodesis (LEAP) (Modified Lemaire). Each group had fifty patients.	They were examined for graft failure, anterolateral rotatory instability with the pivot shift test, and clinical outcomes, which were evaluated with the International Knee Documentation Committee score (IKDC) both subjective and objective.	Patients (n): 100 (50 + 50) Age (Y): 27.5 (mean) Follow up: 24 months	ACLR: 6.3% ACLR + LEAP: 2.1%	Both groups showed a low ACL-graft failure rate, low anterolateral rotatory instability, and a good clinical outcome. Although there was no significant difference in subjective IKDC score between both groups, the failure rate and anterolateral rotatory instability were significantly lower in the ACL-R (4 strands) with LEAP combination group than in the group with the large-diameter (6 strands) graft.	N/D
Feng et al., 2022 [18]	Systematic review and meta-analysis; Level of evidence, 1	PubMed, Embase, and Cochrane Library were searched by two researchers for clinical studies comparing ACLR with (583) and without LEAP (695). Studies with only evidence levels I and II and studies in which anterior lateral ligament reconstruction was performed with grafts were excluded. The risk of bias of the studies was assessed using the Cochrane risk-of-bias and modified Downs & Black tools.	The outcomes included (1) functional outcomes; (2) knee laxity measures; (3) knee injury osteoarthritis and outcome score; and (4) complications. The outcomes of the two groups were extracted, summarized and compared.	Patients (n): 1278 (583 + 695) Age (Y): 22.8 (mean) Follow up: 30 months	ACLR: 11.5% ACLR + LEAP: 3.6%	ACLR combined with LEAP can effectively reduce rotation laxity of the knee joint and reduce the graft failure rate in high-risk patients. However, the effects on the function and activity level of patients cannot be confirmed.	N/D
Castoldi et al., 2020 [16]	Randomized controlled trial; Level of evidence, 2	This study included 121 consecutive knees (120 patients) presenting to a single center with an ACL rupture between 1998 and 1999. In total, 61 knees were randomized to an isolated BTB ACLR, and 60 knees were randomized to a BTB ACLR with an extra-articular lateral tenodesis with gracilis tendon (modified Lemaire). Eighty knees in 79 patients (66%) were available for follow-up at a postoperative mean of 19.4 years (range, 19–20.2). Of those patients, 43 had a clinical examination and completed patient-reported outcome questionnaires, and the other 37 patients were evaluated through the questionnaires alone.	Standard radiographs were available for 45 patients and laximetry (TELOS) for 42 patients. Mean subjective International Knee Documentation Committee score at last follow-up was 81.8, and no differences were noted between the BTB and BTB-LEAP groups ($p = 0.7$). Two-thirds of patients were still participating in pivoting sports.	Patients (n): 80 (38 + 42) Age (Y): 26.2 mean Follow up: 19.4 years (mean)	ACLR: 29% ACLR + LEAP: 13%	There were no significant differences in long-term patient-reported outcomes after ACLR with or without an LEAP. LEAP may increase the risk of lateral compartment osteoarthritis at long-term follow-up. There was a trend toward decreased graft failure risk with the addition of LEAP but this study was underpowered to assess this outcome.	N/D

Table 2. *Cont.*

Publication	Study Design and Level of Evidence	Therapeutic Protocol	Outcomes	Patients' Characteristics	Graft Rupture Rates	Additional Findings	Contra-Lateral YES/NO (Y/N)
Getgood et al., 2020 [4]	Randomized controlled trial; Level of evidence, 1	This is a multicenter, prospective, randomized clinical trial comparing a single-bundle, hamstring tendon ACLR with (291) or without (299) LEAP performed using a strip of iliotibial band. Patients 25 years or younger with an ACL-deficient knee were included and also had to meet at least 2 of the following 3 criteria: (1) grade 2 pivot shift or greater, (2) a desire to return to high-risk/pivoting sports, (3) and generalized ligamentous laxity (GLL).	The primary outcome was ACLR clinical failure, a composite measure of rotatory laxity or a graft rupture. Secondary outcome measures included the P4 pain scale, Marx Activity Rating Scale, Knee injury Osteoarthritis and Outcome Score (KOOS), International Knee Documentation Committee score, and ACL Quality of Life Questionnaire. Patients were reviewed at 3, 6, 12, and 24 months postoperatively.	Patients (n): 590 (291 + 299) Age (Y): 18.9 years Follow up (m): 24 months	ACLR: 11.3% ACLR + LEAP: 3.7%	The number needed to treat with LEAP to prevent 1 patient from graft rupture was 14.3 over the first 2 postoperative years. At 3 months, patients in the ACLR group had less pain as measured by the P4 ($p = 0.003$) and KOOS ($p = 0.007$), with KOOS pain persisting in favor of the ACLR group to 6 months ($p = 0.02$). No clinically important differences in patient-reported outcome measures were found between groups at other time points. The level of sports activity was similar between groups at 2 years after surgery, as measured by the Marx Activity Rating Scale ($p = 0.11$).	N/D
Brinkman et al., 2025 [12]	Retrospective cohort study; Level of evidence, 3	A retrospective review was performed comparing high-risk patients undergoing ACL reconstruction with isolated HA (56), isolated QA (56), or HA + LEAP (47) from August 2013 to January 2023. High-risk patients, as determined by high-grade pivot shift or generalized ligament laxity, with at least a 2-year follow-up, were included.	Lysholm and International Knee Documentation Committee scores were compared at 3, 6, 12, and 24 months postoperatively. Retear rate, postoperative pivot-shift grade, return to sport, and complications were recorded.	Patients (n): 173 (56 + 56 + 47) Age (Y): 18.2 min (mean) Follow up: 24 months	ACLR: HA 17.9%, QA 1.8% ACLR + LEAP: 4.3%	The use of an all-soft tissue QA or HA + LEAP for ACL reconstruction resulted in a lower retear rate and postoperative pivot-shift grade compared to an isolated HA graft in high-risk patients at 2 years postoperatively. There was no difference in the rate of achieving the minimal clinically important difference between the cohorts. The QA and HA + LEAP reconstruction options may improve stability and decrease the failure rate compared with HA reconstruction alone.	N/D
Parmar et al., 2025 [13]	Retrospective comparative study; Level of evidence, 3	A retrospective review of female high school and collegiate soccer players who underwent primary ACLR from 2013 to 2021, with a minimum of 2 years of follow-up, was conducted. Participants were divided into 2 groups: those who received ACLR alone (43) and those who received ACLR with LEAP (90). Generalized ligamentous laxity was defined as a Beighton score ≥4 and was not considered an indication for LEAP. Anterior cruciate ligament (ACL) autografts included the quadriceps, bone-patellar tendon-bone, and hamstrings in both groups.	Patient demographics and physical examination findings, including pivot shift results, were collected. Positive pivot-shift refers to a grade ≥2. Patient outcomes included graft failure (defined as ACL retear), International Knee Documentation Committee score, Lysholm score, return to sport, and complications. Independent t tests, $\chi 2$ tests, and Mann-Whitney U tests were conducted to compare outcomes between the 2 groups. Minimally clinical important difference was calculated from preoperative to final follow-up.	Patients (n): 133 (43 + 90) Age (Y): 17.8 min (mean) Follow up: 24 months min	ACLR: 3% ACLR + LEAP: 4.7%	The addition of LEAP during ACLR in female soccer players with preoperative generalized ligamentous laxity yields graft retear and return-to-sport rates comparable with those of athletes without ligamentous laxity.	N/D

Table 2. *Cont.*

Publication	Study Design and Level of Evidence	Therapeutic Protocol	Outcomes	Patients' Characteristics	Graft Rupture Rates	Additional Findings	Contra-Lateral YES/NO (Y/N)
Lucidi et al., 2025 [20]	Randomized controlled trial; Level of evidence, 1	This study aimed to compare the failure rate, clinical outcomes, and OA incidence of 3 different ACL reconstruction techniques: single-bundle quadrupled hamstring tendon (HT) (20), bone-patellar tendon-bone (BPTB) (19), and over-the-top HT plus LEAP (HT + LEAP) (22). The authors hypothesized that the 3 techniques would have comparable clinical and radiographic outcomes at long-term follow-up.	At the last follow-up (minimum of 20 years), patient-reported outcome measure (PROM) scores, complications, and reoperations were collected, and an objective clinical evaluation was performed, including the measurement of anteroposterior (AP) laxity using an arthrometer and the quantification of the pivot shift (PS) using a triaxial accelerometer. Clinical failure was considered in patients with evidence of a graft rupture or those with a side-to-side difference in AP laxity >5 mm or with a side-to-side difference in the PS >1.5 mm/s^2.	Patients (n): 61 (19, 20, 22) Age (Y): 29.3 (mean) Follow up: 22.9 years min	ACLR: 37% (BPTB) 25% (HT) ACLR + LEAP: 19%	The 3 investigated techniques (BPTB, quadrupled HT, and over-the-top HT plus LEAP) provided comparable good clinical and radiographic outcomes at a mean follow-up time of 23 years. The BPTB group showed a greater prevalence of patellofemoral OA than the HT + LEAP group, while no difference was reported for tibiofemoral OA. The BPTB group revealed a slightly lower Tegner score than the HT + LEAP group, while the HT group showed slightly higher AP laxity than the BPTB group.	N/D
Viglietta et al., 2022 [7]	Cohort study; Level of evidence, 3	The study included 165 consecutive patients treated at a single center by ACLR. A total of 86 patients underwent iACLR (iACLR group) and 79 received combined intra- and extra-articular reconstruction (ACLR + LEAP).	The International Knee Documentation Committee (IKDC), Lysholm, and Tegner activity scores were administered. Knee stability was tested through the Lachman test, the pivot-shift test, and the KT-1000 knee arthrometer test. A positive pivot-shift test (++/+++), laxity on the KT-1000, and referred giving-way episodes or revision ACLR were considered failures. Radiographic results were assessed according to the Fairbank, IKDC, and Kellgren-Lawrence scales. Radiographic evaluation included both the overall tibiofemoral joint and the medial and lateral compartments separately. A univariate and a multivariate logistic regression with penalized maximum likelihood was used to identify risk factors associated with long-term OA.	Patients (n): 165 (86 + 79) Age (Y): 26.1 (mean) Follow up: 15.7 years (mean)	ACLR: 10.4% ACLR + LEAP: 1.2%	A significantly higher risk of long-term OA was found with iACLR than with ACLR combined with the Arnold-Coker modification of the McIntosh extra-articular procedure. Knees with combined ACLR also had a significantly lower OA grade after partial lateral meniscectomy. Additionally, those undergoing combined ACLR had better knee stability and lower graft rupture rates at the long-term follow-up. Partial meniscectomy was the main risk factor negatively associated with OA changes.	N/D
Serna et al.,, 2025 [8]	Retrospective, propensity-matched cohort; Level III evidence.	ACLR alone (CPT 29888) ACLR + LEAP (CPT 29888 + 27427)	5—yr cumulative revision; 2—yr cumulative revision; differences in 5—yr in meniscus surgery, lysis of adhesions, manipulation, or 90—day ED visits	Patients (n) = 1022 per group; Mean age 24.2 y (ACLR + LEAP) vs. 30.0 y (ACLR); Female 46.5%; Overweight/obesity 20.1% vs. 24.9%;	5—yr revision: ACLR + LEAP 2.6% vs. ACLR 4.9%; 2—yr revision: ACLR + LEAP 0.7% vs. ACLR 3.2%	LEAP utilization rose >20% year-on-year after 2017 (except 2020); Only one TKA conversion in ACLR + LEAP group over 5 yrs; No increase in other secondary complications; Coding ensured ipsilateral procedures only.	N/D

Table 2. *Cont.*

Publication	Study Design and Level of Evidence	Therapeutic Protocol	Outcomes	Patients' Characteristics	Graft Rupture Rates	Additional Findings	Contra-Lateral YES/NO (Y/N)
Hopper et al., 2022 [14]	Retrospective cohort study; Level III evidence.	Isolated ACLR (primary hamstring or patellar tendon autograft); ACLR + LEAP (lateral extra-articular procedure)	Graft failure requiring revision; Contralateral ACL rupture; Ipsilateral secondary surgeries	Patients (n) = 342 (166ACLR + 176 ACLR + ALLR professional athletes; mean follow-up 100.2 ± 51.9 months (range 24–215); age subgroup ≤21 vs. >21 years; graft types: hamstring or patellar tendon.	ACLR:15.5%; ACLR + LEAP: 6.0% (p = 0.0105); HR for isolated ACLR 2.678 (95% CI 1.173–4.837; p = 0.0164)	Athletes ≤21 years at >2-fold risk of failure (HR 2.381; 95% CI 1.313–5.463; p = 0.0068); Sex, sport, graft type aren't significant risk factors; Contralateral ACL rupture: 13.2%; Ipsilateral secondary surgeries: 18.1%	Y
Guy et al., 2022 [15]	Retrospective cohort study; Level of evidence III	Isolated ACLR ACLR + LEAP (modified Lemaire or anterolateral ligament reconstruction)	Graft rupture	n = 81 (50 ACLR + 31 ACLR + LEAP) elite alpine skiers; min follow-up 2 y;	ACLR: 34.0%; ACLR + LEAP 6.5% (p = 0.0412)	Age (HR 1.114; p = 0.1157), sex (HR 1.573; p = 0.3743) and graft type (HR 1.417; p = 0.5394) were not associated with a higher risk of graft rupture.	N/D
Mahmoud et al., 2022 [9]	Retrospective matched cohort study; Level III evidence;	ACLR + LEAP (iliotibial band tenodesis via modified Lemaire technique through Kaplan's fibers); Isolated ACLR (standard semitendinosus–gracilis autograft)	PROMs (Lysholm, IKDC, OKS, Tegner), Graft Rupture Rates	Patients (n) = 144 (72 per group); mean age 25 ± 8.5 y; 76% male; median follow-up 10 y (IQR 6.7)	ACLR-LEAP: 5%; ACLR: 11%	PROMs (Lysholm, IKDC, OKS, Tegner) improved significantly post-op in both groups with no significant between-group differences (e.g., Lysholm Δ p = 0.82, IKDC Δ p = 0.07); Few complications: ACLR-LEAP 3 meniscus re-arthroscopies; ACLR 1 DVT, 1 superficial infection, 4 meniscus re-arthroscopies; PROMs exceeded MCID in majority of patients	N/D
Porter et al., 2020 [5]	Prospective randomized controlled trial; Level II evidence; skeletally mature patients with residual pivot shift post-ACLR.	Group A: ACLR alone (no further surgery) Group B: ACLR + Modified Iliotibial Band Tenodesis (MITBT) added intraoperatively	IKDC score; KOOS Sport/Rec; KOOS QoL; Lysholm; Tegner: median; Recurrent ACL ruptures; Meniscal tears; Contralateral ACL ruptures	Patients (n) = 55 randomized (27 A, 28 B); female:male A 15:12, B 17:11; mean age 22.3 ± 3.7 y (A) vs. 21.8 ± 4.1 y (B); pivoting sports; no meniscal repair.	Recurrent ACL ruptures: 14.8% (A) vs. 0% (B); p < 0.001	IKDC score: 90.9 ± 10.7 (A) vs. 94.2 ± 11.2 (B); p = 0.21; KOOS Sport/Rec: 91.5 ± 6.4 vs. 95.3 ± 4.4; p = 0.02; KOOS QoL: 92.0 ± 4.8 vs. 95.1 ± 4.3; p = 0.14; Lysholm: 92.5 ± 4.8 vs. 96.8 ± 8.0; p = 0.004; Tegner: median 7 [6–8] vs. 8 [7–9]; p = 0.03; Recurrent ACL ruptures: 14.8% vs. 0%; p < 0.001; Meniscal tears: 14.8% vs. 3.6%; p = 0.14; Contralateral ACL ruptures: 3.7% vs. 3.6%; p = 0.99; MITBT reduced residual pivot shift: Improved KOOS Sport/Rec, Lysholm, Tegner scores; No difference in contralateral ruptures	Y
Rowan et al., 2019 [10]	Retrospective cohort; propensity-matched case–control; Level III evidence.	ACL reconstruction alone (single-bundle doubled hamstring graft) ACL reconstruction + LEAT (modified iliotibial band tenodesis) based on high-grade pivot shift or ≥2 minor criteria	Post-op Lysholm score; Tegner activity index; Time to return to sport; ACL re-injury (ipsilateral)	Patients (n) = 171 (125 ACLR alone vs. 46 ACLR + LEAT (matched)) Median age 29 vs. 27 years; 54% vs. 59% male; Sports: football, skiing, rugby, hockey, basketball, others; Elite athletes	ACLR: 5%; ACLR + LEAT: 0%	Post-op Lysholm score: median 90 vs. 98; p = 0.005; Tegner activity index: mean 7.54 vs. 8.04; p = 0.003; Time to return to sport: median 8 vs. 6 months; p < 0.001	N/D

5. Discussion

Our systematic review and meta-analysis suggest that adding lateral extra-articular procedures (LEAP) to anterior cruciate ligament reconstruction (ACLR) may be beneficial in reducing the risk of graft failure, particularly in high-risk populations. Across the included studies, encompassing 7336 patients, the pooled analysis showed that ACLR alone was associated with nearly three times the risk of graft rupture compared to ACLR combined with LEAP, with a risk ratio of 2.72 (95% CI: 2.23–3.32; $p < 0.00001$) and negligible heterogeneity ($I^2 = 0\%$) [2–5,8,9]. Individual studies consistently demonstrated lower graft failure rates with LEAP augmentation. For instance, Monaco et al. [6] Anterior Cruciate Ligament Reconstruction with Lateral Extra-Articular Tenodesis Reduces Knee Rotation Laxity and Graft Failure Rate: A Systematic Review and Meta-Analysis reported 0% graft failure in adolescents undergoing ACLR + LEAP compared to 15% in isolated ACLR [2], while Borque et al. [11] observed 3.4% versus 9.5% in elite athletes. Similarly, Getgood et al. [4] found a reduction from 11.3% to 3.7% in young, high-risk patients, and Viglietta et al. [7] demonstrated a long-term decrease in graft rupture from 10.4% to 1.2%. Although a few studies such as Parmar et al. [13] reported slightly higher failure rates in LEAP cohorts, these differences were not statistically significant.

Beyond graft failure, LEAP may improve rotational stability and functional outcomes. Studies reported lower pivot-shift grades and reduced anteroposterior laxity in combined ACLR + LEAP groups, with improved Tegner and Lysholm scores in several cohorts [2,3,5,15,20]. Return-to-sport rates were comparable or superior with LEAP, with Rowan et al. [10] documenting faster return to pivoting sports and higher functional scores. Adverse event profiles were similar between groups, with no significant increase in postoperative stiffness, infection, or contralateral ACL injuries [3,15,16]. Long-term concerns regarding lateral compartment osteoarthritis were inconsistently reported; while Castoldi et al. [16] suggested a trend toward higher osteoarthritis risk after LEAP, other long-term studies found no such association and even reported lower osteoarthritis grades in LEAP groups [7,13,14]. These findings support the notion that the reduction in graft failure may contribute to long-term joint preservation and potentially reduce the risk of post-traumatic osteoarthritis, although further longitudinal studies are needed.

Recent intra-operative findings further underscore the severe long-term consequences of persistent ACL deficiency. Passaretti et al. [21] performed an intra-operative analysis in patients undergoing total knee arthroplasty and found significant correlations between ACL lesions and advanced gonarthrosis, suggesting that unaddressed rotational or translational knee instability may accelerate joint degeneration and lead to end-stage osteoarthritis requiring joint replacement. This evidence reinforces the idea that reducing graft failure and residual instability via adjunct procedures such as LEAP may not only prevent revision surgery, but also contribute to long-term joint preservation.

Potential modifying factors should be considered when evaluating LEAP. Age, participation in pivoting sports, generalized ligamentous laxity, and graft choice may influence outcomes. Adolescents and elite athletes appear to derive the greatest benefit from LEAP [3,4,6,7,11,14], and evidence suggests protective effects across hamstring, quadriceps, and bone-patellar tendon-bone grafts [4,6,12,20].

While the primary focus is on graft protection, clinicians should also consider surgical complexity, operative time, and rehabilitation implications. LEAP is an additional procedure that may increase surgical duration and requires careful technique to avoid lateral overconstraint. Rehabilitation protocols are largely similar to standard ACLR, but close monitoring for lateral knee pain or stiffness is recommended [3,7]. Cost-effectiveness analyses remain limited; however, the potential to reduce revision surgeries may provide long-term economic benefits.

In conclusion, the current evidence suggests that LEAP may be beneficial in reducing graft failure and improving rotational stability in selected high-risk patients without a significant increase in complications. These findings support a selective application of LEAP, guided by patient-specific risk factors, intraoperative assessment, and consideration of modifying factors such as age, sport, and graft type [2,4,6,7,11,21]. Future studies should further investigate long-term joint preservation, cost-effectiveness, and optimal patient selection criteria.

Supplementary Materials: The following supporting information can be downloaded at: https://www.mdpi.com/article/10.3390/jcm14238499/s1, PRISMA Checklist.

Author Contributions: Conceptualization, S.G. and A.M.; methodology, S.P. and A.M.; validation, E.A.; formal analysis, A.M.; investigation, S.P.; data curation, S.P.; writing—original draft preparation, S.P., C.M. and A.M.; writing—review and editing, S.G., S.P., A.M. and C.M.; supervision, E.A. All authors have read and agreed to the published version of the manuscript.

Funding: This research received no external funding.

Institutional Review Board Statement: Not applicable.

Informed Consent Statement: Not applicable.

Data Availability Statement: Data supporting the findings of this study are available from the corresponding author upon reasonable request.

Conflicts of Interest: The authors declare no conflicts of interest.

References

1. Sonnery-Cottet, B.; Carrozzo, A.; Saithna, A.; Monaco, E.; Vieira, T.D.; Musahl, V.; Getgood, A.; Helito, C.P.; Bedi, A.; Bryant, D.; et al. Surgical Treatment and Complications of Lateral Extra-Articular Procedures in the Anterior Cruciate Ligament–Reconstructed Knee: Part II of an International Consensus Statement. *Arthroscopy* **2025**, *41*, 3313–3321. [CrossRef]
2. Nazzal, E.M.; Keeling, L.E.; Ryan, P.M.; Herman, Z.J.; Hughes, J.D. The Role of Lateral Extra-Articular Tenodesis in Anterior Cruciate Ligament Reconstruction and Treatment of Rotatory Knee Instability: A Scoping Review. *Curr. Rev. Musculoskelet. Med.* **2023**, *16*, 235–245. [CrossRef]
3. Heard, M.; Marmura, H.; Bryant, D.; Litchfield, R.; McCormack, R.; MacDonald, P.; Spalding, T.; Verdonk, P.; Peterson, D.; Bardana, D.; et al. No Increase in Adverse Events with Lateral Extra-Articular Tenodesis Augmentation of Anterior Cruciate Ligament Reconstruction—Results from the Stability Randomized Trial. *J. ISAKOS* **2023**, *8*, 246–254. [CrossRef]
4. Getgood, A.M.J.; Bryant, D.M.; Litchfield, R.; Heard, M.; McCormack, R.G.; Rezansoff, A.; Peterson, D.; Bardana, D.; MacDonald, P.B.; Verdonk, P.C.M.; et al. Lateral Extra-Articular Tenodesis Reduces Failure of Hamstring Tendon Autograft Anterior Cruciate Ligament Reconstruction: 2-Year Outcomes From the STABILITY Study Randomized Clinical Trial. *Am. J. Sports Med.* **2020**, *48*, 285–297. [CrossRef]
5. Porter, M.; Shadbolt, B. Modified Iliotibial Band Tenodesis Is Indicated to Correct Intraoperative Residual Pivot Shift After Anterior Cruciate Ligament Reconstruction Using an Autologous Hamstring Tendon Graft: A Prospective Randomized Controlled Trial. *Am. J. Sports Med.* **2020**, *48*, 1069–1077. [CrossRef]
6. Monaco, E.; Carrozzo, A.; Saithna, A.; Conteduca, F.; Annibaldi, A.; Marzilli, F.; Minucci, M.; Sonnery-Cottet, B.; Ferretti, A. Isolated ACL Reconstruction Versus ACL Reconstruction Combined With Lateral Extra-Articular Tenodesis: A Comparative Study of Clinical Outcomes in Adolescent Patients. *Am. J. Sports Med.* **2022**, *50*, 3244–3255. [CrossRef]
7. Viglietta, E.; Ponzo, A.; Monaco, E.; Iorio, R.; Drogo, P.; Andreozzi, V.; Conteduca, F.; Ferretti, A. ACL Reconstruction Combined With the Arnold-Coker Modification of the MacIntosh Lateral Extra-Articular Tenodesis: Long-Term Clinical and Radiological Outcomes. *Am. J. Sports Med.* **2022**, *50*, 404–414. [CrossRef]
8. Serna, J.; Kucirek, N.; Terada-Herzer, K.; Lansdown, D.; Ma, C.B.; Zhang, A.L. Anterior Cruciate Ligament Reconstruction With Lateral Extra-Articular Tenodesis Is Associated With Reduced Risk for Revision Anterior Cruciate Ligament Reconstruction in an Insurance Claims Database. *Arthroscopy* **2025**, *41*, 3425–3434. [CrossRef]
9. Mahmoud, A.; Torbey, S.; Honeywill, C.; Myers, P. Lateral Extra-Articular Tenodesis Combined With Anterior Cruciate Ligament Reconstruction Is Effective in Knees With Additional Features of Lateral, Hyperextension, or Increased Rotational Laxity: A Matched Cohort Study. *Arthroscopy* **2022**, *38*, 119–124. [CrossRef]

10. Rowan, F.E.; Huq, S.S.; Haddad, F.S. Lateral Extra-Articular Tenodesis with ACL Reconstruction Demonstrates Better Patient-Reported Outcomes Compared to ACL Reconstruction Alone at 2 Years Minimum Follow-Up. *Arch. Orthop. Trauma. Surg.* **2019**, *139*, 1425–1433. [CrossRef]
11. Borque, K.A.; Jones, M.; Laughlin, M.S.; Balendra, G.; Willinger, L.; Pinheiro, V.H.; Williams, A. Effect of Lateral Extra-Articular Tenodesis on the Rate of Revision Anterior Cruciate Ligament Reconstruction in Elite Athletes. *Am. J. Sports Med.* **2022**, *50*, 3487–3492. [CrossRef]
12. Brinkman, J.C.; McQuivey, K.S.; Braithwaite, C.; Paul, B.R.; Verhey, J.T.; Haglin, J.M.; Hoffer, A.J.; Economopoulos, S.C.; Economopoulos, K.J. Anterior Cruciate Ligament Reconstruction Using Hamstring Autograft Plus Lateral Extra-Articular Tenodesis and All-Soft Tissue Quadriceps Alone Have Lower Retear Rate and Pivot-Shift Grade but Similar Outcome to Hamstring Autograft Alone in High-Risk Patients. *Arthroscopy* **2025**, *41*, 2988–2995. [CrossRef]
13. Parmar, R.; Tummala, S.V.; Brinkman, J.C.; Economopoulos, K.J. Lateral Extra-Articular Tenodesis With Iliotibial Band in Anterior Cruciate Ligament Autograft Reconstruction for Female Soccer Athletes With Generalized Ligamentous Laxity Yields Graft Failure and Return-to-Sport Rates Comparable With Athletes Without Generalized Laxity. *Arthroscopy* **2025**, *41*, 4136–4144. [CrossRef]
14. Hopper, G.P.; Pioger, C.; Philippe, C.; El Helou, A.; Campos, J.P.; Gousopoulos, L.; Carrozzo, A.; Vieira, T.D.; Sonnery-Cottet, B. Risk Factors for Anterior Cruciate Ligament Graft Failure in Professional Athletes: An Analysis of 342 Patients With a Mean Follow-up of 100 Months From the SANTI Study Group. *Am. J. Sports Med.* **2022**, *50*, 3218–3227. [CrossRef]
15. Guy, S.; Fayard, J.-M.; Saithna, A.; Bahroun, S.; Ferreira, A.; Carrozzo, A.; De Jesus, S.; Bulle, S.; Vieira, T.D.; Sonnery-Cottet, B. Risk of Graft Rupture After Adding a Lateral Extra-Articular Procedure at the Time of ACL Reconstruction: A Retrospective Comparative Study of Elite Alpine Skiers From the French National Team. *Am. J. Sports Med.* **2022**, *50*, 1609–1617. [CrossRef] [PubMed]
16. Castoldi, M.; Magnussen, R.A.; Gunst, S.; Batailler, C.; Neyret, P.; Lustig, S.; Servien, E. A Randomized Controlled Trial of Bone–Patellar Tendon–Bone Anterior Cruciate Ligament Reconstruction With and Without Lateral Extra-Articular Tenodesis: 19-Year Clinical and Radiological Follow-Up. *Am. J. Sports Med.* **2020**, *48*, 1665–1672. [CrossRef]
17. Mao, Y.; Zhang, K.; Li, J.; Fu, W. Supplementary Lateral Extra-Articular Tenodesis for Residual Anterolateral Rotatory Instability in Patients Undergoing Single-Bundle Anterior Cruciate Ligament Reconstruction: A Meta-Analysis of Randomized Controlled Trials. *Orthop. J. Sports Med.* **2021**, *9*, 23259671211002282. [CrossRef]
18. Feng, J.; Cao, Y.; Tan, L.; Liang, J.; He, C.; He, J.; Wu, S. Anterior Cruciate Ligament Reconstruction with Lateral Extra-Articular Tenodesis Reduces Knee Rotation Laxity and Graft Failure Rate: A Systematic Review and Meta-Analysis. *J. Orthop. Surg.* **2022**, *30*, 10225536221095969. [CrossRef]
19. El-Azab, H.; Moursy, M.; Mohamed, M.A.; Elsayed, M. A Comparison of the Outcomes of Anterior Curciate Ligament Reconstruction with Large-Size Graft versus Reconstruction with Average-Size Graft Combined with Extraarticular Tenodesis. *Injury* **2023**, *54*, 976–982. [CrossRef]
20. Lucidi, G.A.; Agostinone, P.; Di Paolo, S.; Dal Fabbro, G.; Serra, M.; Viotto, M.; Grassi, A.; Zaffagnini, S. Long-Term Outcomes After Anterior Cruciate Ligament Reconstruction With 3 Different Surgical Techniques: A Prospective Randomized Clinical and Radiographic Evaluation at a Minimum of 20 Years' Follow-Up. *Orthop. J. Sports Med.* **2025**, *13*, 23259671241302348. [CrossRef]
21. Passaretti, A.; Colò, G.; Bulgheroni, A.; Vulcano, E.; Surace, M.F. Gonarthrosis and ACL Lesion: An Intraoperative Analysis and Correlations in Patients Who Underwent Total Knee Arthroplasty. *Minerva Orthop.* **2025**, *75*, 331–336. [CrossRef]

Journal of
Clinical Medicine

MDPI

Article

Combined ACL and ALL Reconstruction Using Allografts as the ACL Graft Source Reduces Surgical Failure and Improves Graft Maturity Compared with Isolated ACL Reconstruction

Hyun-Soo Moon [1,2], Sungjun Kim [3], Min Jung [1,4], Kwangho Chung [1,5], Se-Han Jung [1,4], Junhee Cho [1,4], Gyunghyun Shin [2] and Sung-Hwan Kim [1,4,*]

1 Arthroscopy and Joint Research Institute, Yonsei University College of Medicine, Seoul 03722, Republic of Korea
2 Department of Orthopedic Surgery, Gangnam Severance Hospital, Yonsei University College of Medicine, Seoul 06273, Republic of Korea
3 Department of Radiology, Gangnam Severance Hospital, Yonsei University College of Medicine, Seoul 06273, Republic of Korea
4 Department of Orthopedic Surgery, Severance Hospital, Yonsei University College of Medicine, Seoul 03722, Republic of Korea
5 Department of Orthopedic Surgery, Yongin Severance Hospital, Yonsei University College of Medicine, Yongin 16995, Republic of Korea
* Correspondence: orthohwan@gmail.com; Tel.: +82-2-2228-2180; Fax: +82-2-363-1139

Abstract

Objectives: This study aimed to perform matched comparisons of the surgical outcomes of combined anterior cruciate ligament (ACL) and anterolateral ligament (ALL) reconstruction with those of isolated ACL reconstruction, in which allografts were used for the ACL. **Methods:** Patients who underwent anatomical ACL reconstruction with or without additional ALL reconstruction between 2017 and 2023 and had a minimum follow-up of 2 years were included and grouped according to whether an additional ALL reconstruction was performed. The cohorts were statistically adjusted using an inverse probability of treatment weighting (IPTW) to control for potential confounders related to surgical indication, including age, activity level, sex, rotational knee laxity, and preoperative osteoarthritic grade. Between-group comparisons were conducted for baseline characteristics, clinical outcomes, knee laxity, and radiologic parameters. **Results:** Fifty-nine patients were included (Group 1: 39 isolated ACL reconstructions; Group 2: 20 combined ACL and ALL reconstructions). Before IPTW adjustment, a significant difference was observed in the preoperative pivot-shift test ($p = 0.008$), which was no longer significant after weighting. Postoperative functional outcomes and knee stability were comparable between groups; however, the incidence of surgical failure was significantly lower in Group 2 both before and after IPTW adjustment ($p = 0.044$ and $p = 0.049$, respectively). Regarding radiologic parameters, the signal-to-noise quotient of the ACL graft was also significantly lower in Group 2, both before and after IPTW adjustment ($p = 0.046$ and $p = 0.038$, respectively). **Conclusions:** In ACL reconstruction using allografts, the addition of ALL reconstruction resulted in more favorable clinical and radiologic outcomes—particularly a lower incidence of surgical failure and greater postoperative graft maturity—compared with isolated ACL reconstruction.

Keywords: anterior cruciate ligament reconstruction; anterolateral ligament reconstruction; allograft; surgical failure; graft maturity

1. Introduction

The addition of anterolateral augmentation procedures, including anterolateral ligament (ALL) reconstruction and lateral extra-articular tenodesis (LET), to anterior cruciate ligament (ACL) reconstruction has been reported to provide significant clinical benefits [1–5]. Combined procedures have demonstrated superior outcomes compared with isolated ACL reconstruction, not only in terms of functional recovery and residual knee laxity but also with respect to graft failure and reoperation rates [1–6]. Consequently, the use of anterolateral augmentation procedures in conjunction with ACL reconstruction has been steadily increasing, with both ALL reconstruction and LET being applied according to surgeon preference and patient characteristics [7–9].

However, most previous studies on combined ACL and anterolateral augmentation procedures have been limited to cases in which autografts were used as the graft source for ACL reconstruction [1–5], and the clinical outcomes of allograft-based procedures remain largely uninvestigated. Allografts have been reported to require a relatively longer period for ligamentization than autografts and may yield less favorable outcomes, particularly in young and active individuals [10–15]. In this regard, graft maturation may be influenced not only by mechanical stability but also by biological healing processes originating from the surrounding soft tissues [16]. Given that the biological behavior of allografts differs from that of autografts, the benefits of anterolateral augmentation observed in autograft-based studies cannot be assumed to translate directly to allograft ACL reconstruction. With the widespread use of allografts in ACL reconstruction worldwide [13,17,18], there remains a need to clarify the clinical outcomes of combined ACL and anterolateral augmentation procedures when ACL reconstruction is performed using allografts. Furthermore, a direct comparison with isolated ACL reconstruction is warranted to better delineate the potential advantages of this combined approach.

Therefore, the purpose of this study was to perform matched comparisons of the surgical outcomes of combined ACL and ALL reconstruction with those of isolated ACL reconstruction, in which allografts were used for the ACL. It was hypothesized that combined ACL and ALL reconstruction would yield superior subjective and objective outcomes compared with isolated ACL reconstruction.

2. Methods

Approval for this study was obtained from the Institutional Review Board of Gangnam Severance Hospital, and the requirement for informed consent was waived owing to the retrospective design of the study (IRB No. 3-2025-0279). A retrospective review of electronic medical records was conducted for patients who underwent surgical treatment for ACL rupture at a single institution by a single senior surgeon between January 2017 and June 2023, which served as the study timeframe for case inclusion. Patients who underwent anatomical ACL reconstruction using the transportal technique were eligible for inclusion, regardless of whether the procedure was performed as an isolated ACL reconstruction or in combination with ALL reconstruction, provided that an allograft was used as the graft source for the ACL. Patients were excluded if they met any of the following criteria: (1) the follow-up period was less than two years; (2) an autograft was used for ACL reconstruction; (3) surgery was performed as a revision procedure; (4) major concomitant procedures such as meniscal allograft transplantation; multi-ligament reconstruction other than ALL reconstruction, or osteotomy; or (5) the available outcome data were insufficient. After applying these criteria, the eligible patients were divided into two groups according to whether ALL reconstruction was performed in addition to ACL reconstruction: Group 1 comprised patients who underwent isolated ACL reconstruction, and Group 2 comprised those who underwent combined ACL and ALL reconstruction (Figure 1).

https://doi.org/10.3390/jcm15020735

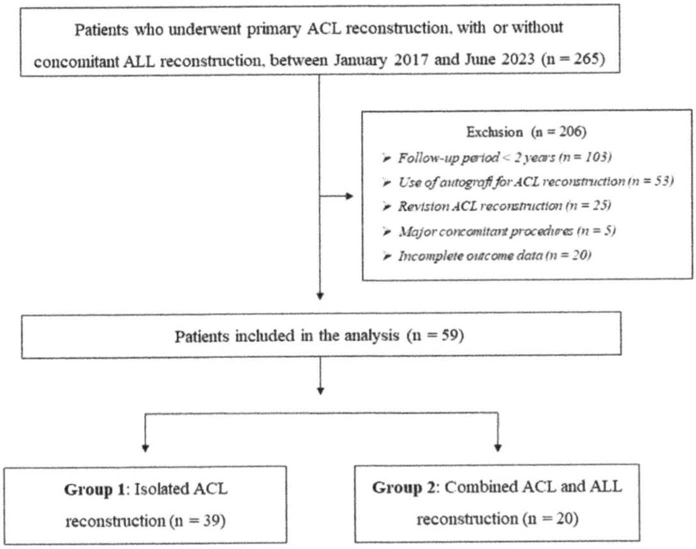

Figure 1. Flowchart of patient selection and grouping.

2.1. Surgical Procedures and Rehabilitation Methods

Before surgery, all patients received detailed counseling regarding the available graft options for ACL reconstruction—including autogenous bone–patellar tendon–bone grafts, autogenous hamstring tendon grafts, and allogeneic tendon grafts—and were informed of the potential advantages and disadvantages of each option [19,20]. The final choice of graft type was made by the patient. For allograft reconstruction, a low-dose γ-irradiated (12.8–12.9 kGy, cobalt-60) tibialis anterior allograft measuring 8–10 mm in diameter was utilized. The graft was thawed at room temperature in a saline solution containing antibiotics, after which both ends were whipstitched with No. 1 Ethibond sutures (Ethicon, Somerville, NJ, USA). The diameter of the tendon was determined by folding the graft over an Ethibond suture to create a double-strand configuration and passing it through a calibrated sizing block (GraftMaster III; Smith & Nephew, Watford, UK). The prepared graft was then pre-tensioned to approximately 80 N for 20 min on a graft-preparation station (GraftMaster III; Smith & Nephew, Watford, UK) [21].

ACL reconstruction began with diagnostic arthroscopy performed through a parapatellar high anterolateral portal to evaluate all knee compartments [22]. Meniscal and/or chondral lesions, if present, were treated appropriately before ligament reconstruction. A tibial tunnel was then created at the anatomic tibial footprint of the ACL, with a diameter matching that of the prepared allograft. An independent femoral tunnel was drilled via a far anteromedial portal at approximately 120° of knee flexion to ensure adequate length and prevent posterior wall blowout [23]. The femoral socket was prepared to match the graft size and extended proximally to accommodate the EndoButton CL (Smith & Nephew, Watford, UK). The graft was inserted and fixed to the femur using the EndoButton, and proper flipping was confirmed. Distal fixation was achieved after pre-tensioning the graft to 80 N and cycling it 20 times. The graft was then secured with a bioabsorbable interference screw and an additional cortical screw with a washer (ConMed Linvatec, Largo, FL, USA) at approximately 10–20° of knee flexion.

At our institution, ALL reconstruction began to be performed actively around 2019. The general surgical indications for performing additional ALL reconstruction in conjunction with ACL reconstruction included the following: (1) young patients with a high

https://doi.org/10.3390/jcm15020735

activity level, (2) grade 2 or 3 pivot shift, and (3) revision ACL reconstruction [24–26]. The ALL reconstruction was performed using either a single-arm or an inverted V-shaped double-arm configuration, with most cases employing the single-arm technique. A tibialis anterior allograft was used, trimmed to approximately 5 mm in diameter, and whipstitched for about 30 mm at one end with No. 2 Ethibond sutures. On the tibial side, a short vertical incision was made just posterior to Gerdy's tubercle. The tibial fixation was aimed midway between Gerdy's tubercle and the anterior margin of the fibular head [27]. After guide pin insertion, a 6 mm tibial tunnel was reamed toward the opposite cortex, with an orientation of 10° axial and −30° coronal [28]. The femoral fixation was targeted at the anatomic origin of the ALL, located just proximal and posterior to the lateral femoral epicondyle [27,29]. A guide pin was inserted distally in the coronal plane, oriented at 0° axial and −40° coronal, to prevent convergence with the ACL femoral tunnel [30], and a closed-socket tunnel approximately 30 mm in length was created. The whipstitched graft end was then secured to the femoral socket with a 4.5–5.5 mm SwiveLock® anchor (Arthrex, Naples, FL, USA). The graft was then passed deep to the iliotibial band and routed through the extra-articular layer from the femur to the tibia. The distal portion of the graft (approximately 30 mm) was whipstitched with No. 2 Ethibond sutures, and the graft was then advanced into the tibial tunnel along the pre-inserted guide pin. Tibial fixation was achieved using a bioabsorbable interference screw while applying gentle traction (~20 N) with the knee in near full extension (10–20° flexion, neutral rotation) [31] (Figure 2).

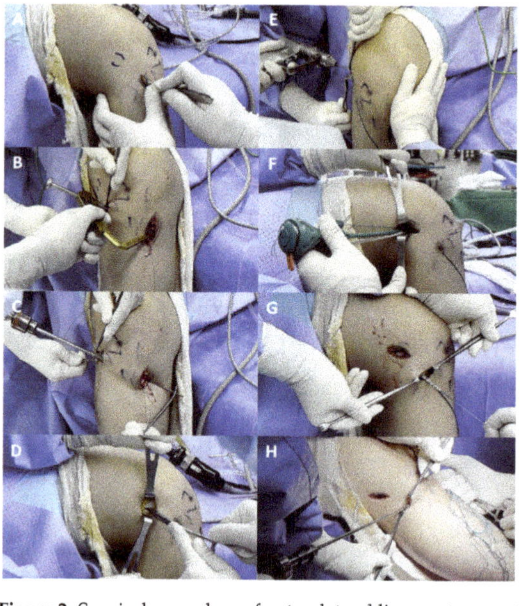

Figure 2. Surgical procedure of anterolateral ligament reconstruction using the single-arm technique: (**A**) A short vertical incision was made midway between Gerdy's tubercle and the anterior margin of the fibular head. (**B**,**C**) A 6 mm tibial tunnel was reamed toward the opposite cortex at an orientation of 10° axial and −30° coronal to minimize the risk of saphenous nerve injury. (**D**) On the femoral side, a small incision was made over the lateral femoral epicondyle, and the point just posterosuperior to the epicondyle was identified beneath the iliotibial band. (**E**) Thereafter, a 5–6 mm diameter, 30 mm deep tunnel was reamed with an orientation of 0° axial and −40° coronal to avoid convergence with the anterior cruciate ligament femoral tunnel. (**F**) The whipstitched graft was fixed to the femoral tunnel with a 4.5–5.5 mm SwiveLock® anchor. (**G**) The graft was passed deep to the iliotibial band and advanced into the tibial tunnel after distal whipstitching. (**H**) Tibial fixation was completed with a bioabsorbable interference screw under gentle traction (~20 N) in near-full extension.

https://doi.org/10.3390/jcm15020735

Postoperative rehabilitation followed a standardized protocol regardless of whether combined ALL reconstruction was performed. Immediately after surgery, patients were allowed crutch-assisted ambulation with tolerable weight-bearing. Early exercises for passive knee range of motion and isometric quadriceps strengthening were encouraged from the first postoperative day. At 6 weeks postoperatively, full weight-bearing ambulation was permitted, and closed kinetic chain exercises were initiated. In cases where meniscal or chondral repair was performed, both weight-bearing and knee range of motion exercises were delayed in accordance with the corresponding rehabilitation protocol for meniscal or cartilage repair. After 6 months, patients were allowed to begin open kinetic chain exercises, jogging, and swimming. Return to sports activities involving pivoting, jumping, or side-stepping was permitted approximately 9 months after surgery.

2.2. Patient Assessment

The evaluation of patients involved conducting clinical assessments, encompassing demographic data, functional scores, and knee laxity, along with intraoperative data and various radiographic parameters. Functional scores used for patient evaluation included the International Knee Documentation Committee (IKDC) subjective, Lysholm, and Tegner activity scores [32,33]. The assessment of knee laxity was conducted for both anterior-posterior (AP) and rotational laxity. AP laxity of the knee was measured using a KT-2000 arthrometer (MEDmetric, San Diego, CA, USA) under maximum manual force [34], as well as with the manual Lachman test. The anterior tibial translation of the affected knee was measured using a KT-2000 arthrometer and compared with that of the contralateral knee; the side-to-side difference (SSD) was recorded for analysis. Rotational laxity of the knee was evaluated through the manual pivot shift test and recorded as follows: grade 0 (absent = normal), grade 1 (glide = nearly normal), grade 2 (jump = abnormal), and grade 3 (transient lock = severely abnormal). The assessments of functional scores and knee laxity were based on records conducted independently of this study when patients visited outpatient clinics. In this study, the analysis was performed using records from the preoperative phase, postoperative 2-years, and the final follow-up. Surgical failure after ACL reconstruction was defined as the presence of any of the following findings indicative of unfavorable surgical outcomes during follow-up: (1) graft re-tear confirmed by magnetic resonance imaging (MRI); (2) AP knee laxity graded as 2 or 3, based on KT-2000 arthrometer measurements or the manual Lachman test; or (3) rotational knee laxity graded as 2 or 3 on the manual pivot-shift test [35–37]. Although surgical failure did not necessarily correspond to the need for revision surgery at our institution—since the decision for revision was also influenced by patient characteristics and the severity of subjective symptoms—this definition was adopted to comprehensively capture all potential cases associated with unsatisfactory postoperative outcomes.

Intraoperative data were analyzed with respect to the diameter of the ACL graft and the intra-articular status of the meniscus and articular cartilage, as documented in records completed immediately after surgery. The condition of the meniscus was assessed separately for the medial and lateral compartments and categorized as functional, nonfunctional, or repaired. A meniscus was regarded as functional when no pathologic tear was present or when a limited partial meniscectomy had been performed for lesions not compromising its biomechanical integrity [38]. A nonfunctional meniscus referred to cases with a history of prior subtotal meniscectomy or the presence of extensive, irreparable tears [38]. Tibiofemoral articular cartilage was classified as intact, low-grade lesion, high-grade lesion, or treated with a cartilage repair procedure. Lesions corresponding to International Cartilage Repair Society grades 1–2 were considered low-grade, whereas those graded 3 or higher were defined as high-grade defects.

https://doi.org/10.3390/jcm15020735

Radiologic assessment was conducted using both plain radiographs and MRI. On plain radiographs, the degree of osteoarthritis was evaluated on standing AP knee views according to the Kellgren–Lawrence grading system. The posterior tibial slope and lateral femoral condyle ratio were measured on lateral knee views, and the hip–knee–ankle (HKA) angle was determined on full-length weight-bearing lower extremity AP radiographs [39–42]. Radiographic osteoarthritis grade and HKA angle were assessed at three time points: preoperatively, 2 years postoperatively, and at the final follow-up. MRI evaluation included an assessment of ACL graft maturity. One year after surgery, 3.0-T MRI scans were obtained using either an Achieva system (Philips Healthcare, Best, The Netherlands) or a Discovery 750w system (GE Healthcare, Waukesha, WI, USA). Turbo spin-echo T2-weighted sequences with a slice thickness of 3 mm were used for the analyses. Graft signal intensity (SI) was measured at the proximal, middle, and distal thirds of the graft according to the method described by Tashiro et al. [43]. The signal-to-noise quotient (SNQ) was then calculated to quantify graft maturity using the following formula: SNQ = (SI of ACL graft—SI of posterior cruciate ligament)/SI of the background [43]. Radiologic measurements were independently performed on a picture archiving and communication system (PACS) workstation by two orthopedic surgeons experienced in radiologic assessment of the knee. Both observers were blinded to all clinical data and to each other's measurements. For continuous variables, the mean of the two measurements was used for analysis, whereas for categorical variables, any disagreement was resolved through discussion. If consensus could not be achieved, the final decision was made in consultation with the senior author.

2.3. *Statistical Analysis*

All statistical analyses were performed with SAS version 9.4 (SAS Institute Inc., Cary, NC, USA). In initial between-group comparisons, normality of continuous variables was assessed using the Shapiro–Wilk test. Variables satisfying normality assumptions were compared using Student's *t*-test, whereas the Mann–Whitney U test was applied for non-normally distributed variables. Categorical variables were compared using Pearson's chi-square test, or Fisher's exact test when more than 20% of cells had an expected frequency of ≤5. Because treatment allocation (isolated ACL reconstruction vs. combined ACL + ALL reconstruction) was determined historically rather than randomized, we addressed confounding by surgical indication using an inverse probability of treatment weighting (IPTW) based on a propensity score [44]. The propensity model included factors related to the surgical indication for ALL reconstruction—age, activity level, sex, and rotational knee laxity—and additionally incorporated preoperative radiographic osteoarthritis grade as a prognostic covariate. IPTW was then applied to create a weighted pseudo-population in which these baseline covariates were balanced across groups [44]. Covariate balance before and after IPTW was assessed using standardized mean differences, with values < 0.2 considered acceptable and indicative of minimal residual imbalance [45]. After IPTW adjustment, between-group comparisons were conducted using weighted Student's *t*-tests for continuous variables and the Rao–Scott chi-square test for categorical variables, both of which appropriately account for the weighting scheme and the resulting pseudo-population created by IPTW. Interobserver reliability for radiographic measurements of continuous variables was evaluated using intraclass correlation coefficients (ICC) with 95% confidence intervals. Statistical significance was defined as $p < 0.05$.

3. Results

A total of 59 patients were included in this study (Group 1: 39 isolated ACL reconstructions; Group 2: 20 combined ACL and ALL reconstructions), and between-group comparisons were performed for variables included in the propensity model for IPTW.

https://doi.org/10.3390/jcm15020735

In the initial comparison, a statistically significant difference was observed in the preoperative pivot-shift test ($p = 0.008$); however, no significant difference was noted after IPTW, indicating that the overall balance of covariates was improved following weighting (Table 1).

Table 1. Comparison of covariates used for IPTW.

Variable [b]	Overall Cohort				After IPTW [a]			
	Group 1 (N = 39)	Group 2 (N = 20)	*p* Value	SMD	Group 1 (N = 42.9)	Group 2 (N = 28.3)	*p* Value	SMD
Covariates used for IPTW								
Age, years	32.7 ± 16.1	31.5 ± 11.9	0.943	0.084	33.3 ± 16.7	33.3 ± 10.2	>0.999	<0.001
Pre-injury Tegner activity score	5.9 ± 1.8	6.3 ± 1.6	0.667	0.208	6.0 ± 1.7	6.0 ± 1.5	0.961	0.014
Sex [c]			0.493	0.193			0.685	0.14
Male	28	16			31.0	18.6		
Female	11	4			11.9	9.7		
Preoperative Pivot-shift, grade [c]			0.008				0.913	
1	5	1		0.277	4.5	4.2		0.133
2	25	6		0.727	22.9	13.6		0.104
3	9	13		0.932	15.5	10.5		0.016
Preoperative KL grade [c]			0.347				0.174	
0	33	18		0.162	37.9	26.5		0.185
1	4	1		0.199	3.5	1.3		0.146
2	2	0		0.329	1.5	0		0.167
3	0	1		0.324	0	0.5		0.189

IPTW, inverse probability of treatment weighting; KL, Kellgren–Lawrence; SMD, standardized mean difference. [a] Adjusted for the following covariates: age, pre-injury Tegner activity score, sex, preoperative pivot-shift test, and preoperative Kellgren–Lawrence grade. [b] Values are presented as mean ± standard deviation unless otherwise indicated. [c] Values are presented as the number of patients.

Regarding clinical outcomes, no significant between-group differences were observed in any functional scores at the preoperative, 2-year postoperative, or final follow-up assessments. However, the incidence of surgical failure, as defined in this study, was significantly lower in Group 2 than in Group 1, and this difference was consistently observed both before and after IPTW adjustment ($p = 0.044$ for the initial comparison; $p = 0.049$ after IPTW application) (Table 2). For knee laxity, no significant between-group differences were observed either before or after IPTW application, except for the preoperative pivot-shift test in the initial comparison ($p = 0.008$) (Table 3).

Comparisons of radiologic parameters and intraoperative data were also performed. No significant between-group differences were observed in preoperative radiologic parameters or intraoperative findings. Among the postoperative assessments, most parameters showed no significant differences between groups; however, SNQ of the ACL graft evaluated by MRI at 1 year postoperatively was significantly lower in Group 2, and this finding was consistent both before and after IPTW adjustment ($p = 0.046$ for the initial comparison; $p = 0.038$ after IPTW application) (Table 4). The interobserver ICCs for the continuous radiological parameters ranged from 0.845 to 0.918.

https://doi.org/10.3390/jcm15020735

Table 2. Comparison of demographic data and clinical outcomes.

Variable [b]	Overall Cohort			After IPTW [a]		
	Group 1 (N = 39)	Group 2 (N = 20)	p Value	Group 1 (N = 42.9)	Group 2 (N = 28.3)	p Value
Demographic data						
Age, years	32.7 ± 16.1	31.5 ± 11.9	0.943	33.3 ± 16.7	33.3 ± 10.2	>0.999
Pre-injury Tegner activity score	5.9 ± 1.8	6.3 ± 1.6	0.667	6.0 ± 1.7	6.0 ± 1.5	0.961
Sex			0.493			0.685
Male/Female	28/11	16/4		31.0/11.9	18.6/9.7	
Affected side [c]			0.787			0.536
Right/Left	20/19	11/9		23.2/19.7	12.6/15.7	
Body Mass Index, kg/m^2	23.8 ± 3.0	25.0 ± 3.0	0.088	23.7 ± 2.9	24.8 ± 2.8	0.213
Postoperative MRI [c]			0.156			- [e]
Yes/No	34/5	20/0		35.3/7.7	28.3/0	
Follow-up duration, year	4.1 ± 1.6	3.5 ± 1.4	0.179	4.1 ± 1.6	3.2 ± 1.4	0.06
Preoperative						
IKDC subjective score	54.2 ± 16.9	49.7 ± 19.2	0.359	53.9 ± 16.9	46.1 ± 16.8	0.091
Lysholm score	62.4 ± 25.1	68.4 ± 12.2	0.553	60.7 ± 23.9	67.7 ± 13.8	0.226
Tegner activity score	1.4 ± 1.0	1.8 ± 1.2	0.266	1.4 ± 1.0	1.7 ± 1.0	0.204
Postoperative 2-years						
IKDC subjective score	77.2 ± 14.5	74.4 ± 13.5	0.374	77.4 ± 14.5	73.7 ± 14.1	0.399
Lysholm score	87.9 ± 11.6	82.0 ± 14.0	0.125	87.5 ± 11.1	82.4 ± 15.3	0.267
Tegner activity score	3.7 ± 2.0	3.9 ± 1.5	0.702	3.7 ± 2.1	3.7 ± 1.4	0.994
Final follow-up						
IKDC subjective score	76.3 ± 16.3	75.9 ± 14.7	0.854	74.4 ± 17.5	73.1 ±14.5	0.783
Lysholm score	85.7 ± 12.8	85.7 ± 12.8	0.891	84.1 ± 13.5	82.5 ± 13.6	0.698
Tegner activity score	3.7 ± 1.9	3.8 ± 1.4	0.714	3.6 ± 1.8	3.6 ± 1.3	0.996
Surgical failure [c,d]			0.044			0.049
Yes/No	11/28	1/19		14.0/28.9	2.0/26.3	
Revision surgery [c,d]			>0.999			0.767
Yes/No	3/36	1/19		4.2/38.8	2.0/26.3	

IPTW, inverse probability of treatment weighting; MRI, magnetic resonance imaging; IKDC, International Knee Documentation Committee. [a] Adjusted for the following covariates: age, pre-injury Tegner activity score, sex, preoperative pivot-shift test, and preoperative Kellgren–Lawrence grade. [b] Values are presented as mean ± standard deviation unless otherwise indicated. [c] Values are presented as the number of patients. [d] Defined as cases identified during the follow-up period. [e] p value could not be estimated due to a computational limitation caused by zero frequency in one category.

Table 3. Comparisons of knee laxity.

Variable [b]	Overall Cohort			After IPTW [a]		
	Group 1 (N = 39)	Group 2 (N = 20)	p Value	Group 1 (N = 42.9)	Group 2 (N = 28.3)	p Value
Preoperative						
SSD in ATT, MM	8.1 ± 2.1	6.7 ± 3.3	0.409	8.0 ± 2.0	7.0 ± 2.7	0.111
Lachman test, grade [c]			0.325			0.435
1/2/3	0/37/2	0/17/3		0/41.3/1.7	0/26.0/2.3	
Pivot-shift test, grade [c]			0.008			0.913
1/2/3	5/25/9	1/6/13		4.5/22.9/15.5	4.2/13.6/10.5	
Postoperative 2-years						
SSD in ATT, MM	2.2 ± 2.7	2.1 ± 2.1	0.972	2.3 ± 2.7	2.2 ± 1.9	0.796
Lachman test, grade [c]			0.8			0.557
0/1/2	24/13/2	14/5/1		26.1/15.2/1.6	20.1/6.2/2.0	
Pivot-shift test, grade [c]			0.713			0.313
0/1/2/3	27/10/1/1	16/3/1/0		28.5/11.0/1.6/1.9	23.0/3.3/2.0/0	
Final follow-up						

https://doi.org/10.3390/jcm15020735

Table 3. *Cont.*

Variable [b]	Overall Cohort			After IPTW [a]		
	Group 1 (N = 39)	Group 2 (N = 20)	*p* Value	Group 1 (N = 42.9)	Group 2 (N = 28.3)	*p* Value
SSD in ATT, MM	2.9 ± 2.7	1.9 ± 1.7	0.109	3.3 ± 2.9	1.9 ± 1.8	0.055
Lachman test, grade [c]			0.237			0.102
0/1/2	18/15/6	14/5/1		17.2/18.1/7.7	20.5/5.9/2.0	
Pivot-shift test, grade [c]			0.529			0.293
0/1/2	21/14/4	14/5/1		21.4/15.8/5.8	20.7/5.6/2.0	

IPTW, inverse probability of treatment weighting; SSD, side-to-side difference; ATT, anterior tibial translation; MM, manual maximum. [a] Adjusted for the following covariates: age, pre-injury Tegner activity score, sex, preoperative pivot-shift test, and preoperative Kellgren–Lawrence grade. [b] Values are presented as mean ± standard deviation unless otherwise indicated. [c] Values are presented as the number of patients.

Table 4. Comparison of radiological parameters and intraoperative data.

Variable [b]	Overall Cohort			After IPTW [a]		
	Group 1 (N = 39)	Group 2 (N = 20)	*p* Value	Group 1 (N = 42.9)	Group 2 (N = 28.3)	*p* Value
Preoperative						
KL grade [c]			0.347			0.174
0/1/2/3	33/4/2/0	18/1/0/1		37.9/3.6/1.5/0	26.5/1.3/0/0	
Hip–Knee–Ankle angle, °	0.1 ± 3.7	0.7 ± 2.1	0.467	0.06 ± 3.6	0.7 ± 2.2	0.399
Posterior Tibial Slope, °	7.8 ± 2.3	8.0 ± 3.0	0.785	7.7 ± 2.1	8.6 ± 3.1	0.249
Lateral femoral condyle ratio, %	66.6 ± 3.0	66.5 ± 3.0	0.933	66.8 ± 2.9	66.2 ± 2.9	0.534
Intraoperative data						
Graft diameter, mm	8.7 ± 0.6	9.0 ± 0.5	0.123	8.7 ± 0.6	8.9 ± 0.6	0.392
Medial meniscus [c]			0.892			0.826
Functional/Non-functional/Repair	26/2/11	12/1/7		28.3/1.8/12.9	18.1/0.5/9.7	
Lateral meniscus [c]			0.106			0.351
Functional/Non-functional/Repair	33/0/6	13/0/7		36.8/0/6.2	21.3/0/7.0	
Tibiofemoral joint cartilage [c]			0.999			0.545
Intact or low-grade lesion/High-grade lesion/Repair	36/1/2	18/1/1		39.3/0.8/2.8	27.0/0.8/0.5	
Postoperative 1-year						
ACL Graft maturity, SNQ [d]	28.1 ± 62.2	5.1 ± 4.4	0.046	28.1 ± 61.2	4.6 ± 4.3	0.038
Postoperative 2-years						
KL grade [c]			0.38			0.324
0/1/2/3	29/8/2/0	15/2/2/1		33.2/8.2/1.5/0	21.6/3.0/3.2/0.5	
Hip–Knee–Ankle angle, °	0.0 ± 3.4	−0.1 ± 2.4	0.816	0.4 ± 3.4	0.3 ± 2.8	0.924
Final follow-up						
KL grade [c]			0.454			0.449
0/1/2/3	24/13/2/0	10/7/2/1		26.9/14.6/1.5/0	14.6/10.0/3.2/0.5	
Hip–Knee–Ankle angle, °	0.0 ± 3.4	−0.3 ± 2.5	0.762	0.5 ± 3.4	0.4 ± 3.2	0.978

IPTW, inverse probability of treatment weighting; KL, Kellgren–Lawrence; ACL, anterior cruciate ligament; SNQ, signal-to-noise quotient. [a] Adjusted for the following covariates: age, pre-injury Tegner activity score, sex, preoperative pivot-shift test, and preoperative Kellgren–Lawrence grade. [b] Values are presented as mean ± standard deviation unless otherwise indicated. [c] Values are presented as the number of patients. [d] Data available for patients who underwent 1-year postoperative MRI (34 in Group 1 and 20 in Group 1).

https://doi.org/10.3390/jcm15020735

4. Discussion

The principal finding of this study was that, in ACL reconstruction performed using allografts, the addition of ALL reconstruction resulted in more favorable clinical outcomes compared with ACL reconstruction alone. Patients who underwent the combined procedure demonstrated a lower incidence of surgical failure and improved graft maturity during the follow-up period. These findings suggest that, for patients for whom ACL reconstruction with allografts is planned, combined ALL reconstruction is recommended when performing ACL reconstruction in appropriately indicated cases.

The advantages of combined ACL and ALL reconstruction have been well established. The addition of ALL reconstruction to ACL reconstruction provides superior biomechanical stability of the knee joint compared with isolated ACL reconstruction and has been shown to yield distinct clinical benefits [1–6,46]. However, most previous studies have focused on cases in which autografts were used for ACL reconstruction, and limited information is available regarding procedures performed with allografts [1–5]. It has been theoretically recognized that autografts and allografts differ in several aspects, including the ligamentization process—which encompasses graft incorporation and revascularization—as well as in their mechanical properties [11,12,15]. Although a recent large cohort study has suggested that the graft source is not directly associated with clinical outcomes after ACL reconstruction [47], the potential disadvantages of allografts warrant careful consideration when interpreting postoperative results. Given the increasing adoption of ALL reconstruction in clinical practice [7], further investigation is warranted to clarify how combined ALL reconstruction influences the outcomes of ACL reconstruction using allografts, thereby prompting the design of the present study.

In this study, when allografts were used as the graft source for ACL reconstruction, the incidence of surgical failure was significantly lower in patients who underwent combined ACL and ALL reconstruction than in those who underwent isolated ACL reconstruction. Although no significant differences were observed when each parameter—functional scores and postoperative knee laxity—was analyzed separately, the reduced rate of surgical failure in the combined reconstruction group may indicate a clinically meaningful advantage of adding ALL reconstruction. These findings are consistent with previous studies using autografts for ACL reconstruction [1–5], despite variations in the definition of surgical failure across studies. Furthermore, although the difference did not reach statistical significance, patients who underwent combined reconstruction tended to exhibit less residual anteroposterior laxity postoperatively. Overall, these results suggest that the addition of ALL reconstruction to ACL reconstruction may confer potential clinical benefits, even when allografts are used as the graft source.

Beyond the clinical outcomes, this study demonstrated a difference in ACL graft maturity between the two groups. Patients who underwent additional ALL reconstruction exhibited significantly lower SNQ values of the ACL graft compared with those who received isolated ACL reconstruction, indicating a relatively greater degree of graft maturation. The SNQ of the ACL graft measured on MRI has been reported to correlate with the graft's mechanical properties, showing a negative correlation with load to failure, tensile strength, and stiffness [48]. Accordingly, patients who underwent the combined procedure exhibited more advanced graft maturation and healing. This finding may be explained by the stress-sharing effect of the reconstructed ALL, which could reduce mechanical stress on the ACL graft during the healing period, thereby preventing microdamage or overstretching and promoting graft maturation. Beyond this mechanical explanation, the addition of ALL reconstruction may also have influenced biological healing responses from surrounding soft tissues, such as vascular ingrowth and cellular migration described in epiligament-related healing mechanisms, thereby contributing to the observed differences

https://doi.org/10.3390/jcm15020735

in graft maturation [16,49]. Although such biological processes were not directly evaluated in the present study, interpretation of our findings within the framework of the epiligament theory may provide a complementary biological context [16,49]. The difference in graft maturity observed between the two groups may, in turn, have contributed to the disparity in the incidence of surgical failure in this study. Although previous studies investigating the effect of anterolateral augmentation procedures, including ALL reconstruction, on ACL graft healing have reported conflicting results [50–52], it should be noted that the present study differed from most prior reports in that allografts were used as the graft source for ACL reconstruction, whereas autografts were predominantly used in previous investigations. Taken together, these findings suggest that combined ACL and ALL reconstruction may yield more favorable outcomes than isolated ACL reconstruction, not only in subjective but also in objective assessments.

As previously discussed, the clinical advantages of adding ALL reconstruction to ACL reconstruction have been well established. However, the present study holds particular significance as it is, to our knowledge, the first to analyze this combined procedure specifically in the context of allograft-based ACL reconstruction. By employing matched comparisons, this study provides a balanced comparison that minimizes confounding related to surgical indications and baseline characteristics. These findings may serve as meaningful clinical evidence supporting the potential benefits of performing combined ACL and ALL reconstruction when allografts are used as the graft source.

This study has several limitations. First, as this was a retrospective study, the potential risks of selection and information bias could not be fully eliminated. Second, the number of patients included in this study was relatively small, which may have introduced limited statistical power and increased susceptibility to sampling-related bias, including variability in data distribution for certain outcomes. However, because the analysis was limited to patients who underwent ACL reconstruction using allografts at a single institution, this limitation was inevitable. Furthermore, the statistical power of the outcome comparisons was dependent on the IPTW rather than the absolute sample size, given that the analysis was conducted using an IPTW-based pseudo-population. Third, the patients were grouped historically according to whether an additional ALL reconstruction was performed, and this grouping inherently reflected differences in the original surgical indications. Although the potential confounding effect of surgical indication was minimized by performing a matched analysis that controlled for related covariates, the possibility of residual confounding cannot be entirely excluded. Fourth, changes in clinical practice over the study period may have introduced unmeasured sources of variability. While the single-surgeon, single-center design ensured technical consistency, it may limit the generalizability of the findings and introduce selection bias. Finally, the SNQ, which was identified as a clinically relevant variable in this study, was measured only once at 1 year postoperatively. Considering that the ligamentization process of allografts may extend beyond 1 year, serial MRI evaluations would be required for a more precise assessment of graft maturity.

5. Conclusions

In ACL reconstruction using allografts, the addition of ALL reconstruction resulted in more favorable clinical and radiologic outcomes—particularly a lower incidence of surgical failure and greater graft maturity at 1 year postoperatively—compared with isolated ACL reconstruction.

Author Contributions: The project was coordinated by S.-H.K.; H.-S.M. drafted the manuscript, together with M.J., K.C., and S.-H.J.; H.-S.M. and S.-H.K. generated the concept of the study. The acquisition of data and analysis was done by J.C. and G.S., and S.K. provided supervision and guidance throughout the research process. The design of the study and interpretation of data were all

https://doi.org/10.3390/jcm15020735

done jointly by all authors. H.-S.M. revised the final draft critically for important intellectual content and approved the version to be submitted. All authors have read and agreed to the published version of the manuscript.

Funding: This research received no external funding.

Institutional Review Board Statement: This study was ethically approved by the institutional review board from Gangnam Severance Hospital (ID Number: 3-2025-0279, approval date: 27 October 2025).

Informed Consent Statement: The requirement for informed consent was waived owing to the retrospective design of the study.

Data Availability Statement: The datasets analyzed during the current study are available upon reasonable request.

Conflicts of Interest: The authors declare that they have no conflicts of interest.

References

1. Sonnery-Cottet, B.; Haidar, I.; Rayes, J.; Fradin, T.; Ngbilo, C.; Vieira, T.D.; Freychet, B.; Ouanezar, H.; Saithna, A. Long-term graft rupture rates after combined acl and anterolateral ligament reconstruction versus isolated acl reconstruction: A matched-pair analysis from the santi study group. *Am. J. Sports Med.* **2021**, *49*, 2889–2897. [CrossRef]
2. Pioger, C.; Gousopoulos, L.; Hopper, G.P.; Vieira, T.D.; Campos, J.P.; El Helou, A.; Philippe, C.; Saithna, A.; Sonnery-Cottet, B. Clinical outcomes after combined acl and anterolateral ligament reconstruction versus isolated acl reconstruction with bone-patellar tendon-bone grafts: A matched-pair analysis of 2018 patients from the santi study group. *Am. J. Sports Med.* **2022**, *50*, 3493–3501. [CrossRef]
3. Pettinari, F.; Carrozzo, A.; Saithna, A.; Ali, A.A.; Alayane, A.; Barosso, M.; Vieira, T.D.; Sonnery-Cottet, B. Effect of lateral extra-articular procedures combined with acl reconstruction on the rate of graft rupture in patients aged older than 30 years: A matched-pair analysis of 1102 patients from the santi study group. *Am. J. Sports Med.* **2024**, *52*, 1765–1772. [CrossRef]
4. Mercurio, M.; Cofano, E.; Gasparini, G.; Galasso, O.; Familiari, F.; Sanzo, V.; Ciolli, G.; Corona, K.; Cerciello, S. Isolated acl reconstruction versus combined acl and anterolateral ligament reconstruction: Functional outcomes, return to sport, and survivorship: An updated meta-analysis of comparative studies. *Am. J. Sports Med.* **2025**, *53*, 971–980. [CrossRef]
5. Shatrov, J.; Freychet, B.; Hopper, G.P.; Coulin, B.; El Helou, A.; An, J.S.; Vieira, T.D.; Sonnery-Cottet, B. Radiographic incidence of knee osteoarthritis after isolated acl reconstruction versus combined acl and all reconstruction: A prospective matched study from the santi study group. *Am. J. Sports Med.* **2023**, *51*, 1686–1697. [CrossRef] [PubMed]
6. Lai, S.; Zhang, Z.; Li, J.; Fu, W.L. Comparison of anterior cruciate ligament reconstruction with versus without anterolateral augmentation: A systematic review and meta-analysis of randomized controlled trials. *Orthop. J. Sports Med.* **2023**, *11*, 23259671221149403. [CrossRef] [PubMed]
7. Hollyer, I.; Sholtis, C.; Loughran, G.; Raji, Y.; Akhtar, M.; Smith, P.A.; Musahl, V.; Verdonk, P.C.M.; Sonnery-Cottet, B.; Getgood, A.; et al. Trends in lateral extra-articular augmentation use and surgical technique with anterior cruciate ligament reconstruction from 2016 to 2023, an acl study group survey. *J. ISAKOS* **2024**, *9*, 100356. [CrossRef] [PubMed]
8. Ra, H.J.; Kim, J.H.; Lee, D.H. Comparative clinical outcomes of anterolateral ligament reconstruction versus lateral extra-articular tenodesis in combination with anterior cruciate ligament reconstruction: Systematic review and meta-analysis. *Arch. Orthop. Trauma. Surg.* **2020**, *140*, 923–931. [CrossRef]
9. Öktem, H.; Jamil, Y.; Sever, S.N. Mapping the anterolateral ligament of the knee: A bibliometric analysis. *Knee Surg. Relat. Res.* **2025**, *37*, 21. [CrossRef]
10. Bottoni, C.R.; Smith, E.L.; Shaha, J.; Shaha, S.S.; Raybin, S.G.; Tokish, J.M.; Rowles, D.J. Autograft versus allograft anterior cruciate ligament reconstruction: A prospective, randomized clinical study with a minimum 10-year follow-up. *Am. J. Sports Med.* **2015**, *43*, 2501–2509. [CrossRef]
11. Cusumano, A.; Capitani, P.; Messina, C.; de Girolamo, L.; Viganò, M.; Ravasio, G.; Facchini, F.; Sconfienza, L.M.; Zerbi, A.; Schoenhuber, H.; et al. Different timing in allograft and autograft maturation after primary anterior cruciate ligament reconstruction does not influence the clinical outcome at mid-long-term follow-up. *Knee Surg. Sports Traumatol. Arthrosc.* **2022**, *30*, 2281–2290. [CrossRef] [PubMed]
12. Moretti, L.; Bizzoca, D.; Cassano, G.D.; Caringella, N.; Delmedico, M.; Moretti, B. Graft intra-articular remodeling and bone incorporation in acl reconstruction: The state of the art and clinical implications. *J. Clin. Med.* **2022**, *11*, 6704. [CrossRef] [PubMed]
13. Paul, B.R.; Robaina, J.; Parmar, R.; Carter, T.; Shah, A. Myths and facts about allograft use in anterior cruciate ligament reconstruction: A detailed review of the literature. *JBJS Rev.* **2025**, *13*, e25. [CrossRef] [PubMed]

https://doi.org/10.3390/jcm15020735

14. Kaeding, C.C.; Aros, B.; Pedroza, A.; Pifel, E.; Amendola, A.; Andrish, J.T.; Dunn, W.R.; Marx, R.G.; McCarty, E.C.; Parker, R.D.; et al. Allograft versus autograft anterior cruciate ligament reconstruction: Predictors of failure from a moon prospective longitudinal cohort. *Sports Health* **2011**, *3*, 73–81. [CrossRef]
15. Scheffler, S.U.; Schmidt, T.; Gangéy, I.; Dustmann, M.; Unterhauser, F.; Weiler, A. Fresh-frozen free-tendon allografts versus autografts in anterior cruciate ligament reconstruction: Delayed remodeling and inferior mechanical function during long-term healing in sheep. *Arthroscopy* **2008**, *24*, 448–458. [CrossRef]
16. Georgiev, G.P.; Telang, M.; Landzhov, B.; Olewnik, Ł.; Slavchev, S.A.; LaPrade, R.F.; Ruzik, K.; Tubbs, R.S. The novel epiligament theory: Differences in healing failure between the medial collateral and anterior cruciate ligaments. *J. Exp. Orthop.* **2022**, *9*, 10. [CrossRef]
17. Tibor, L.; Chan, P.H.; Funahashi, T.T.; Wyatt, R.; Maletis, G.B.; Inacio, M.C. Surgical technique trends in primary acl reconstruction from 2007 to 2014. *J. Bone Jt. Surg. Am.* **2016**, *98*, 1079–1089. [CrossRef]
18. Lee, D.W.; Lee, S.; Ro, D.H.; Han, H.S. Satisfactory clinical outcomes of revision anterior cruciate ligament reconstruction using quadriceps tendon-patellar bone allograft. *Clin. Orthop. Surg.* **2025**, *17*, 91–99. [CrossRef]
19. Malige, A.; Baghdadi, S.; Hast, M.W.; Schmidt, E.C.; Shea, K.G.; Ganley, T.J. Biomechanical properties of common graft choices for anterior cruciate ligament reconstruction: A systematic review. *Clin. Biomech.* **2022**, *95*, 105636. [CrossRef]
20. Haybäck, G.; Raas, C.; Rosenberger, R. Failure rates of common grafts used in acl reconstructions: A systematic review of studies published in the last decade. *Arch. Orthop. Trauma. Surg.* **2022**, *142*, 3293–3299. [CrossRef]
21. Pilia, M.; Murray, M.; Guda, T.; Heckman, M.; Appleford, M. Pretensioning of soft tissue grafts in anterior cruciate ligament reconstruction. *Orthopedics* **2015**, *38*, e582–e587. [CrossRef]
22. Kim, S.J.; Kim, H.J. High portal: Practical philosophy for positioning portals in knee arthroscopy. *Arthroscopy* **2001**, *17*, 333–337. [CrossRef]
23. Kim, S.H.; Kim, S.J.; Choi, C.H.; Kim, D.; Jung, M. Optimal condition to create femoral tunnel considering combined influence of knee flexion and transverse drill angle in anatomical single-bundle acl reconstruction using medial portal technique: 3d simulation study. *BioMed Res. Int.* **2018**, *2018*, 2643247. [CrossRef] [PubMed]
24. Sonnery-Cottet, B.; Daggett, M.; Fayard, J.M.; Ferretti, A.; Helito, C.P.; Lind, M.; Monaco, E.; de Pádua, V.B.C.; Thaunat, M.; Wilson, A.; et al. Anterolateral ligament expert group consensus paper on the management of internal rotation and instability of the anterior cruciate ligament—Deficient knee. *J. Orthop. Traumatol.* **2017**, *18*, 91–106. [CrossRef] [PubMed]
25. Weber, A.E.; Zuke, W.; Mayer, E.N.; Forsythe, B.; Getgood, A.; Verma, N.N.; Bach, B.R.; Bedi, A.; Cole, B.J. Lateral augmentation procedures in anterior cruciate ligament reconstruction: Anatomic, biomechanical, imaging, and clinical evidence. *Am. J. Sports Med.* **2019**, *47*, 740–752. [CrossRef] [PubMed]
26. Jung, S.H.; Park, J.S.; Jung, M.; Chung, K.; Ha, T.H.; Choi, C.H.; Kim, S.H. Combined anterolateral ligament reconstruction results in better knee stability and more satisfactory subjective outcomes in non-athlete patients undergoing revision anterior cruciate ligament reconstruction. *J. Clin. Med.* **2024**, *13*, 4087. [CrossRef]
27. Claes, S.; Vereecke, E.; Maes, M.; Victor, J.; Verdonk, P.; Bellemans, J. Anatomy of the anterolateral ligament of the knee. *J. Anat.* **2013**, *223*, 321–328. [CrossRef]
28. Jung, S.H.; Jung, M.; Chung, K.; Moon, H.S.; Kim, S.; Lee, S.H.; Choi, C.H.; Kim, S.H. Optimal anterolateral ligament tibial tunnel orientation to prevent acl tunnel collision and saphenous nerve injury. *Orthop. J. Sports Med.* **2025**, *13*, 23259671251327414. [CrossRef]
29. Katakura, M.; Koga, H.; Nakamura, T.; Araki, D.; Nagai, K.; Nishida, K.; Kuroda, R.; Muneta, T. Biomechanical effects of additional anterolateral structure reconstruction with different femoral attachment sites on anterior cruciate ligament reconstruction. *Am. J. Sports Med.* **2019**, *47*, 3373–3380. [CrossRef]
30. Moon, H.S.; Choi, C.H.; Seo, Y.J.; Lee, Y.; Jung, M.; Park, J.H.; Kim, S.H. The orientation of the all femoral tunnel to minimize collision with the acl tunnel depends on the need or not of far-cortex drilling. *Knee Surg. Sports Traumatol. Arthrosc.* **2022**, *30*, 3805–3817. [CrossRef]
31. Kolin, D.A.; Apostolakos, J.; Fabricant, P.D.; Jivanelli, B.; Yen, Y.M.; Kramer, D.E.; Kocher, M.S.; Pennock, A.T.; Nepple, J.J.; Willimon, S.C.; et al. Knee flexion angle of fixation during anterolateral ligament reconstruction or lateral extra-articular tenodesis: A systematic review and meta-analysis of lateral extra-articular reinforcement techniques performed in conjunction with acl reconstruction. *Orthop. J. Sports Med.* **2024**, *12*, 23259671241231254. [CrossRef] [PubMed]
32. Irrgang, J.J.; Anderson, A.F.; Boland, A.L.; Harner, C.D.; Neyret, P.; Richmond, J.C.; Shelbourne, K.D. Responsiveness of the international knee documentation committee subjective knee form. *Am. J. Sports Med.* **2006**, *34*, 1567–1573. [CrossRef] [PubMed]
33. Briggs, K.K.; Lysholm, J.; Tegner, Y.; Rodkey, W.G.; Kocher, M.S.; Steadman, J.R. The reliability, validity, and responsiveness of the lysholm score and tegner activity scale for anterior cruciate ligament injuries of the knee: 25 years later. *Am. J. Sports Med.* **2009**, *37*, 890–897. [CrossRef]
34. Myrer, J.W.; Schulthies, S.S.; Fellingham, G.W. Relative and absolute reliability of the kt-2000 arthrometer for uninjured knees. Testing at 67, 89, 134, and 178 n and manual maximum forces. *Am. J. Sports Med.* **1996**, *24*, 104–108. [CrossRef] [PubMed]

https://doi.org/10.3390/jcm15020735

35. Grassi, A.; Kim, C.; Marcheggiani Muccioli, G.M.; Zaffagnini, S.; Amendola, A. What is the mid-term failure rate of revision acl reconstruction? A systematic review. *Clin. Orthop. Relat. Res.* **2017**, *475*, 2484–2499. [CrossRef]
36. Moon, H.S.; Jung, M.; Choi, C.H.; Chung, K.; Jung, S.H.; Byun, J.; Kim, J.G.; Lee, S.; Kim, S.H. Modifiable and non-modifiable risk factors affecting surgical failure after revision acl reconstruction: A cohort study. *Knee Surg. Relat. Res.* **2024**, *36*, 37. [CrossRef]
37. Ifarraguerri, A.M.; Graham, G.D.; White, A.B.; Berk, A.N.; Gachigi, K.K.; Siparsky, P.N.; Trofa, D.P.; Piasecki, D.P.; Fleischli, J.E.; Saltzman, B.M. Two-stage revision anterior cruciate ligament reconstruction reduces failure risk but leads to lesser clinical outcomes than single-stage revision after primary anterior cruciate ligament graft failure: A retrospective cohort study. *Knee Surg. Relat. Res.* **2025**, *37*, 5. [CrossRef]
38. Tischer, T.; Andriolo, L.; Beaufils, P.; Ahmad, S.S.; Bait, C.; Bonomo, M.; Cavaignac, E.; Cristiani, R.; Feucht, M.J.; Fiodorovas, M.; et al. Management of anterior cruciate ligament revision in adults: The 2022 esska consensus part iii-indications for different clinical scenarios using the rand/ucla appropriateness method. *Knee Surg. Sports Traumatol. Arthrosc.* **2023**, *31*, 4662–4672. [CrossRef]
39. Pfeiffer, T.R.; Burnham, J.M.; Hughes, J.D.; Kanakamedala, A.C.; Herbst, E.; Popchak, A.; Shafizadeh, S.; Irrgang, J.J.; Debski, R.E.; Musahl, V. An increased lateral femoral condyle ratio is a risk factor for anterior cruciate ligament injury. *J. Bone Jt. Surg. Am.* **2018**, *100*, 857–864. [CrossRef]
40. Moon, H.S.; Choi, C.H.; Jung, M.; Lee, D.Y.; Eum, K.S.; Kim, S.H. Medial meniscal posterior horn tears are associated with increased posterior tibial slope: A case-control study. *Am. J. Sports Med.* **2020**, *48*, 1702–1710. [CrossRef]
41. Iseki, Y.; Takahashi, T.; Takeda, H.; Tsuboi, I.; Imai, H.; Mashima, N.; Watanabe, S.; Yamamoto, H. Defining the load bearing axis of the lower extremity obtained from anterior-posterior digital radiographs of the whole limb in stance. *Osteoarthr. Cartil.* **2009**, *17*, 586–591. [CrossRef] [PubMed]
42. Park, J.; Chaar, O.; Narayanakurup, J.; Abdelhamead, A.S.A.; Ro, D.H.; Kim, S.E. Do knee alignment patterns differ between middle eastern and east asian populations? A propensity-matched analysis using artificial intelligence. *Knee Surg. Relat. Res.* **2025**, *37*, 11. [CrossRef] [PubMed]
43. Tashiro, Y.; Gale, T.; Sundaram, V.; Nagai, K.; Irrgang, J.J.; Anderst, W.; Nakashima, Y.; Tashman, S.; Fu, F.H. The graft bending angle can affect early graft healing after anterior cruciate ligament reconstruction: In vivo analysis with 2 years' follow-up. *Am. J. Sports Med.* **2017**, *45*, 1829–1836. [CrossRef] [PubMed]
44. Austin, P.C.; Stuart, E.A. Moving towards best practice when using inverse probability of treatment weighting (iptw) using the propensity score to estimate causal treatment effects in observational studies. *Stat. Med.* **2015**, *34*, 3661–3679. [CrossRef]
45. Austin, P.C. Balance diagnostics for comparing the distribution of baseline covariates between treatment groups in propensity-score matched samples. *Stat. Med.* **2009**, *28*, 3083–3107. [CrossRef]
46. Kelly, S.R.; Cutter, B.M.; Huish, E.G., Jr. Biomechanical effects of combined anterior cruciate ligament reconstruction and anterolateral ligament reconstruction: A systematic review and meta-analysis. *Orthop. J. Sports Med.* **2021**, *9*, 23259671211009879. [CrossRef]
47. Zhu, S.; Ma, R.; Qiao, R.; Zhang, J.; Hu, Y. The results of anterior cruciate ligament reconstruction with allograft versus autograft: A systematic review and meta-analysis. *Eur. J. Orthop. Surg. Traumatol.* **2025**, *35*, 337. [CrossRef]
48. Weiler, A.; Peters, G.; Mäurer, J.; Unterhauser, F.N.; Südkamp, N.P. Biomechanical properties and vascularity of an anterior cruciate ligament graft can be predicted by contrast-enhanced magnetic resonance imaging. A two-year study in sheep. *Am. J. Sports Med.* **2001**, *29*, 751–761.
49. Georgiev, G.P.; Yordanov, Y.; Olewnik, Ł.; Tubbs, R.S.; LaPrade, R.F.; Ananiev, J.; Slavchev, S.A.; Dimitrova, I.N.; Gaydarski, L.; Landzhov, B. Do the differences in the epiligament of the proximal and distal parts of the anterior cruciate ligament explain their different healing capacities? Quantitative and immunohistochemical analysis of cd34 and α-sma expression in relation to the epiligament theory. *Biomedicines* **2024**, *12*, 156. [CrossRef]
50. Cavaignac, E.; Mesnier, T.; Marot, V.; Fernandez, A.; Faruch, M.; Berard, E.; Sonnery-Cottet, B. Effect of lateral extra-articular tenodesis on anterior cruciate ligament graft incorporation. *Orthop. J. Sports Med.* **2020**, *8*, 2325967120960097. [CrossRef]
51. Rojas, G.; Perelli, S.; Ibanez, M.; Formagnana, M.; Ormazabal, I.; Monllau, J.C. Effect of modified lemaire anterolateral extra-articular tenodesis on the magnetic resonance imaging maturity signal of anterior cruciate ligament hamstring graft. *Am. J. Sports Med.* **2021**, *49*, 2379–2386. [CrossRef]
52. Yau, W.P.; Lin, W. Evaluation of graft maturation by mri in anterior cruciate ligament reconstruction with and without concomitant anterolateral ligament reconstruction. *Orthop. J. Sports Med.* **2024**, *12*, 23259671231223976. [CrossRef]

MDPI AG
Grosspeteranlage 5
4052 Basel
Switzerland
Tel.: +41 61 683 77 34

Journal of Clinical Medicine Editorial Office
E-mail: jcm@mdpi.com
www.mdpi.com/journal/jcm

www.ingramcontent.com/pod-product-compliance
Lightning Source LLC
Chambersburg PA
CBHW062045220926
51850CB00010B/2666

* 9 7 8 3 7 2 5 8 7 5 8 5 6 *